ELECTRORETINOGRAMS

Edited by **Gregor Belušič**

Electroretinograms
Edited by Gregor Belušič

Published by InTech
Janeza Trdine 9, 51000 Rijeka, Croatia

Publishing Process Manager Romina Krebel

Technical Editor Teodora Smiljanic

Cover Designer InTech Design Team

Additional hard copies can be obtained from orders@intechopen.com

Electroretinograms, Edited by Gregor Belušič
p. cm.
ISBN 978-953-307-383-5

For EU product safety concerns:
IN TECH d.o.o., Prolaz Marije Krucifikse Kozulić 3, 51000 Rijeka, Croatia,
info@intechopen.com or visit our website at intechopen.com.

Meet the editor

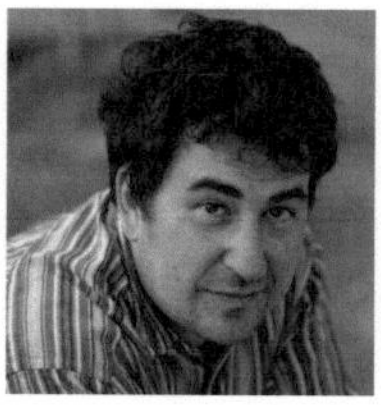

Gregor Belušič, born in 1972, received his Ph.D. degree in Biological sciences from the University of Ljubljana, Slovenia, in 2003. His research interests include comparative physiology of insect visual systems and vision in transgenic Drosophila, and his primary research techniques include ERG and intracellular recording. He has been collaborating with the groups of Prof. Paulsen (University of Karlsruhe), Prof. Huber (University of Hohenheim), and Prof. Stavenga (University of Groningen), with whom he has published articles on insect vision. He is currently employed as a teaching assistant at Biotechnical Faculty, Ljubljana, Slovenia, leading courses in Animal and Human Physiology and Neurobiology. The Human Physiology practicals include an extensive course in human electroretinography in collaboration with the group of Prof. Hawlina at the Eye Clinic, University Medical Centre Ljubljana. He has been awarded the ADInstruments Macknight Progressive Educator award by the American Physiological Society in 2011 for innovations in physiology teaching.

Contents

Preface

The function of the visual pathways can be objectively examined by means of several non-invasive electrophysiological assays, including the electrooculogram (EOG), the visual evoked potential (VEP), and the electroretinogram (ERG). ERG is the time course of the voltage difference across the eye or across the retina elicited by light stimulation. It is a very well studied bioelectrical signal, which has been extensively used in the clinic and in the research laboratory for a very long time. The timeline of discovery in electroretinography spans back to 1849, when the standing voltage across the eye has been first discovered in the isolated frog eye by DuBois-Reymond. ERG from the same preparation was first recorded in 1865 by Holmgren and described again in 1873 by Dewar and McKendrick. Dewar succeeded in recording the first human ERG in 1877, and the first human ERG was published by Kahn and Löwenstein in 1924. Subsequently, advances in the recording instrumentation enabled researchers to analytically approach the electroretinography. Thus, the cellular origin of the different components of the ERG, still in use nowadays, was identified in the vertebrate animal models and in the human eye in the years between 1933 and 1947 by the Nobel laureate Ragnar Granit. At about the same time, Riggs (1941) introduced the scleral contact electrode. The advancements in recording techniques and the progress in ERG analysis soon led to the application of the ERG into the clinical routine by Karpe (1945). Since then, the advances in stimulation, signal recording and signal analysis allowed the researchers to introduce more sophisticated and powerful ERG methods, such as the pattern ERG, multifocal ERG, or scotopic threshold response, which all together yield information about the functional state of all types of retinal excitable cells. ERG is now an indispensable part of the repertoire of the clinical and research methods, not only in the diagnostics of the human visual system disease, but also in the diagnostics of other neurological and system diseases, and in the basical biomedical research in the human, in the vertebrate and in the invertebrate animal models.

This book brings together several review and original research articles on the recent state of certain electoretinographical methods, of the ERG in certain human diseases and of the ERG in certain animal models. The first, methodological part, contains review chapters on the standard methods of the human ERG testing, the normative data in the human ERG, the advanced spatial, temporal and spectral methods of stimulation in the human ERG, and a chapter on the multifocal ERG signal analysis. For a more comprehensive treatment of human ERG, the reader should refer to the web site of the International Society for the Clinical Electrophysiology of Vision, www.iscev.org, where a list of the relevant literature on the subject is available. The second part on the ERG in human disease contains a general review chapter, a contribution on the use of ERG in the framework of an interdisciplinary approach to a hereditary degenerative disease, and a review of the ERG as a clinical assay in a disease of a non-retinal origin, the diabetes. The third part of the book brings three chapters on the ERG in the standard vertebrate models – mouse, rat and macaque, and a chapter on the most important invertebrate model of eye disease, the fruitfly.

Gregor Belušič
University of Ljubljana,
Biotechnical faculty,
Department of Biology
Ljubljana, Slovenia

Part 1

Methodology of Human ERG

1

Electroretinography

Kyle Wolpert and Stephen Tsang
Bernard and Shirlee Brown Glaucoma Laboratory
Department of Ophthalmology, Columbia University
USA

1. Introduction

Electroretinography is a mainstay of clinical ophthalmic diagnostic testing. The electroretinogram, or ERG, provides an objective, quantitative measure of retinal function and allows the clinician to monitor the function of rod cells, cone cells, and ganglion cells in each eye. It uses electrodes placed on the cornea or adjacent to the orbit to monitor changes in the electrical potential of the eye in response to specific stimuli. Careful manipulation of the stimulus and testing conditions allows the clinician to investigate different cell types and layers of the retina. The ability to distinguish between different cell layers and cell types means that ERGs can be used to discern between myriad inherited retinal disorders and dystrophies that may otherwise prove clinically indistinguishable.

Several different types of ERG test provide specific information about the patient's visual function. The full-field ERG, or ffERG, is the most common form of electroretinographic testing. It provides an assessment of general retinal function and can distinguish between the various cell types, revealing the function of photoreceptors, bipolar cells, ganglion cells and amacrine cells, but cannot provide specific information about individual sectors of the retina. That information is provided by the multi-focal ERG, or mfERG, which measures the response in each of a large number of small sectors, typically either 61 or 103, of the retina. It thus provides a map that allows the clinician to locate specific areas of malfunction. The pattern ERG, or PERG, measures the response to a temporally changing pattern of contrast at a constant level of luminance, providing information about ganglion cells and generalized macular function. The electro-oculogram, or EOG, measures changes in the resting potential of the eye during adaptation to dark and light states, revealing function of the retinal pigment epithelium.

2. Basic principle

2.1 Electrical impulses of neurons

Photoreceptors and downstream neurons in the retina maintain a non-neutral electrical "resting potential" by manipulating the intracellular and extracellular concentrations of positive sodium, potassium, and calcium ions and negative chloride ions, as well as larger electronegative molecules.

Human rod cells present a model system of phototransduction. The chromophore, or light-sensing pigment, in rods is 11-*cis*-retinal, which is bound to an apoprotein called opsin, forming rhodopsin. When a photon strikes 11-*cis*-retinal, the added energy causes it to isomerize into all-trans-retinal (Burns and Baylor, 2001; Stryer, 1991; Tsang et al., 1996; Yarfitz and Hurley, 1994). This conformational change causes rhodopsin to activate transducin, a heterotrimeric G protein (Arshavsky et al., 2002; Fung et al., 1981; Tsang et al., 1996). Activated transducin binds to the inhibitory subunits of phosphodiesterase 6 (PDE6), thereby de-inhibiting it. The newly active PDE6 hydrolyzes cyclic Guanosine monophosphate (cGMP), reducing intracellular cGMP levels and closing cGMP-gated cationic channels (CNG) in the rod cellular membrane (Lagnado and Baylor, 1992; Stryer, 1991; Tsang and Gouras, 1996; Yarfitz and Hurley, 1994). This reduces the influx of NA^{+} and Ca^{2+} into the cell, thereby hyperpolarizing it.

The hyperpolarization of the cell causes it to cease transmitting glutamate across synapses to bipolar cells, inducing changes in their polarization. Bipolar cells transmit this signal either directly to ganglion cells, each of which has an axon proceeding out of the orbit along the optic nerve, or to amacrine cells, which then activate ganglion cells or alter the output of other bipolar cells. Photoreceptors, bipolar cells, and amacrine cells operate via graded potentials, but ganglion cells generate action potentials in response to incoming signals from bipolar and amacrine cells; these action potentials help to propagate the information along the optic nerve. The function of each of these cell types can be measured using precise electroretinographic techniques.

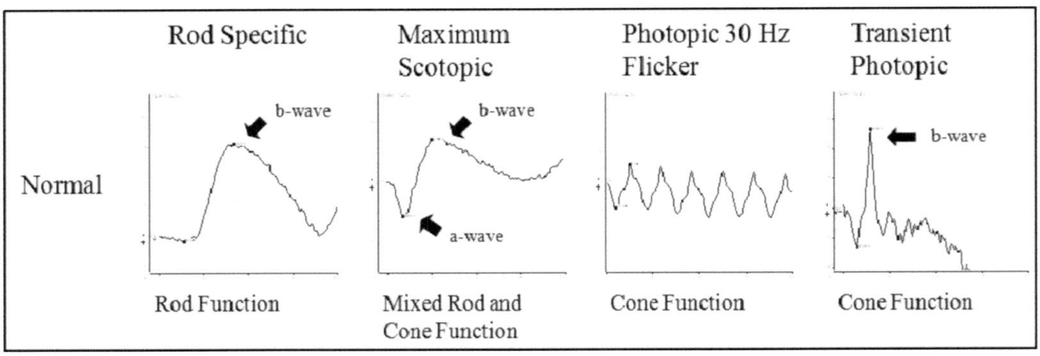

Fig. 1. Normal ERG Tracings. The a-wave and b-wave are noted where applicable.

2.2 Wave components explanation

The typical ERG waveform (see figure 1, Maximum Scotopic) is the sum result of activity in the photoreceptors and bipolar cells, with some contribution from Müller cells. The initial negative deflection, known as the a-wave, is the result of early signals from the rod and cone photoreceptors. The subsequent rise towards the positive peak, known as the b-wave, is created primarily by slower signals from the rod and cone bipolar cells. The ascending slope from the a-wave to the peak of the b-wave typically shows several small oscillations; these are called the oscillatory potentials, or OPs, and reveal the function of the amacrine cells. Other components that become apparent only under certain conditions are beyond the scope of this chapter.

2.3 Sources of variability

Because ERG measurements can vary greatly, it is important to minimize sources of variability whenever possible. Different variables of the test itself, including stimulus duration and intensity, electrode resistance and type, and the length of dark adaptation can all induce substantial changes in the recorded potential. The International Society for Clinical Electrophysiology of Vision, or ISCEV, has developed publically available, specific standards to promote consistent ERG results and to preserve comparability between different testing centers. However, a number of factors unrelated to the hardware can also affect the recorded potential. ERGs measure the response to light, so the pupil should be maximally dilated every time an electroretinogram is performed; changes in pupil dilation can reduce the potential. Systemic blood pressure and local blood flow can affect ERG amplitude, so drugs that alter either of these should be noted. Patients also experience a diurnal change in signal amplitude as a result of circadian physiological changes including blood pressure and rod outer-segment disc shedding, so testing should be performed at approximately the same time. Certain anesthetics can affect the b-wave amplitude, so they should be noted as well. Ocular movement can generate interference in ffERG testing and strongly affects the results of spatially specific tests such as the mfERG, so the patient's fixation should be closely monitored by the clinician.

3. Hardware

The two most important pieces of hardware for obtaining an ERG are the light stimulus and the electrodes. The standard light stimulus for full-field ERGs is the Ganzfeld stimulator, a spherical device with hole to fit the patient's head that ensures the even distribution of the light stimulus.

The standard ERG setup includes several electrodes. Typically a reference electrode is placed on the skin in the middle of the forehead. Grounding electrodes for each eye are placed on the earlobes. Two different types of recording electrodes are commonly used, each with its own advantages and disadvantages. Each requires that the patient be given a topical anesthetic to prevent difficulty of electrode insertion and discomfort during the test. The strongest response signal is provided by Burian-Allen electrodes, which consist of a contact lens with a conducting surface around the edge. These electrodes reduce the negative effects of eye movements and blinking, but because the lens tends to blur the patient's vision, they are not inherently well-suited for pattern ERGs or multifocal ERGs, both of which require sensitivity to geographic distribution of the stimulus. A cheaper, more comfortable alternative to the Burian-Allen electrode is the Dawson-Trick-Litzkow, or DTL, electrode. The DTL electrode consists of a fine, single-thread silver wire that spans the eye, resting on the surface of the cornea. DTL electrodes are more comfortable for patients and therefore more suited for long tests, but they promote greater eye movement and they produce a 10-20% weaker signal than contact lens electrodes. A similar alternative is the Hawlina-Konec electrode, also called HK or metal loop electrode, which consists of a metal loop that is shaped to fit into the conjunctival sac. Much of the metal is coated in Teflon to facilitate comfort, but patches remain un-insulated to ensure recording sensitivity. These electrodes are less sensitive to movement artifacts than DTL electrodes but they produce a weaker response amplitude. Another alternative is the cotton wick electrode, first introduced by Sieving and colleagues in 1978 (Sieving et al., 1978). These electrodes consist of a cotton wick, rather than metal wire, which rests on the cornea. The use of cotton eliminates recording artifacts from the photovoltaic effect, in which light striking a metal generates a voltage potential. Because of difficulty with use, cotton wick electrodes are not widely used in clinical practice, but recent research has validated their potential for ERG testing in animal research (Chekroud et al., 2011). Because they do not interfere with central vision, DTL, metal loop, and cotton wick electrodes are ideal for full-field and pattern ERG recordings.

4. Types of ERG

4.1 Full-field

4.1.1 Purpose

The full-field ERG is the most commonly performed, and best-understood, electroretinographic test. It consists of a full-field light stimulus, typically generated in a Ganzfeld stimulator. It can demonstrate differences between the right and left eyes, differentiate between rod, cone, and bipolar cell disorders, and show functional deficits resulting from systemic conditions or advanced degenerations. However, it is not sensitive to localized dysfunctions such as those caused by lesions or small scotomas.

4.1.2 Protocol

The testing protocol as stipulated by the ISCEV standards includes 5 different tests to be performed. After 20 minutes of dark adaptation, the electrodes are applied under dim red light in order to prevent rod photoreceptor activation. If dark adaptation occurs in a dark room, rather than through the use of eye patches or a mask, the electrodes may be applied before adaptation begins. The full-field ERG can be performed using any of the common types of electrodes. The standards set forth by the ISCEV should be followed when performing an ERG.

After dark adaptation and electrode application, the five standard tests are performed in a specific order. The first three tests are performed directly following dark adaption and consist of light flashes against a dark background. This enables them to detect the rod response. The last two tests are performed against a light background, which cancels out the rod response, allowing the cone response to be isolated. First is the dark-adapted, or scotopic, dim ERG to measure rod responses. The stimulus is dim (0.01 $cd*s*m^{-2}$) in order to prevent cone stimulus, thereby allowing the rod response to be isolated and quantified. Second is the dark-adapted (scotopic) bright ERG to measure combined rod and cone function. This and the following tests use a bright stimulus (3.0 $cd*s*m^{-2}$) in order to stimulate both rods and cones. Following the second test, the patient must be light-adapted for ten minutes. Third is the scotopic bright oscillatory potential. Fourth is the light-adapted, or photopic, bright ERG to measure cone response. Fifth is the photopic bright flicker ERG at 30 Hz. During each test, fixation must be monitored to ensure proper measurement, and after each test, artifacts from disruptions such as blinking should be removed from the data before averaging the results.

4.2 Multi-focal

4.2.1 Purpose

The multifocal ERG provides some spatial sensitivity, allowing the clinician to simultaneously measure the retinal response from each of a large number of sections on the retina. The mfERG is an important clinical tool both because it can detect localized abnormalities and because it provides a means to assess central and peripheral function separately.

The most common patterns test either 61 or 103 different hexagonal elements, with central elements that are much smaller than peripheral elements because the receptive fields are larger in the periphery. The tested area typically spans 20-30 degrees to each side of the fovea. During the test, approximately half of the elements are illuminated at any given time, but each follows a distinct, pseudorandom "m-sequence" (Sutter, 1991) pattern of bright and dark states. Because the electrodes are placed on the cornea and offer no spatial resolution by themselves, the response generated is not truly a series of individual response elements but rather the result of mathematical calculation. The signal from the electrodes is amplified and then analyzed by complex software that determines the response to each spatial element by analyzing the response at the time points when the element was illuminated.

The results of the mfERG test can be displayed in several ways. The standard trace array is an array of the waveforms from each element, organized spatially as are the elements themselves. This allows general trends in the amplitudes of the waveforms to be observed and compared. Another method of presenting the data is a 3-dimensional plot, referred to as a topographic density plot, in which the relative wave amplitudes are quantified and presented as a color-coded map of hexagons in which the height represents the wave amplitude.

A number of artifacts can make mfERG interpretation difficult and should be avoided if possible. Electrical noise from ambient surfaces or the electrical power source (typically 50 or 60 Hz) is easily discernible as regular oscillations rather than typical wave forms on the trace array, but on the topographic map they can be misinterpreted as physiologic responses. Small errors of ocular movement or poor fixation can cause the elements to average with their neighbors, reducing the available resolution. Large movement errors produce abnormal signals and should be removed prior to data analysis. The hexagonal elements are not uniformly sized; they are smaller in the central region to provide greater resolution and sensitivity. One result of this configuration is that relatively low levels of noise can cause larger disturbances centrally than peripherally because they are averaged out over a larger area in the periphery. Thus small noise levels often create artificially high central peaks on the topographic map. Electrodes that interfere with central vision should not be used; others, such as DTL electrodes, are preferable. Contact lens electrodes can be effectively used for mfERG testing provided that they are calibrated to the patient's refraction. The standards set forth by the ISCEV should be followed when performing an mfERG.

Summation of all the responses to the mfERG generates a waveform similar to that of the ffERG maximum response, and the signals share the same sources, but the two traces represent very different measurements. The full-field ERG shows the direct response to changes in luminance, whereas the multifocal ERG is a mathematically derived representation of the response to changes in contrast. As such, while the summation of the mfERG shows features similar to the a-wave and b-wave, they are labeled differently to reflect the difference. The initial negative deflection resembling the a-wave is referred to as N1 (for the first negative deflection), the large secondary, positive deflection is referred to as P1 (for the first positive deflection), and a subsequent negative deflection is referred to as N2 (the second negative deflection).

4.3 Pattern

4.3.1 Purpose

The pattern ERG provides a useful measure of macular function and generalized bipolar cell function. The pattern ERG aids the clinician in interpreting the results of the visual evoked potential test (VEP; not covered in this chapter), as the PERG can distinguish between the contributions of impaired macular function and impaired optic nerve function to a reduced VEP waveform.

4.3.2 Stimulus

The stimulus for the PERG is subject to certain constraints. The test measures response to contrast changes, not luminance changes, so the overall luminance of the stimulator must remain constant. Furthermore, any spatial irregularities would contribute to local luminance changes, so it must be spatially regular, fully symmetrical, and centered on the fovea. The most common spatial pattern is a checkerboard stimulus composed of white and black squares (see figure 2). However, there are two options for the temporal pattern of stimulation. The first and simplest to calibrate is referred to as reversal stimulation and consists of alternating white and dark squares in the aforementioned checkerboard pattern; e.g. the central square would be white, then change to black, then back to white. The alternative, referred to as onset stimulation, consists of an even, grey background, which then switches to the checkerboard pattern. This temporal stimulation is difficult to calibrate, as the average luminance of the grey background must be exactly the same as the average luminance of the checkerboard pattern. Any imbalance in luminance between the two states of the stimulation pattern will lead to uneven modulation of the on- and off- pathways in the retina, creating an unusual waveform. As with the mfERG, the electrodes used should not interfere with central vision; as such, DTL or metal loop electrodes are ideal. The standards set forth by the ISCEV should be followed when performing a PERG.

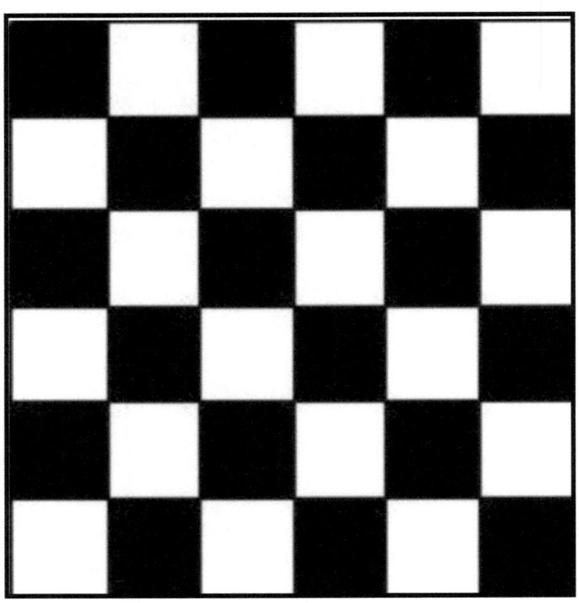

Fig. 2. Sample of an appropriate PERG stimulus. Note the symmetry around the center, sharp contrast between squares, and even luminance levels when averaged over any section of the pattern. In a reversal test, the pattern would reverse such that the top-left square would be white, and then reverse back to black; this would stimulate the retina at each reversal, or twice per cycle.

The source of the PERG waveform was determined with a series of experiments. After the first PERG recordings by Riggs and others in 1964 (Riggs et al., 1964), Sieving and Steinberg attempted to locate the electrical source by measuring electric potential with an electrode in various layers of the cat retina (Sieving and Steinberg, 1987). They determined that the source was located in the proximal layers of the retina, rather than the distal photoreceptors responsible for much of the ffERG response. Later experiments examined patients with unilateral optic nerve atrophy and knocked out animal ganglion cell activity with various means, including tetrodotoxin (which blocks action potentials), and determined that ganglion cells are the primary source of the PERG response (Bach et al., 1992; Harrison et al., 1987; Maffei and Fiorentini, 1981; Maffei et al., 1985; Menger and Wässle, 2000; Miller et al., 2002; Sherman, 1982; Viswanathan et al., 2000).

5. EOG

The electro-oculogram, or EOG, provides a measurement of the standing potential of the eye in light- and dark-adapted states. The value of the resting potential itself is of little clinical relevance, but the ratio between the light and dark values can be diagnostically important. This potential is primarily generated in the retinal pigment epithelium (RPE). Because the resting potential of the eye is the result of polarity of the eye itself, the EOG test procedure consists of the patient alternating between a fixation point to the right and a fixation point to the left, thereby alternating the polarity of the eye with respect to electrodes placed on the medial and lateral canthi. A ground electrode is placed on the forehead. The alternating horizontal ocular motion is performed periodically during an initial period of 15 minutes of light adaptation, then regularly during 15 minutes in the dark, then regularly during another 15-minute period of light-adaptation. The sequence of light and dark adaptations provides a measure of the speed with which the patient adapts to each state.

After the light is turned off, the difference in potential between the poles of the eye steadily decrease, reaching a minimum "dark trough" after roughly 8 to 12 minutes. Once the light is turned on, the potential difference increases steadily until it reaches a "light peak" after approximately 6 to 9 minutes. The ratio of the light peak to the dark trough is the primary metric obtained in the EOG. Substantial variability exists between testing centers, patients, and even multiple tests in a single patient, but a ratio of approximately 1.8 or higher is considered normal, while a light peak to dark trough ratio of 1.6 or less is considered abnormal. The standards set forth by the ISCEV should be followed when performing an EOG.

The light rise, light peak, and dark trough are the result of slow changes in the state of ion channels in the retinal pigment epithelium. As such, the EOG provides a clinical measure of RPE function. However, the clinical relevance of the EOG is limited by the length of the test.

6. Diagnosis/prognosis

Electroretinography is an important test with both diagnostic and prognostic applications. It can help to diagnose a patient with various visual symptoms including nyctalopia, photophobia, field defects, and reduced visual acuity, and it can be of use when the symptoms seem incompatible. It can also help determine the significance of fundus abnormalities and provide an early diagnosis for patients with a family history of inherited retinal disease. Furthermore, electrophysiology can help to assess the post-retinal, intracranial visual pathway. ERG testing is especially significant because it provides an objective, quantifiable evaluation of visual function, unlike tests such as microperimetry that require reliable patient input.

7. Toxicity and vitamin deficiency

Numerous toxic compounds diminish retinal function and can be assessed and monitored with ERG testing. For example, vigabatrin, an anti-epileptic that functions by inhibiting GABA transaminase, causes irreversible retinal damage in approximately ten percent of patients. Patients taking vigabatrin are typically required to participate in regular electroretinographic recording to monitor retinal function. A decreased b-wave to a-wave ratio is an early indicator of retinal damage in patients taking vigabatrin. Such patients also tend to show a reduced 30-Hz flicker amplitude and a loss of the oscillatory potentials in the maximum response.

An early symptom of vitamin A deficiency, rare in the western world but common in third-world countries, is night blindness. Rhodopsin, the light-sensitive protein in rod cells, consists of 11-*cis*-retinal bound to the apoprotein opsin. 11-*cis*-retinal is an aldehyde of vitamin A, so reduced intake of the vitamin leads to a scarcity of the photopigment, causing night blindness. Vitamin A deficiency can be suggested by an undetectable scotopic ERG and maximum response, even with increased luminance, in conjunction with minimally reduced 30-Hz flicker and photopic responses. Visual function can be largely restored within a week of treatment.

In instances of suspected damage to the visual pathway, combined ffERG and PERG testing can elucidate the site of the damage. An ERG abnormality would indicate photoreceptor dysfunction; combined ffERG and PERG abnormalities may indicate bipolar dysfunction; VEP abnormality would suggest dysfunction late in the visual pathway.

8. Stationary rod dysfunction

Stationary rod dysfunctions including congenital stationary night blindness (CSNB) can be assessed via ffERG testing. CSNB is an inherited condition affecting rod cells, thereby preventing night vision. It typically stems from a signaling deficit between rod cells and their post-synaptic bipolar cells, but variants affecting rod phototransduction exist as well. Cases of CSNB have been observed to follow autosomal dominant, autosomal recessive, and X-linked recessive inheritance patterns. Patients with autosomal dominantly inherited CSNB often have normal visual acuity and no myopia, but autosomal recessive and X-linked forms of the disease often confer reduced visual acuity and myopia.

Cases of CSNB vary widely in their electrophysiological presentation. Some patients show only rod-specific scotopic reduction, while many others experience an electronegative b-wave on the maximum scotopic test as well (see figure 3). The transient photopic b-wave is delayed in some patients.

9. Stationary cone dysfunction

Patients with congenital achromatopsia (referred to as "monochromats" because they see shades of grey) can be classified into two separate groups. Typical (rod) monochromats show symptoms similar to those of progressive cone dystrophies, such as photophobia, decreased visual acuity, and poor color perception. Although they typically have normal fundus appearance, they often have characteristic ffERG recordings with extinguished cone function response, reduced maximum response, and relatively normal scotopic rod response (see figure 4). Atypical (cone) achromatopsia is a rare disorder thought to originate in the post-bipolar cell transmission of color vision, as it often presents a nearly normal photopic ERG response.

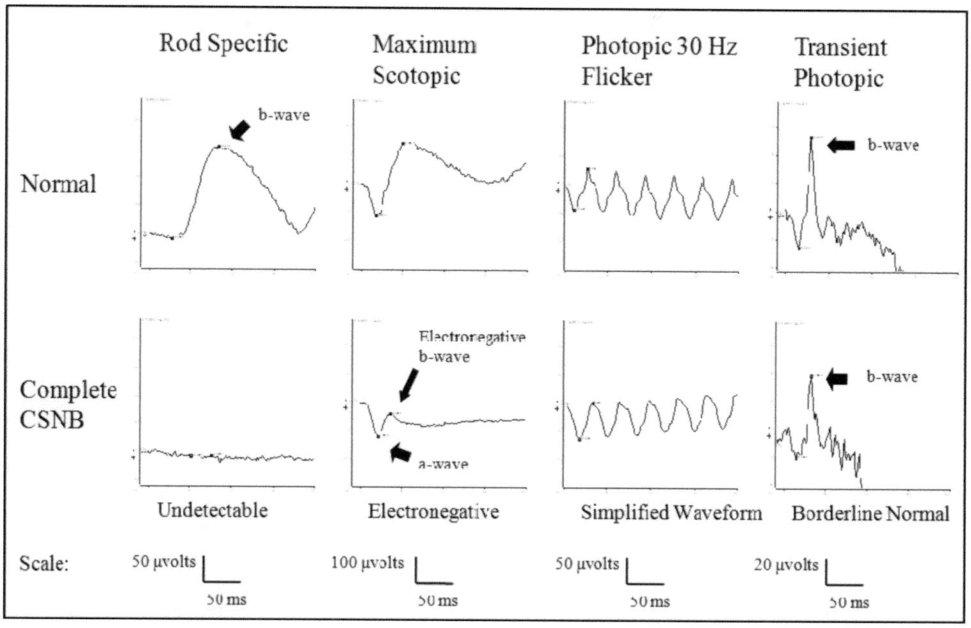

Fig. 3. ERG tracings from a normal patient and a patient with congenital stationary night blindness. Note the undetectable rod response and electronegative maximum response.

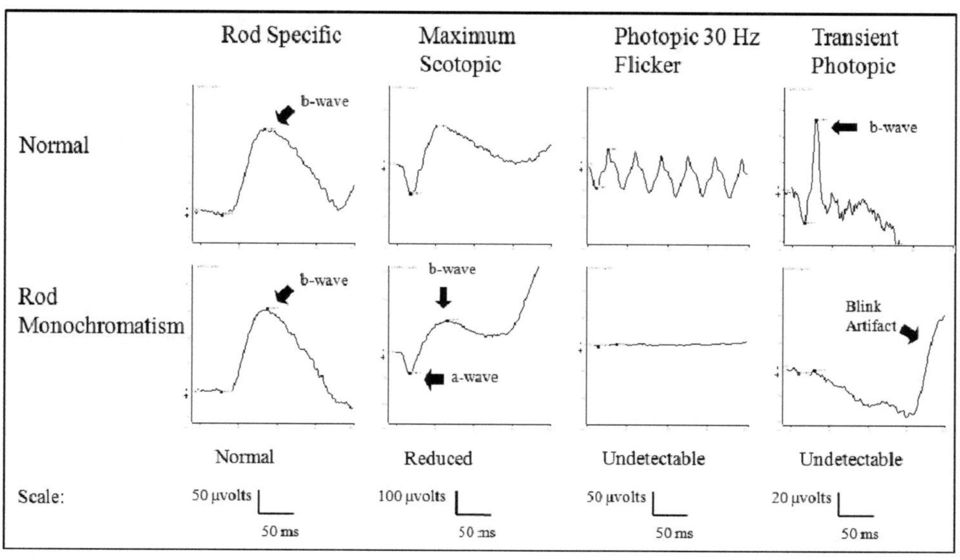

Fig. 4. ERG tracings from normal patient and from patient with rod monochromatism. Note the undetectable 30 Hz flicker and transient photopic responses.

10. Progressive retinal dysfunction

The electroretinogram is an essential diagnostic and prognostic tool for patients with progressive retinal degenerations such as retinitis pigmentosa (RP) or Leber's Congenital Amaurosis (LCA). The degree of amplitude reduction in the various tests of the ffERG can help to differentiate between rod-cone and cone-rod degenerations.

Rod-cone degenerations such as RP are characterized by progressive photoreceptor loss, with cone death secondary to rod death. As such, patients often present with reduced or extinguished night vision, followed by reduced daytime visual acuity or visual field defects. Cone death in RP often begins in the periphery and develops into a progressively constricting ring around the macula. As such, patients often develop tunnel vision, followed in time by blurred then extinguished central vision. While the progression of the ring constriction can be monitored with autofluorescent fundus imaging, the degree of visual function is typically assessed with the ffERG.

Retinitis pigmentosa is characterized by pigmentation of the peripheral retina and reduced rod function (leading to early night blindness). Patients with early-stage RP tend to show greatly reduced or even extinguished scotopic rod response and some decrease in maximum response amplitude, corresponding to the early loss of rod photoreceptors. As the diseases progresses, the maximal ERG, 30-Hz flicker, and photopic responses also steadily diminish as cone cells die (see figure 5). An implicit time delay is often seen, which demonstrates generalized dysfunction.

Retinitis pigmentosa is a heterogeneous disease that has been associated with mutations in 34 different genes (see table 1). The specific gene affected in a given patient dictates the inheritance pattern. Autosomal recessive cases account for approximately 60 percent of total RP cases and have been associated with mutations in 17 different genes. Autosomal dominant inheritance defines approximately 15 to 35 percent of cases and is associated with 15 known mutations. The X-linked form of RP is associated with just three genes and accounts for approximately 5 to 18 percent of total cases.

The autosomal dominant form of RP (adRP) tends to be milder and progress more slowly than the other forms. Patients with adRP often present with reduced visual acuity in late adulthood and may progress to legal blindness by the age of 70 or 80. In early adulthood, such patients are often funduscopically indistinguishable from normal patients. However, the scotopic ERG response may be reduced years earlier than other symptoms appear.

Autosomal recessive RP (arRP) typically is more severe, progresses more quickly, and presents earlier than adRP. Patients often notice reduced visual acuity in their early 20s and may progress to legal blindness by the age of 50.

Sex-linked RP (XLRP) is the most severe form of retinitis pigmentosa. It often presents in the first two decades of life and may progress to legal blindness by the age of 25. Female carriers of XLRP that are over the age of 60 can show a characteristic tapeto-like sheen on autofluorescent images and may show a diminished scotopic response on ffERG.

The full-field ERG is an essential clinical tool for diagnosing and monitoring retinitis pigmentosa. The 30 Hz flicker amplitude can be used to estimate the length of time that a patient will retain useful vision, based on an assumed loss of approximately 10 percent each year with no treatment (Berson, 2007). This provides an approximate prognosis after a single visit. However, repeated visits over several years are important to examine the rate of visual decline and develop a more accurate prognosis. Because of its early diagnostic potential, the ffERG is also important for genetic counseling. ERG testing is often much cheaper than genetic screening, and it provides an opportunity for would-be parents with a family history of RP to determine if they carry the mutant gene. Full-field ERG testing can also help determine early in a patient's life whether they will develop symptoms in later decades. This allows patients to plan accordingly, as unexpected vision loss severely disrupts the patient's well-being.

Disease	**Gene**	**Protein**
adRP, arRP, CSNB	*RHO*	Rhodopsin
adRP	*HPRP3*	Pre-mRNA splicing factor 3
	PRPF8	Pre-mRNA processing factor 8
	PRPF13	Pre-mRNA processing factor 13
	PRPF31	Pre-mRNA processing factor 31
	RP17	RP17
	CRX	Cone-rod otx-like homeobox
	FSCN2	Fascin
	ROM1	Retinal outer segment protein 1
	NRL	Neural retinal leucine zipper
	IMPDH1	Inosine monophosphate dehydrogenase 1
	RP9	RP9
arRP	*CNGA1*	Alpha subunit of rod cGMP-gated channel
	CNGB1	Beta subunit of rod cGMP-gated channel
	PDE6A	Alpha subunit of PDE
	PDE6B	Beta subunit of PDE
	USH2A	Usherin
	LRAT	Lecithin retinol acyltransferase
	RGR	RPE-retinal G protein-coupled receptor
	RLBP1	Cellular retinaldehyde-binding protein 1
	RPE65	Retinal pigment epithelium-specific 65 kD protein
	CRB1	Crumb's homolog 1
	CERKL	Ceramide kinase-like protein
	TULP1	Tubby-like protein 1
	MERTK	C-mer proto-oncogene receptor tyrosine kinase
	RP22	RP22
	RP25	RP25
	RP28	RP28
	RP29	RP29
XLRP	*RP6*	RP6
	RP23	RP23
	RP24	RP24
Stargardt	*ABCA4*	Rim
VMD	*RDS*	Peripherin 2
	VMD2	Bestrophin

Table 1. Genes known to be associated with congenital retinal dysfuction.

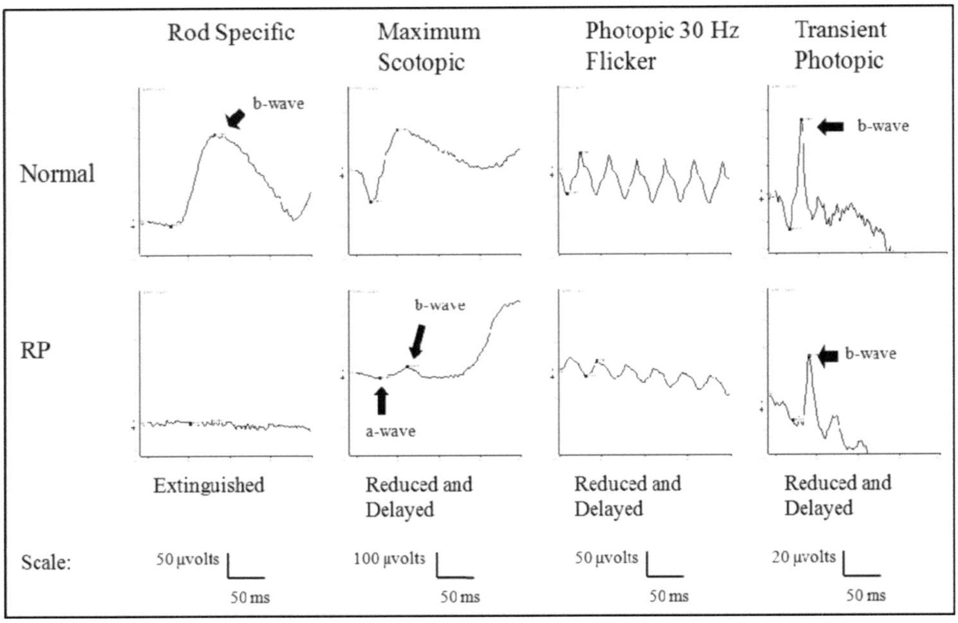

Fig. 5. ERG tracing from a normal patient and from a patient with retinitis pigmentosa. Note extinguished rod response and diminished cone response.

11. Central dystrophies

Central dystrophies such as Stargardt disease (STGD) can show a reduced or extinguished PERG even with no discernible reduction in the full-field ERG. In these diseases, full-field ERG results may still respond to very advanced disease progression and can be useful for categorizing the disease state. Pattern ERG results are far more clinically relevant, as they can be used to track the disease progression and monitor the success of potential therapies.

11.1 Stargardt

Stargardt disease is a progressive cone-rod disease known to be associated with mutations in the ABCA4 gene. It often presents in the first two decades of life and progresses rapidly, although it often reaches a plateau before extinguishing vision. Though not a universal system, some clinicians classify the disease into three distinct groups, according to the photoreceptor responses as measured by full-field ERG (see figure 6). Group 1 Stargardt disease is classified by relatively unaffected rod and cone function on ffERG, although such patients often have severely impaired central vision and diminished or undetectable PERG recording. Group 2 Stargardt disease is marked by diminished cone function but unaffected rod function. Group 3Stargardt disease shows diminished or extinguished rod and cone function on ffERG. While the disease is often considered to be progressive, the group classification can be misleading, as the disease often plateaus and therefore will not necessarily progress, for example, from Group 1 to Group 2.

11.2 Vitelliform macular dystrophy

Vitelliform macular dystrophy (VMD) is a progressive disorder marked by vitelliform ("egg-like") lesions in the macula that presents in children and middle-age adults. The early-onset form of the disease, known as Best disease, is inherited in an autosomal dominant fashion and tends to be more severe than the adult-onset form. Patients with vitelliform macular dystrophy often experience progressive loss of central vision, progressing to central blindness and a visual acuity of approximately 20/100. As the vision deteriorates, the central lesion tends to atrophy and scarred and fibrotic. Two genes are associated with vitelliform macular dystrophy: *VMD2* and *RDS*. Best disease is associated with *VMD2* but both mutations are associated with adult-onset vitelliform dystrophy.

Patients with Best vitelliform macular dystrophy maintain normal peripheral vision and as such, full-field ERG results are typically normal. However, Best disease can be definitively diagnosed by a diminished light-peak to dark-trough ratio in an EOG.

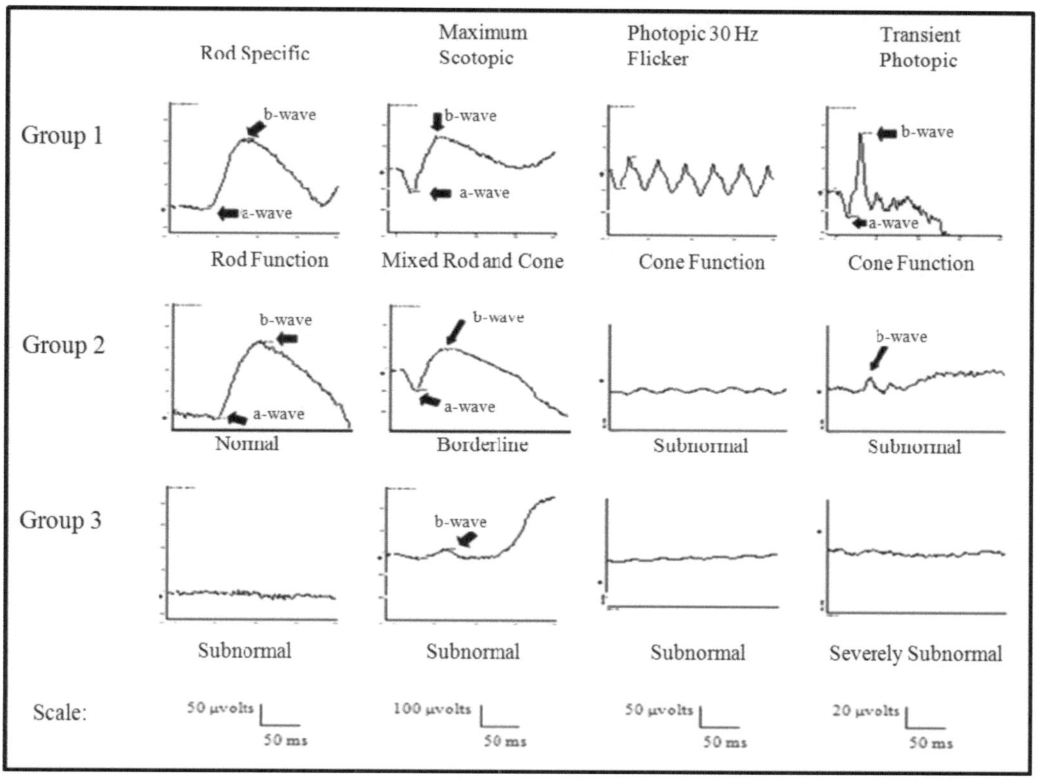

Fig. 6. Representative ERG tracings from Group 1, Group 2, and Group 3 Stargardt patients. Note normal function in Group 1; reduced cone response in Group 2; and nearly extinguished cone response and diminished rod response in Group 3.

11.3 AMD

Age-related macular degeneration (AMD) is a common progressive degeneration of the macula. Its incidence is expected to double within a decade, affecting 20 percent of all Americans between the ages of 65 and 75. AMD typically presents as blurry central vision between the ages of 60 and 70 (Friedman et al., 2004). The vision loss progresses in the central retina but does not expand outside of the macula. Because it is contained within the macula, the full-field ERG often shows normal overall function. There may a slight drop in cone response amplitude, but the implicit time, which typically signals generalized function, is normal. However, the pattern ERG, which measures macular funciton, is markedly reduced.

Patients with AMD are typically classified as having either "dry" or "wet" AMD depending on whether they show signs of neovascularization. Wet, or neovascular, AMD can be treated with several different methods. Elevated levels of vascular endothelial growth factor, or VEGF, lead to the formation of new blood vessels. As such, subretinal injection of anti-VEGF therapeutics can stop or slow the neovascular development and prevent further loss of vision. An alternative is photodynamic therapy. In photodynamic therapy, a high-energy laser is used to coagulate the retina in a number of small spots around the neovascular area. This initiates chemical changes in the retina that prevent further neovascularization. After either treatment, PERG recording on follow-up visits can measure the degree of recovery or monitor further vision loss.

12. Conclusion

Electrophysiological recording is a valuable asset for the clinician. Because ERG tests can measure the function of different cell types and cell layers, they can aid the clinician in distinquishing between symptomatically similar diseases. Furthermore, because they provide an objective measure of retinal function, they can help clinicians evaluate very young patients, very old patients, and others that may otherwise be difficult to diagnose. The quantitative results that ERG tests provide make them useful as tools for both prognosis and disease monitoring. Because of the importance of accurate data and the large number of sources of variability, it is essential that all ERG testing be performed according to the standards established and regularly reviewed by the Internation Society for Clinical Electrophysiology of Vision, or ISCEV.

13. Acknowledgement

We would like to thank Luz Amaro-Quireza, O.D., and Vivienne Greenstein, M.D., for their help.

14. References

Arshavsky, V.Y., Lamb, T.D., & Pugh, E.N. Jr. (2002). G proteins and phototransduction. *Annual Review of Physiology*. 2002; 64:153-87.

Bach, M., Gerling, J., & Geiger, K. (1992). Optic atrophy reduces the patter-electroretinogram for both fine and coarse stimulus patterns. *Clinical Vision Sciences*. 1992; 7:327-333.

Berson, E.L. (2007). Long-term visual prognoses in patients with retinitis pigmentosa: the Ludwig von Sallmann lecture. *Experimental Eye Research*. 2007; 85(1):7-14.

Burns, M.E. & Baylor, D.A.. (2001). Activation, deactivation, and adaptation in vertebrate photoreceptor cells. *Annual Review of Neuroscience*. 2001; 24:779-805. Review.

Chekroud, K., Arndt, C., Basset, D., Hamel, C.P., Brabet, P., & Pequignot, M.O. (2011). Simple and efficient: validation of a cotton wick electrode for animal electroretinography. *Ophthalmic Research*. 2011;45(4):174-9.

Friedman, D.S., O'Colmain, B.J., Munoz, B., Tomany, S.C., McCarty, C., de Jong, P.T., Nemesure, B., Mitchell, P., & Kempen, J. (2004). Prevalence of age-related macular degeneration in the United States. *Archives of Ophthalmology.* Apr 2004, 122(4):564-572.

Fung, B.K., Hurley, J.B., & Stryer, L. (1981). Flow of information in the light-triggered cyclic nucleotide cascade of vision. *Proceedings of the National Academy of Sciences U S A.* 1981 Jan; 78(1):152-156.

Harrison, J.M., O'Connor, P.S., Young, R.S.L., Kincaid, M., & Bentley, R. (1987). The pattern ERG in man following surgical resection of the optic nerve. *Investigative Ophthalmology & Visual Science.* 1987; 28:492-499.

Hood, D.C., Frishman, L.J., Viswanathan, S., Robson, J.G., & Ahmed, J. (1999). Evidence for a ganglion cell contribution to the primate electroretinogram (ERG): Effects of TTX on the multifocal ERG in macaque. *Visual Neuroscience.* 1999; 16:411-416.

Lagnado, L. & Baylor, D. (1992). Signal flow in visual transduction. *Neuron.* 1992 Jun;8(6):995-1002.

Maffei, L. & Fiorentini, A. (1981). Electroretinographic responses to alternating gratings before and after section of the optic nerve. *Science.* 1981; 211:953-954.

Maffei, L., Fiorentini, A., Bisti, S., & Holländer, H. (1985). Patten ERG in the monkey after section of the optic nerve. *Experimental Brain Research.* 1985; 59:423-425.

Menger, N. & Wässle, H. (2000). Morphological and physiological properties of the A17 amacrine cell of the rat retina. *Visual Neuroscience.* 2000; 17:769-780.

Miller, R.F., Stenback, K., Henderson, D., & Sikora, M. (2002). How voltage-gated ion channels alter the functional properties of ganglion and amacrine cell dendrites. *Archives Italiennes de Biologie.* 2002; 140:347-359.

Riggs, L.A., Johnson, E.P., & Schick, A.M.L. (1964). Electrical Responses of the human eye to moving stimulus patterns. *Science.* 1964; 144:567

Sherman, J. (1982). Simultaneous pattern-reversal electroretinograms and visual evoked potentials in diseases of the macula and optic nerve. *Annals of the N Y Academy of Sciences.* 1982; 388:214-226.

Sieving, P.A., Fishman, G.A., & Maggiano, J.M. (1978). Corneal wick electrode for recording bright flash electroretinograms and early receptor potentials. *Archives of Ophthalmology.* 1978 May; 96(5):899-900.

Sieving, P.A. & Steinberg, R.H. (1987). Proximal retinal contribution to the intraretinal 8-Hz pattern ERG of cat. *Journal of Neurophysiology.* 1987; 57(1):104-20.

Stryer, L. (1992). Molecular mechanism of visual excitation. *Harvey Lectures.* 1991-1992; 87:129-43. Review.

Sutter, E.E. (1991). The fast m-transform: a fast computation of cross-correlations with binary m-sequences. *Journal of the Society for Industrial and Applied Mathematics.* 1991; 20:686–694.

Tsang, S.H., Gouras, P., Yamashita, C.K., Kjeldbye, H., Fisher, J., Farber, D.B., & Goff, S.P. (1996). Retinal degeneration in mice lacking the gamma subunit of the rod cGMP phosphodiesterase. *Science.* 1996 May 17; 272(5264):1026-9.

Viswanathan, S., Frishman, L.J., & Robson, J.G. (2000). The uniform field and pattern ERG in macaques with experimental glaucoma: Removal of spiking activity. *Investigative Ophthalmology & Visual Science*. 2000; 41:2797-2810.

Yarfitz, S. & Hurley, J.B. (1994). Transduction mechanisms of vertebrate and invertebrate photoreceptors. *Journal of Biological Chemistry*. 1994 May 20; 269(20):14329-32.

2

Electroretinograms and Normative Data

Rustum Karanjia[1], Martin W. ten Hove[2] and Stuart G. Coupland[1]
[1]The Ottawa Eye Institute, University of Ottawa
[2]Queen's University, Kingston
Canada

1. Introduction

Electroretinography (ERG) is an important clinical tool that provides an objective quantitative measure of retinal function. Decreased a and b wave amplitudes and prolonged latencies correlate to reductions in retinal function that may be the result of toxicity, ischemic damage, or retinal dystrophy (Fishman et al. 2001, Ophthalmology monographs). Furthermore, since the different components of the ERG waveform correspond to the different layers of the retina, one is able to attribute changes in the ERG to damage to specific retinal layers. This data can be a useful surrogate for retinal health, for example establishing safety profiles for drugs under clinical development.

Since 1989 the International Society for Clinical Electrophysiology of Vision (ISCEV) has provided standards for the recording of ERGs. These documents provide a framework for the clinical electrophyisologist to obtain "standard" ERG recordings (Marmor 1989). The variety of permissible ERG instruments and their individual calibration requirements contributes to significant inter-laboratory variability. This variability is recognized in the ISCEV standards and partly addressed by stating "it is incumbent on the manufactures and users to verify that full-field stimulation meets the requirements of this standard." Placing the onus for compliance on the manufactures but leaving the clinical electrophyisologist to determine if the recording standards are indeed met.

ERG standards have extended beyond the a- and b-wave of the full field flash ERG. The pattern ERG (PERG) is the electroretinal response to a pattern reversing stimulus such as bar gratings or checkerboard pattern. The PERG primarily reflects ganglion cell function and since it is viewed on display monitors it largely represents ganglion cell function within the macula. The peak and trough components of the PERG have been formally defined as the N35, P50 and N95 which represent the polarity (Negativity or Positivity) and the mean latency of occurrence. The ISCEV has produced standards for the recording and reporting of the PERG (Holder et al. 2007).

While the PERG provides a single waveform which represents the electroretinal response of the entire macular region, the clinical multifocal electroretinogram (mERG) provides information of local retinal function. The mERG is recorded typically displaying the local retinal response of 61 or 103 local regions within the central 45° of the posterior pole. The responses represent localized cone-driven ERGs obtained in the light adapted state. While the waveform morphology of the mERG is similar to the fullfield ERG the electroretinal generator sites of the trough and peak are not equivalent so it is incorrect to use the 'a-wave' and 'b-wave' labels for the mERG. Rather, the major features of the mERG waveform are labelled based on polarity and order of appearance, namely, the N1, P1 and N2 components. Unlike fullfield flash ERGs which can be seen in response to single flashes, the mERGs are highly processed responses obtained to over 16,000 presentations and subject to more technical artifacts including eye movement, head tilt, poor refractive capability, and poor fixation. There are ISCEV standards for the recording and reporting of mERG (Hood et al. 2008) that also deal with the identification of artifacts and their solution.

The ISCEV Standards Committee are also reviewing and examining other ERG techniques, parameters and waveforms such as On-Off response and Photopic Negative Response (PhNR) and will be developing guidelines and standards for recording and reporting these electroretinal responses.

The expert consensus panel that authored the 2008 ISCEV standards also recognised that older ERG recording equipment may not comply with some of the current stimulus parameters, including background illumination level and flash stimulus levels, but they expressed their hope that manufacturers would strive to update their protocols and comply with the most recent standard. The instrument manufacturers are indeed making modifications as they bring out new equipment models. The panel tacitly stated that since updating non-compliant equipment takes time, publication of data from laboratories that do not fully comply with the current standards is permissible provided they clearly indicate all variances from the ISCEV protocol. This poses a challenge for any organisation attempting to interpret ERG recordings between centers or over time as recordings techniques and standards are continually changing

Two significant sources of variability are the background luminance and the intensity of the stimulus flash. The most recent ISCEV standards chose to define the stimulus intensity and background luminance as single values rather than acceptable ranges (Marmor et al. 2009, 118:69-77). They also recognize that differences between equipment and calibration fluctuations would cause minor variability in the strength of the stimulus and thus provide for a tolerance of ± 10% as an acceptable amount of fluctuation in the standard.

The ISCEV standards provide a good framework for the establishment of an ERG recording system but they are by no means all encompassing. Compliance with ISCEV standards at two different sites does not mean recordings of the same patient at two different time points are directly comparable. This difficulty in obtaining reproducible ERG tests at different centers has hindered the utility of ERG testing in drug development and clinical trials.(Chambers 2011)

There are several challenges encountered in comparing and compiling data between different test sites that are important considerations and affect the clinical utility of ERG both for individual patients and in clinical trials. The following sections highlight some of these challenges and offer suggestions to overcome or decrease inter-site and inter-test variability in ERG recordings.

2. Equipment issues

It is the responsibility of the clinical electrophysiologist to ensure that their laboratory complies with the published ISCEV standards. The standard states "it is necessary that all electrophysiologists master the technical requirements of their chosen electrode, to ensure proper impedance, to ensure that waveforms are comparable to standard ERGs, and to define both normal values and variability for their own laboratory." Essential to the adherence to the ISCEV standards is a thorough understanding of the implications of variability at all points in the stimulus - recording loop along with implications of fluctuations in the environment. In this section we review some of the challenges faced in recording ERGs and minimizing inter-site and inter-test variability.

2.1 The light source problem

Differences in standardized luminance pose a major challenge to comparing ERGs between clinical testing centers. The main problem is an inherent property of the most common light source, the xenon flash tube. In xenon flash tubes there is instability produced by arc-wander which can give rise to random fluctuations of a few percent in light output (Robson 1998). All Xenon tubes produce less light as they age necessitating frequent radiometric calibration. Unfortunately, due to manufacturing tolerances the working standard of radiometry equipment provides an overall uncertainty of about 10% (Ryer 1997). This measurement error would be multiplied between sites potentially providing a significantly greater amount of inter-site variability. One possible solution to this issue is the recent change to light emitting diodes (LEDs) for the ERG stimulus source.

While LEDs do not have the luminous efficacy of xenon flash tubes they are still a promising light source for electroretinography since they can be precisely controlled with regards to intensity and flash duration. LEDs show remarkable flash-to-flash stability with less than 1% variation in light intensity(Robson 2005). In addition, long term output change is around 1% after 2000 hours of continuous output at an ambient operating temperature of +55°C(Coupland 2004a). In the late 1990's several investigators began using LED stimulator systems for clinical electroretinography in the laboratory and for intra-operative monitoring. In 2000, a light-emitting diode flash stimulator became commercially available, the Espion ColorBurst™ and Espion ColorDome™ (Diagnosys LLC, Littleton, MA). These systems have now been employed as the stimulus for ERG recording systems and have significantly reduced inter-test and inter-site variability.

2.2 Electrode issues

There are many designs of ERG recording electrodes available, including contact lens, gold foil, gold wire, corneal wick, wire loops, microfibers, as well as skin electrodes. The clinical ERG is obtained with an electrode placed at some distance from the neural elements producing the signals of interest. The electrical current originates in the retinal circuitry around the eyeball and orbit, with both spatial and temporal variations. The ERG signals are conducted from their retinal generator sites through various tissues to the surface electrode. Each electrode type has its own characteristic impedance, recording characteristics, and inherent artefacts(Coupland 2004a).

In 2006 an international survey of ERG electrode use amongst ISCEV members was conducted via email(Coupland 2006a). Members were asked which electrode system they used most often and their second choice of electrode system. Over 80% of respondents used two or more different ERG electrodes in their clinical practice. The majority of respondents (52%) use the contact lens electrode as their first choice for clinical electroretinography. The second and third most popular choices were the DTL fibre electrode (36%) and the lid hook electrode (12%) respectively. There were no respondents who use skin electrodes as their electrode of first choice in all their patients.

Of the 80% of respondents who used a second ERG electrode, lid hook electrodes were chosen by 44%; whereas, 21% of these respondents used DTL fibers or contact lens electrodes as their second choice. A small number of respondents (12%) indicated they used a skin electrode as their second choice; all of these respondents were involved in testing paediatric patients.

Respondents were also asked why they preferred the ERG electrode they were using. Those using contact electrodes preferred better signal-to-noise, quality and consistency of recorded ERGs, the durability and convenience of the lid speculum were also considered important. Those respondents choosing the lid hook electrode preferred better patient acceptance, good ERG recording results, the unaltered optical quality provided by lid hook electrodes and their ease of use. Those respondents expressing preference for DTL-fiber electrodes were impressed with patient acceptance, the electrode's ease of use, the unaltered optical quality provided, the fact that it cannot be blinked out, the electrode is disposable, and that no sterilization is needed. Skin electrodes were preferred because of ease of use, patient comfort, and the fact that no sterilization was needed.

As illustrated by this study the choice of recording electrode is varied amongst the members of ISCEV. Furthermore, when asked whether clinicians were using the best ERG electrode recording system, 72% of respondents expressed agreement; whereas, 20% of respondents weren't sure and 8% of respondents felt they were not using the best electrode available. The chief impediments to changing to a better ERG electrode recording system were listed as the cost and time needed to collect new normative data, the time for training staff to use the new electrode effectively, and the inability to find consistent supplies of disposable microfiber electrodes.

The signal to noise ratio, impedence and sensitivities for each of these electrode systems differ considerably (Coupland 2006a). As highlighted by this study it was felt that changing the electrode significantly changed the recordings, to the point where the clinical electrophyisologist felt it was necessary to recreate the normal database. If comparisons are made between recordings from different sites or at different times it is important that same electrode system is used to allow these comparisons to be valid. This difference is amplified between sites where not only the electrodes are different but the entire recording systems are different.

2.3 Calibration issues

The Calibration Standard Committee of the ISCEV has provided guidelines for the calibration of stimulus and recording parameters used in clinical electrophysiology of vision (Brigell et al. 2003, 107:185-193). The document is concerned with both the calibration of the visual stimulus including protocols for the measurement of luminous flash intensity, mean luminance, contrast and visual angle of pattern stimuli. The photometric measurement of luminance levels used for stimulation of the rods is most accurately specified in scotopic units. Unfortunately, few photometers have scotopic correction filters available and the suggested ISCEV standard is a photopic photometric calibration of the stimulus. This allows only an approximation of the rod flash luminance. In our clinical experience many clinical laboratories do not have appropriate technology or familiarity with both photopic and scotopic photometric calibration. The use of automated calibration routines can be usefully applied to optoelectronic (i.e. light emitting diode) stimulators and at least one manufacturer has incorporated internal calibration of their LED stimulator. While the ISCEV standard requires the calibration of Ganzfeld strobe flash and background luminance is performed at least every 6 months, in reality the frequency of calibration varies widely across different laboratories. Some equipment manufacturers have provided internal reminders to prompt users to perform calibration, this is particularly useful if internal automated calibration systems are provided.

The ISCEV standards also provide guidelines for the calibration of electrophysiological recording systems and include protocols for the measurement of electrode impedance and amplifier calibration(Brigell, Bach, Barber, Moskowitz, and Robson 2003, 107:185-193). The calibration of amplifiers is particularly challenging since most manufacturers do not provide a standard calibrator to pass a known signal through the system to measure the system output. Suitable signal generators must be capable of producing low amplitude output using both sine wave and square wave pulses. The use of both sine wave and square wave calibration signals allows detection of unwanted harmonic distortion and assesses the filtering characteristics of the amplifiers themselves(Brigell, Bach, Barber, Moskowitz, and Robson 2003, 107:185-193). The ISCEV standards committee is presently communicating with equipment manufacturers to develop appropriate standardized calibrators.

With increasing use and popularity of optoelectronic stimulation, internal calibration is essential because the luminous intensity of an LED is temperature dependent. This means that as temperature linearly increases or decreases, the light intensity of an LED exponentially decreases or increases respectively. Red and amber LEDs are more sensitive to temperature effects than blue and green LEDs. Some ERG systems (e.g. Diagnosys LLC, Lowell, MA) utilizing an LED stimulator provide the user with the ability to perform internal calibration of the LED system once the system is turned on or it can be evoked every time a new test is selected. Presently, the ISCEV standards do not address calibration of LED systems, but this should be rectified in the next revision of the standards.

2.4 Conclusions

The ISCEV standards provide a good basis for creation of an ERG recording system. However it is incumbent on the electrophyisologist managing the recording laboratory to ensure that the equipment is properly and regularly calibrated and that the recording technique is standardised and conforms to ISCEV standards.

3. Normative data

Dorland's Medical Dictionary defines Normal as "agreeing with the regular and established type."(Dorland 2003) Typically in medicine this is taken as the mean ± 95% confidence intervals for a given population. Thus an ERG response for a given type of stimulation would be normal if it fell with-in the 95 % confidence intervals for that type of recording. The challenge however is defining the 95% confidence intervals for ERG.

The need to establish a new normative database as indicated in Coupland's 2006 survey of ISCEV members is a major hindrance to changing or updating any electrophysiological system(Coupland 2006a). To date few companies supply a normative database which can negate the need to carry out on site testing to establish site specific guides for normative values. This is contrary to most diagnostic equipment utilized in ophthalmology and is in part due to the inherent variability in recording systems identified above. Population specific factors such as age, race, pupil size, axial length, and diurnal variation, impact the ability to establish a normative database; these issues are addressed in this section.

3.1 Age factors

The effect of age on ERG parameters has been well demonstrated(Birch and Anderson 1992, 110:1571-1576;Peterson 1968:Suppl-77;Weleber 1981, 20:392-399). Birch and Anderson(Birch and Anderson 1992, 110:1571-1576) for instance described ERGs in 270 normal subjects recorded under the ISCEV standard and ranging in age from newborn to 79 years. The mean log amplitude of both rod and cone responses increased from birth reaching its maximum at around 25 years and then showed a progressive decline with age. While the exact factors causing the decrease in ERG amplitude in the elderly are not well understood, it is likely that preretinal media changes, reduction in photopigment optical density with age, or bipolar and/or Müller cell degeneration with aging could account for such age-related amplitude reduction (1992).

Similar changes are observed at the other end of the age spectrum. Both scotopic and photopic ERGs are recordable at birth. There is a rapid increase in b-wave amplitude during the first 4 months in the neonatal period. By 6 months of age, b-wave scotopic sensitivity has become equivalent to that of adults(Fulton 1988, 69:101-109). Development of normal, rod-mediated vision in human infants is primarily based on studies of electroretinal function, and psychophysical adaptation to bleaching lights as well as adaptation to steady background lights. Presently, it is thought that early postnatal development of human scotopic function reflects the reorganization of the inner retinal circuitry(Fulton 1988, 69:101-109).

As with most diagnostic tests in medicine, it is important to compare any ERG recording with age matched normal subjects - but this significantly increases the number of ERG recordings required to establish a normative database. This task becomes even more monumental when one takes into consideration ethnic diversity.

3.2 Ethnic diversity

Coupland et al., (2006b) described an international study of the ERG in normals using the same ERG equipment and protocol at two centers in the Peoples Republic of China and in Canada. It is assumed that any observed differences in ERG parameters would likely reflect true population differences rather than variations resulting from instrumentation or methodology. Two similar aged populations were recruited and identical recording methodology was employed. Interestingly, there were no significant differences observed in a- and b-wave peak latency (i.e. implicit time) between the two groups; however, there were statistically significant differences in b-wave amplitude observed for the scotopic rod, scotopic mixed rod-cone, photopic cone and 30 Hz flicker ERGs, with amplitudes being significantly larger in the Canadian subjects. They proposed that the observed b-wave amplitude differences observed were due to increased axial length in Chinese eyes as evidenced by increased mean (myopic) refractive error. This study demonstrated a correlation between axial length and b-wave amplitudes and implicit times suggesting individuals with pathological myopia may result in falsely abnormal values if these factors are not reflected in the normative database.

3.3 Gender

Gender differences in ERG b-wave amplitude have been noted by several investigators (Birch and Anderson 1992, 110:1571-1576;Peterson 1968:Suppl-77). Peterson (Peterson 1968:Suppl-77) first noted that females had statistically significant larger b-wave amplitude in all ages from 10 to 50 years. A similar small but statistically significant affect of gender was also demonstrated by Birch and Anderson(Birch and Anderson 1992, 110:1571-1576) showing slightly smaller amplitude which they and others thought likely due to greater axial length in males. Thus comparing a female subject to a normative database of males would not be valid.

3.4 Pupil size

Retinal illumination is proportional to pupil area. Coupland (2004) reported dilated pupil size in 400 consecutive patients between ages 10 and 90 years and found the dilated pupil size varied from 4 to 9.5 mm and was significantly correlated with age ($p<0.001$) (Figure 1). Since there was significant variation in dilated pupil size with age in the clinical population, the affect of this was studied in a small group of patients in which dilated pupil size could be strictly controlled through a set of custom made soft contact lenses with artificial pupil sizes of 4 and 6 mm (Figure 2). ERGs obtained to a photopic ISCEV standard flash were measured in subjects against their normal fully dilated pupil and then through a 4 mm and 6 mm artificial pupil. Variability of dilated pupil size can significantly affect amplitude and implicit time obtained using standard flash ERG.

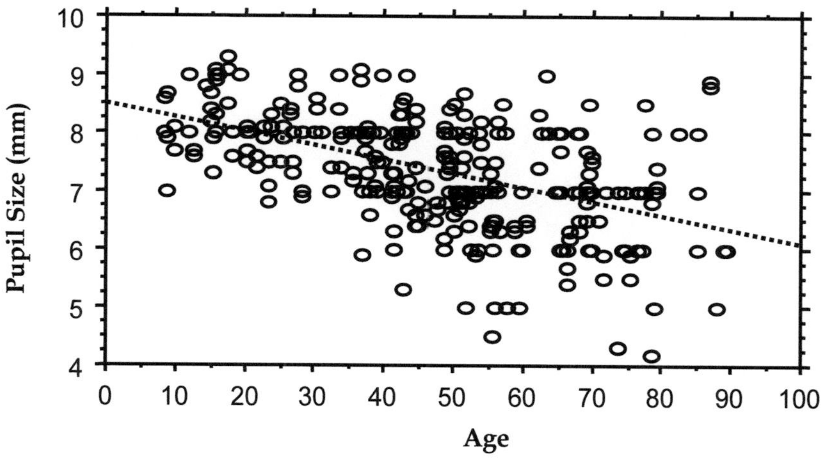

Fig. 1. Dilated Pupil size decreases with increasing age (Line of best fit = 8.487-0.24 x Age; R^2=0.228). Adapted from Coupland (2004).

3.5 Diurnal variation in ERG

Birch et al.(Birch, Berson, and Sandberg 1984, 25:236-238) described the range of diurnal variation for the rod b-wave amplitude to beapproximately a 13% reduction occurring 1.5 hours after the onset of daylight. Interestingly, this time period corresponds to the point of maximum rod outer segment disc shedding. ERG b-waves become largest by midday. In a larger study of circadian rhythm on the dark-adapted ERG, Nozaki et al.,(Nozaki, Wakakura, and Ishikawa 1983, 27:346-352) reported that a-wave amplitude showed no circadian rhythm. B-wave amplitudes were also noted to be lowest around 6 a.m. and highest at midday. B-wave amplitude showed no direct correlation with corticosteroid levels but did show correlation with dopamine β-hydroxylase. Melatonin level has also been found to affect the ERG (Fufiange et al. 2002). Significant inverse correlation was found between salivary melatonin level and ERG b-wave amplitude; when melatonin levels were highest, the ERG b-wave amplitude was lowest(Rufiange, Dumont, and Lachapelle 2002, 43:2491-2499). These findings suggest that the ERG recordings in patients during clinical trials, to monitor patient improvement or progression, are best performed at approximately the same time of day.

A

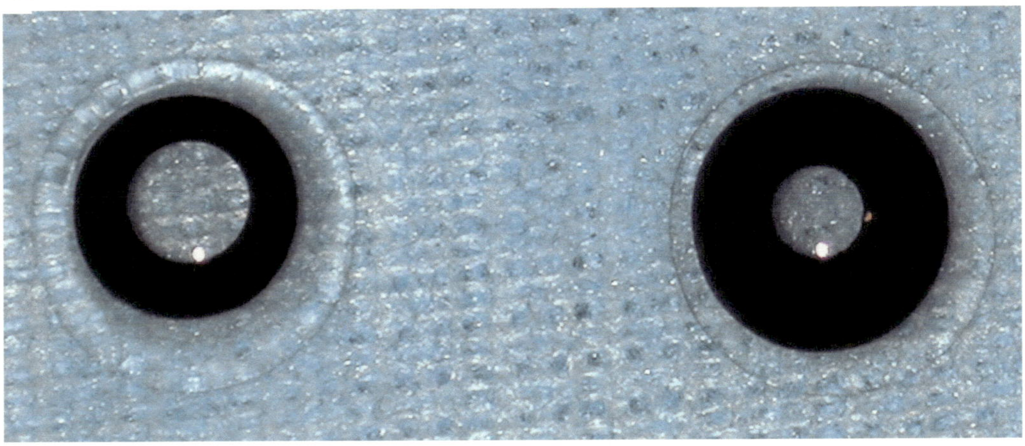

B
Pupil Size

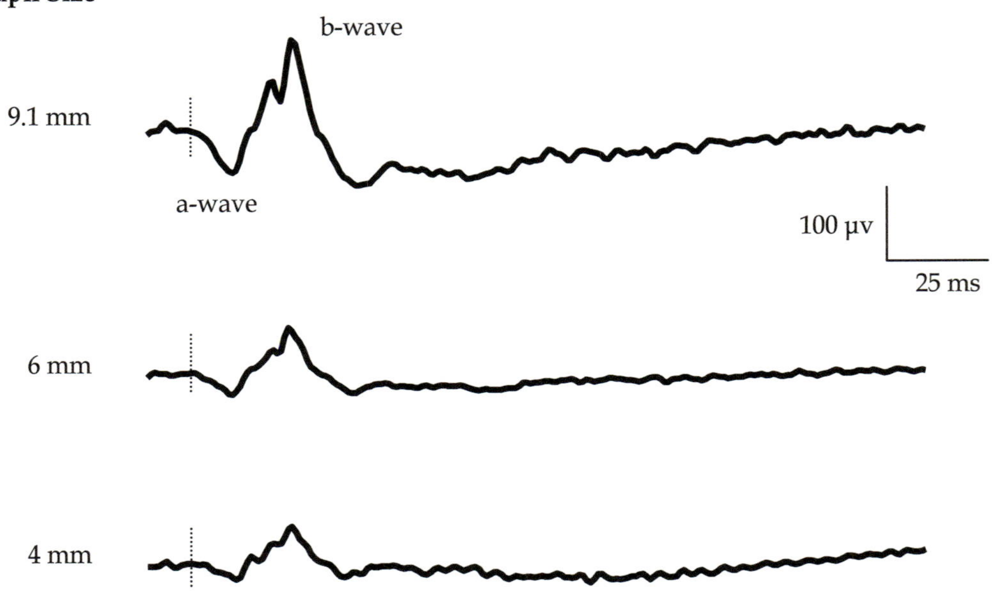

Fig. 2. B-wave amplitude decreases with decreasing pupil size. A: Contact lens with standardized apertures were used to simulate a fixed sized pupil in dilated normal individuals. B: the ERG responses to a standard flash (3 cd·s/m^2) in these experiments show a decrease in the b-wave amplitude of >40% in these normal individuals with decreasing pupil size. Adapted from Coupland (2004).

3.6 Recording conditions

The effects of environmental conditions on the recording equipment have been outlined above. These conditions also affect the subject and can adversely impact the quality of the recordings obtained. In a study looking at optimization of visual evoked potentials (VEP), Karanjia et al.,(Karanjia, Brunet, and ten Hove 2009, 36:89-92) were able to demonstrate that use of a recumbent position improved the signal to noise ratio for the recordings. Failure to attend to patient positioning can artificially alter the quality and amplitude of all types of electrophysiological recordings and thus must be consistently addressed during the recording of ERGs.

3.7 Conclusions

This information demonstrates the need for appropriately selecting subjects for a normative database. Databases which are homogenous for one ethnic group, of a single age group or refractive state may not accurately reflect the normative data range for individual subjects who do not match those demographics. Furthermore, consistency in recording time and technique is essential as variation in pupil size from inadequate dilatation may artificially alter the amplitude of the recording. Thus, it is important that the subject be comfortable and tested under consistent conditions including the time of day.

As illustrated in Coupland's survey (2006a) the need for site specific normative databases is a serious impediments to the individual laboratory adapting new recording equipment or techniques. Establishing a new normative database is labour intensive, time-consuming and expensive. The solution, it might seem, would be a cooperative multicenter collaboration for normative ERG data collection. The advantages would include a reduction in cost, resources and testing time to those participant sites. The challenges posed by recording at different sites is addressed in the following section.

4. Multicenter recordings

Conflicting findings between testing sites have been published since the early days of ERG. For example Sabates et al.,(Sabates, Hirose, and McMeel 1983, 101:232-235) looked at the b/a wave ratio as a surrogate of inner retinal function in patients with central retinal vein occlusion (CRVO). This study was based on the understanding that the a-wave represents outer retinal function and thus the neurons responsible for this component of the ERG would be supported by choroidal circulation, whereas the b-wave is representative of the neuronal activity of the inner retina, supplied by the central retinal artery and thus more likely to be damaged in a CRVO. Sabates found that a b/a ratio of less than one was correlated with a higher likely hood of a patient having neovascularisation of the iris (NVI) as a result of the CRVO.

Sabates's finding was refuted by Johnson et al.,(Johnson et al. 1988, 106:348-352) found that b/a ratios were greater than unity in 8 out of 9 patients who subsequently developed NVI when a maximal stimulus amplitude luminance was utilized. While Johnson and Sabates results appear to be at odds with each other it is important to note that several key difference existed between Sabates and Johnsons recording systems.

Differences in the luminance for both sets of experiments coupled with differences in the type of recording electrode, Ganzfeld stimulator, and recording equipment only compounded any difference in the signals recorded at the two sites. These issues make it virtually impossible to directly compare data collected in the two studies and similar limitations still exist today when trying to compare or compile data from multiple sites.

Over two decades has passed since Sabates's and Johnson's studies and a basic ERG protocol has been standardized for certain responses since 1989(Marmor 1989, 73:299-302). This ERG standard has since been updated three times, most recently in 2008(Marmor et al. 2009, 118:69-77) and in theory would allow for comparison of recordings throughout the world. The guidelines include recommendations for commercial recording instrumentation to allow for the recording of the standard five ERG responses and in conjunction with numerous commercially available electro-diagnostic systems. Given the number of manufactures of stimulus and recording equipment and number of permissible recording techniques, the number of possible combinations and subsequent variability, remains very large.

A:

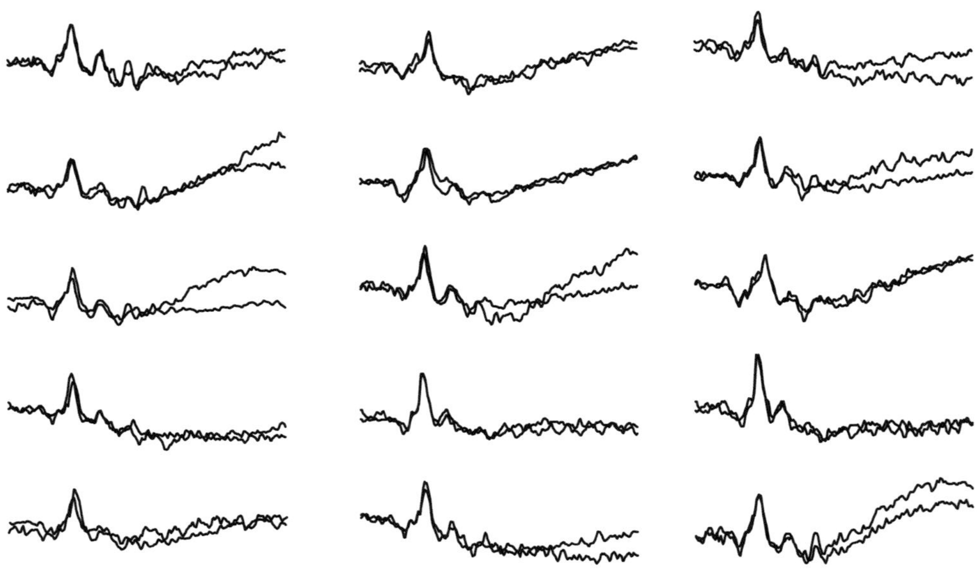

B:

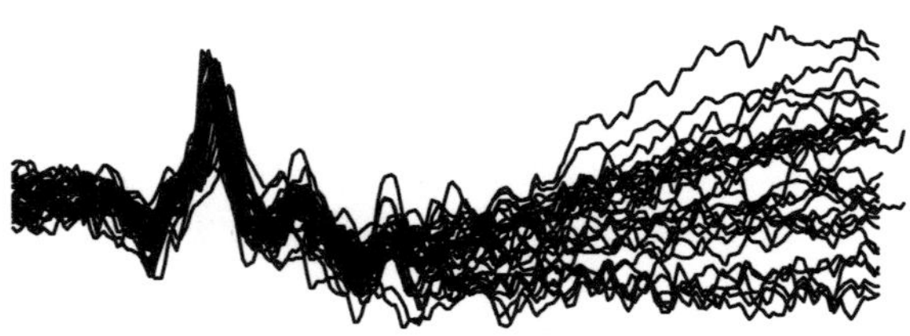

Fig. 3. Fifteen serial ERG recordings from 15 Espion e^2 (Diagnosys LLC, Lowell, MA) electrodiagnostic instruments. ERGs were recorded to 3 cd·s/m^2 flash through undilated pupils in a single subject, ND using DTL-Plus Diagnosys LLC, Lowell, MA) microconductive fiber electrode. A: ERGs were repeated at each site to demonstrate replicability. B: Overlay of all recordings demonstrates consistent A and B wave response amplitudes and latencies across all recordings. (*The authors would like to thank Natalie Doran and Diagnosys LLC for providing the ERGs used in this illustration.)*

The greatest impediment to collaborative multicenter data collection is this inter-site variability in ERG recording parameters. In order to utilize multi-site data collection the two main sources of inter-site variance; differences in recording methodology and differences in standardized stimulus luminance; would need to be addressed. Inter-site variability resulting from differences in recording methods (e.g. different recording electrodes, filter settings, adaptation time, inter-flash intervals etc.) can be largely controlled through standardization. When a single recording system and protocol is used a consistent ERG recording can be obtained at different test centres (Figure 3). All fifteen sets of recordings were done on a single subject and show consistent a- and b-wave amplitude and latency. In order for ERGs to have a use in clinical trials recordings between test centres need to be consistent. Figure 3 clearly illustrates that this is possible provided the appropriate care and protocols, as discussed below, are in place.

4.1 ERG and clinical trials

The strength of ERG recordings as a primary or secondary endpoint lies in the quantitative objective nature of the recordings. Yet the clinical significance of decreased ERG amplitudes or delay is not always clear in clinical trials setting.

The US FDA Center for Drug Evaluation and Research is responsible for monitoring the drug development process as well as approving new drug products and monitoring adverse events after approval has been granted. ERG is first used in preclinical studies on drugs that are intended to affect electrophysiology, bind with melanin, or cause retinal lesions (Chambers 2011). In clinical studies ERGs are used as outcome measures to assess therapeutic efficacy as well as monitor potential retinal toxicity when demonstrated ERG abnormalities have been shown in animal studies. In human clinical trials ERG is often used as a secondary endpoint although it has been used as a primary endpoint in a recent safety study(Cordell et al. 2009, 127:367-373). FDA does not usually set ERG testing standards and generally accepts the ISCEV standards(Chambers 2011). To date changes greater than 40% in b-wave amplitude from baseline have been accepted as clinically significant(Cordell, Maturi, Costigan, Marmor, Weleber, Coupland, Danis, McGettigan, Antoszyk, Klise, and Sides 2009, 127:367-373).

4.2 ERG and multicenter clinical trials

ERG has the potential to provide objective information on retinal function and thus is highly desirable in clinical trials. The difference in recording technique and equipment, however, make interpretation between centers a major challenge to the clinical utility of ERG.

New clinical trials may soon be obligated by the FDA to include ERG as one of the outcome measures if a medication is intended to directly affect the electrophysiology of cells or if there has been demonstrated ERG abnormality in animal studies(Chambers 2011). Given this FDA mandate for ERG testing as part of new drug development the ability to record from subjects at different centers during a multicenter clinical trial is becoming a necessity. To date there is one multicenter clinical trial which utilized ERG as a primary endpoint and it provides an excellent case study on how to address the challenges of multicenter ERG recordings(Cordell, Maturi, Costigan, Marmor, Weleber, Coupland, Danis, McGettigan, Antoszyk, Klise, and Sides 2009, 127:367-373).

4.3 Standardized multicenter clinical trial

Cordell et al.,(Cordell, Maturi, Costigan, Marmor, Weleber, Coupland, Danis, McGettigan, Antoszyk, Klise, and Sides 2009, 127:367-373) were mandated to look at potential for retinal toxicity for tadalafil or sildenafil by the FDA, in a post market Phase IV clinical trial conducted at 15 US clinics using standardized ERG equipment and protocols. ERG was selected as the primary measure of retinal toxicity in this clinical trial as it provided objective quantities measure of retinal function. Subjects were recruited at 15 centers within the United States mandating that ERG testing be conducted at all 15 centers. In order to overcome the technical limitations to multicenter recordings all centers used the same standardized equipment, the same ERG protocol, and a single normative data set with a single website based ERG reading center. In the process they have established guidelines which address the challenges of multicenter ERG recordings with a variety of technical and logistical solutions for the use of ERG in future clinical trials.

4.3.1 Personnel and training

Consistency of outcome across multiple testing sites can only be ensured through appropriate training and consistent monitoring of ERG outcomes to maintain quality assurance standards and this is one of the roles of the ERG reader. It is critical that all sites submit standardized ERG tests on normal subjects and empirically demonstrate consistency before receiving certification for multicenter trials.

Appropriately trained technologists are critical for multicenter ERG clinical trials. Preferably, all centers should be trained by the same trainer to ensure consistency of technique. On-site visit during patient testing confirms performance consistency at the individual site. In the Cordell et al., (2009) study, all 15 sites received centralized training on the east and west coasts (Washington DC and Scottsdale Arizona). In addition, all 15 sites received individualized on-site refresher training all within a 4-week period following centralized training. Reproducibility and consistency of ERGs obtained on individual non-clinical trial patients at multiple sites were assessed through a centralized web-based ERG reading center. Through the use of standardised training and protocols this study was able to demonstrate that ERG is a viable method of compiling objective multicenter data with low levels of inter-site variability.

4.3.2 Role of ERG reader

The ERG reviewer or ERG reader performs two vital roles in clinical trials using ERGs as clinical endpoints. The primary role is to monitor quality and consistency in reproducibility of ERGs submitted from clinical sites. It is essential that ERGs have quality assurance review in order that they are interpreted correctly. Technical artefact such as power mains interference, eye blink and eye movement, high frequency noise, electrical spiking, and other myogenic interference can produce spurious changes in waveform morphology which could be incorrectly interpreted. The secondary role of the ERG reader is to determine if there have been objective quantitative or subjective qualitative changes in ERG findings over time. It is critical that the ERG reader be blind to both patient identification and experimental clinical trial condition. This reduces the degree of bias as does the reliance on statistical criteria for determining ERG change.

When multiple ERG readers are used in large clinical trials a process for conflict resolution is necessary. In order to maintain consistency of quality of ERG interpretation it is essential that all readers review all waveforms or all those waveforms that are deemed to fall outside of normal limits and agree that significant changes in ERG amplitude and timing have occurred. It is essential that criteria for determining ERG change be determined before the clinical trial begins.

Multicenter recording protocols such as the one employed in Cordell et al., (2009) benefited from having a centralised electronic database of all the recordings. This allowed multiple readers to assess the complete set of data and make independent evaluations of the ERGs. Conflicting interpretations were then reassessed as a group using the predetermined criteria established prior to the commencement of recruitment. The acceptance of this clinical trial by the FDA provides tacit approval of the methodology employed in Cordell et al., (2009).

4.4 Conclusions

As an objective measure of retinal function ERG is poised to play a major role in clinical trails. Cordell et al., (2009) provides a framework by which one can run a successful multicenter clinical trial that utilizes ERG as a primary endpoint. Their success was dependent on standardization of not just the recording equipment but the training and personnel, both technicians and ERG readers, involved in the trial.

5. References

Birch DG, and Anderson JL. 1992. Standardized full-field electroretinography. Normal values and their variation with age. *Arch. Ophthalmol.* 110 (11): 1571-1576.

Birch DG, Berson EL, and Sandberg MA. 1984. Diurnal rhythm in the human rod ERG. *Invest Ophthalmol. Vis. Sci.* 25 (2): 236-238.

Brigell M, Bach M, Barber C, Moskowitz A, and Robson J. 2003. Guidelines for calibration of stimulus and recording parameters used in clinical electrophysiology of vision. *Doc. Ophthalmol.* 107 (2): 185-193.

Chambers WA. 2011. Electroretinography: The FDA's Viewpoint.

Cordell WH, Maturi RK, Costigan TM, Marmor MF, Weleber RG, Coupland SG, Danis RP, McGettigan JW, Jr., Antoszyk AN, Klise S, and Sides GD. 2009. Retinal effects of 6 months of daily use of tadalafil or sildenafil. *Arch. Ophthalmol.* 127 (4): 367-373.

Coupland SG. 2004 A proposal to adopt retinal illuminance as an ISCEV standard for clinical electroretinography. Paper presented at 9th Annual Chinese Symposium for Clinical Visual Electrophysiology, at Chengdu, China.

Coupland SG, Wu D, Li M, 2005. International Multicenter Normative ERG Database Using the ISCEV Standard. International Society for Clinical Electrophysiology of Vision (ISCEV) Annual Meeting, Glasgow, Scotland August 22-27th, 2005.

Coupland SG. 2006a. Electrodes for Visual Testing. In *Principles and Practice of Clinical Electrophysiology of Vision,* eds JR Heckenlively and GB Arden Cambridge: MIT Press.

Coupland SG. 2006b. International Multicenter Normative ERG Database Using the ISCEV Standard. Paper presented at Annual Meeting of Association for Research in vision and Ophthalmology (ARVO), at Ft. Lauderdale.

Droland WAN. 2003. *Dorland's Illustrated Medical Dictionary*. Philidelphia, PA: Saunders.

Fishman FA, Birch DG, Holder GE, and Brigell MG. 2001. Electrophysiologic Testing. *Ophthalmology* 2nd Supplement.

Fulton AB. 1988. The development of scotopic retinal function in human infants. *Doc. Ophthalmol.* 69 (2): 101-109.

Holder GE, Brigell MG, Hawlina M, Meigen T, Vaegan, and Bach M. 2007. ISCEV standard for clinical pattern electroretinography--2007 update. *Doc. Ophthalmol.* 114 (3): 111-116.

Hood DC, Bach M, Brigell M, Keating D, Kondo M, Lyons JS, and Palmowski-Wolfe AM. 2008. ISCEV guidelines for clinical multifocal electroretinography (2007 edition). *Doc. Ophthalmol.* 116 (1): 1-11.

Johnson MA, Marcus S, Elman MJ, and McPhee TJ. 1988. Neovascularization in central retinal vein occlusion: electroretinographic findings. *Arch. Ophthalmol.* 106 (3): 348-352.

Karanjia R, Brunet DG, and ten Hove MW. 2009. Optimization of visual evoked potential (VEP) recording systems. *Can. J. Neurol. Sci.* 36 (1): 89-92.

Marmor MF. 1989. An international standard for electroretinography. *Doc. Ophthalmol.* 73 (4): 299-302.

Marmor MF, Fulton AB, Holder GE, Miyake Y, Brigell M, and Bach M. 2009. ISCEV Standard for full-field clinical electroretinography (2008 update). *Doc. Ophthalmol.* 118 (1): 69-77.

Nozaki S, Wakakura M, and Ishikawa S. 1983. Circadian rhythm of human electroretinogram. *Jpn. J. Ophthalmol.* 27 (2): 346-352.

Peterson H. 1968. The normal B-potential in the single-flash clinical electroretinogram. A computer technique study of the influence of sex and age. *Acta Ophthalmol. (Copenh)*: Suppl-77.

Robson JG. 1998. Light Sources. In *Vision Research: a practical guide to laboratory methods,* Oxford University Press.

Robson JG. 2005. Personal Communication. ed SG Coupland.

Rufiange M, Dumont M, and Lachapelle P. 2002. Correlating retinal function with melatonin secretion in subjects with an early or late circadian phase. *Invest Ophthalmol. Vis. Sci.* 43 (7): 2491-2499.

Ryer A. 1997. *Light Measurement Handbook.* Newburyport MA: International Light Inc.

Sabates R, Hirose T, and McMeel JW. 1983. Electroretinography in the prognosis and classification of central retinal vein occlusion. *Arch. Ophthalmol.* 101 (2): 232-235.

Weleber RG. 1981. The effect of age on human cone and rod ganzfeld electroretinograms. *Invest Ophthalmol. Vis. Sci.* 20 (3): 392-399.

3

Objective Assessment of Local Retinal Function by Focal Macular and Multifocal Electroretinograms

Kei Shinoda[1,2], Celso Soiti Matsumoto[1] and Hisao Ohde[2,3]
[1]*Teikyo University*
[2]*Keio University*
[3]*Makuhari Ode Eye Clinic*
Japan

1. Introduction

There are two clinically methods to record electroretinographic (ERG) responses from focal areas of the retina; the focal macular ERGs (fmERGs) (Hirose et al., 1977; Miyake et al., 1989a; Miyake 1998) and multifocal ERGs (mfERGs).(Sutter &Tran 1992;Sutter et al., 1999; Hood &Greenstein 2003) Each technique has advantages and disadvantages. For example, fmERGs can be used to assess the function of different layers of localized areas of the retina, while mfERGs can be used to assess the function of different localized areas of the macula. These two techniques have been extensively investigated to determine their abilities to detect and assess functional alterations in different retinal areas in different retinal diseases. The results of these studies combined with the morphological findings of the same retinas determined by optical coherence tomography (OCT) have led to significant advances in the diagnosis and treatment of macular diseases. This chapter reviews the findings made by these two techniques, and show how they have advanced the diagnosis and therapy of macular diseases.

2. Focal macular electroretinograms (fmERGs)

Full-field scotopic and photopic ERGs are mass responses elicited by diffuse illumination of the entire retina. Because the total number of cones in the macula represents only 9% of the total cone population, (Crucio et al., 1990) full-field photopic ERGs are not suited for detecting focal lesions in the macular area or in determining the pathogenesis of macular diseases. Although the full-field ERGs can be normal in eyes with some types of macular diseases, it is often non-recordable when only the macular function is preserved such as in patients with retinitis pigmentosa (RP). Thus, the fmERG was developed to evaluate macular function in patients with similar conditions.

2.1 Principles of eliciting and recording fmERGs

fmERGs are elicited by presenting a small, 5° to 15°, stimulus on the macula and recording the response from the stimulated area. Background illumination is used to depress the sensitivity of the area surrounding the stimulus and thus eliminate contamination from stray light responses. It is essential to monitor the location of the stimulus on the fundus during the recordings, particularly in eyes with poor fixation, to assure that only the macula is stimulated. Miyake et al developed the first stimulating and recording system for fmERGs in 1981, and thereafter extensive information has been collected on the physiological and pathological properties of the macula in both normal subjects and patients with different types of macular diseases.(Miyake 1998, 2006) Their recording system for fmERGs was based on a fundus camera into which a focal stimulus system was integrated. Another system to record fmERGs was developed by Matsumoto et al.(Choshi et al., 2003;Yamada et al., 2006) Their system is based on a slit-lamp microscope, and both the focal stimulus and fundus observation systems were integrated into the slit-lamp. With both systems, the examiner records the ERGs while monitoring the stimulus on the fundus either by an infrared television fundus camera or a slit-lamp-mounted infrared CCD camera. The optical system is designed to have the stimulus light and background illumination installed either into the fundus camera or the slit-lamp. The low amplitude fmERGs can be recorded by summating the responses with a computer with a signal averaging program.

2.2 Waveform of fmERGs

The waveform and components of the fmERGs are similar to those of the conventional full-field photopic ERGs. Thus, the same methods used to analyze full-field photopic ERGs can be used to analyze the different components of the fmERGs. By analyzing individual components of the fmERGs, a layer-by-layer analysis of the retina can be made in the macular area. fmERGs recorded from a normal subject displaying the different components are shown in Figures 1 and 2. The a- and b-waves, oscillatory potentials (OPs), photopic negative response (PhNR), on and off components elicited by the long duration stimuli, and 30 Hz flicker responses can be separately analyzed.

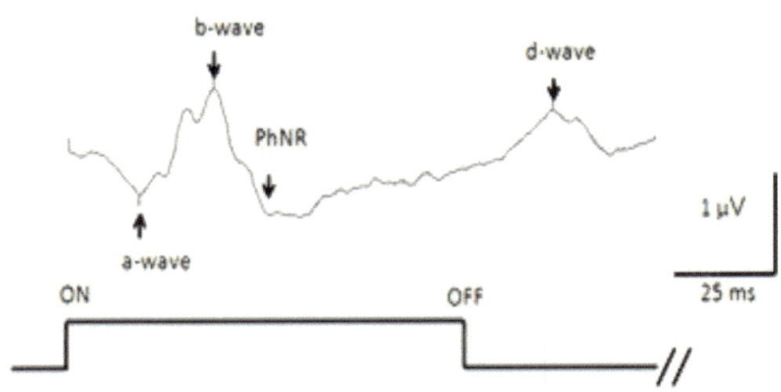

Fig. 1. Waveform of focal macular ERG elicited by a long duration stimulus.

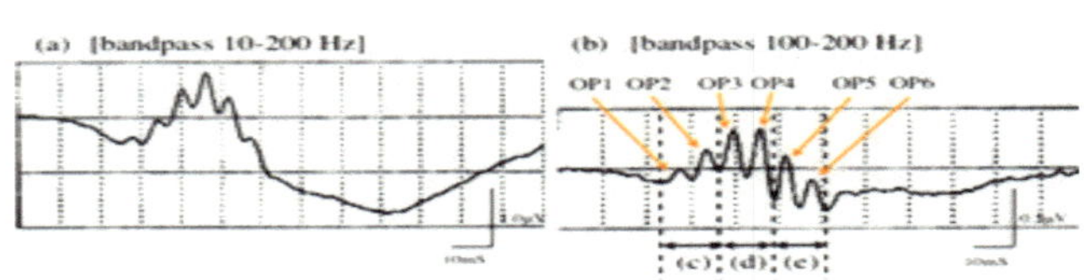

Fig. 2. Oscillatory potentials of focal macular ERGs elicited by a 10° diameter flash from a LED.

2.3 Focal rod ERGs

Although fmERGs are generally used to evaluate cone function, some techniques to record focal rod ERGs have been established. Because a background illumination to eliminate the responses elicited by stray light cannot be used, light scatter is a problem for eliciting focal responses. Sandberg et al showed that small rod responses could be elicited by a relatively large test spot of 30-40 degrees which was distinguishable from a larger but slower stray light response.(Sandberg et al., 1996) The ERGs elicited by stray light can also be eliminated by subtracting the response from a dimmer rod-matched full-field flash.
Another technique used to record focal rod responses is the use of double-flashes to stimulate a 40 degree area that can isolate focal rod a-waves (Nusinowitz et al., 1995) or by using a small blue light (λ_{max} = 470 nm) stimuli after dark-adaptation.(Choshi et al., 2003) Thus far, the clinical use of each technique to record scotopic responses from a focal area is limited.

2.4 Characteristics of fmERGs in normal subjects

Analyses of the fmERGs in normal humans showed several important characteristics. A nasal-temporal asymmetry was found in the OPs of the fmERGs (Fig. 3; Miyake et al., 1989a) When a semicircular stimulus is used to elicit fmERGs from the temporal and nasal sectors of the macula, no significant differences were observed in the amplitudes and implicit times of the a-waves and b-waves. However, the amplitudes of the OPs were significantly larger when the nasal retina was stimulated than when the temporal retina was stimulated. (Miyake et al., 1989a) The amplitude of the focal ERGs recorded with circular stimulus was approximately the same as the sum of the amplitudes of the temporal and nasal ERGs.

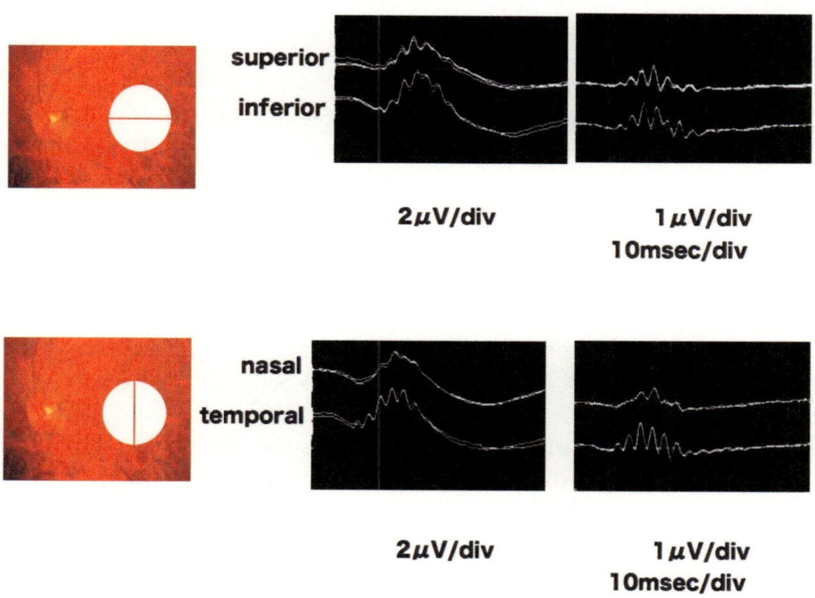

Fig. 3. Comparison of focal macular ERGs using semicircular stimuli on the superior and inferior (Upper), and on the nasal and temporal (Lower) macular areas. The OPs in the temporal macular sector are significantly larger than those in the nasal macula.

Another interesting feature of the fmERGs is that the implicit time of each component is relatively constant for different intensities (Figure 4).

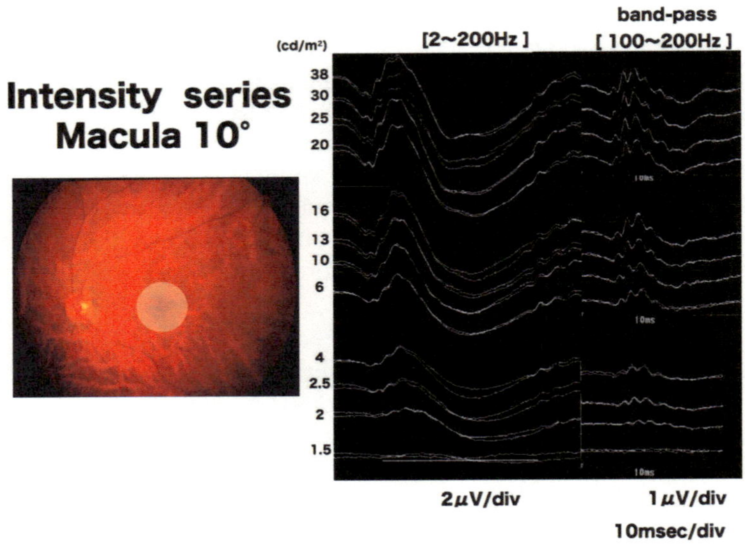

Fig. 4. Focal macular ERGs elicited by different stimulus intensities from a normal subject. The stimulus duration is 100 ms and the luminance of the constant background illumination is 3.0 cd/m^2. An increase in the amplitudes of each component is observed with increasing luminances but the implicit times appear to be constant.

3. Multifocal ERGs (mfERGs)

The second method to examine focal areas of the retina is by mfERGs. The techniques for recording and analyzing the mfERGs were developed by Sutter and Tran in 1992.(Sutter & Tran 1992) With this method, focal ERGs can be recorded simultaneously from multiple retinal locations during a single recording session using cross-correlation techniques. Unlike the fmERGs, there are still questions about how this method works and what it measures.

3.1 Principles of mfERGs

The principles, recording methods, and clinical applications of mfERGs are described in the International Society of Clinical Electrophysiology of Vision (ISCEV) guideline.(Hood et al., 2008) The recording methods for mfERGs are similar to that of full-field ERGs. Typically, the pupil is dilated and a ground electrode is attached to the forehead. A bipolar contact-lens electrode is used as the recording electrode although other electrodes such as the DTL electrode, gold-foil electrode, and other types can be used. The recordings are performed under light-adapted conditions to assess cone functions.

The stimuli are created on a video monitor and consist of a number of hexagonal elements driven at a 75-Hz frame rate (Fig. 5). The sizes of the hexagons are scaled with eccentricity to elicit focal retinal responses of approximately equal amplitude at all locations in normal subjects. At any given moment, about 50% of the hexagons are at a high luminance (white) and the other hexagons are at a low luminance (black). The pattern appears to be a random flicker, but each element follows a fixed, predetermined maximum-length sequence (m-sequence) so that the overall luminance of the screen over time is relatively stable. Maintaining stable central fixation during the recordings is critical to ensure accuracy of the topographical ERG information. This is one of the disadvantages of mfERGs compared to fmERGs. A central fixation target such as a circle, cross, or "X", whose size can be changed according to the visual acuity, is created on the monitor. The recording time depends on the m-sequence and stimulation rate. Most investigators use a series of recording segments of approximately 30-s duration. Any segment containing a substantial artifact can be discarded and repeated.

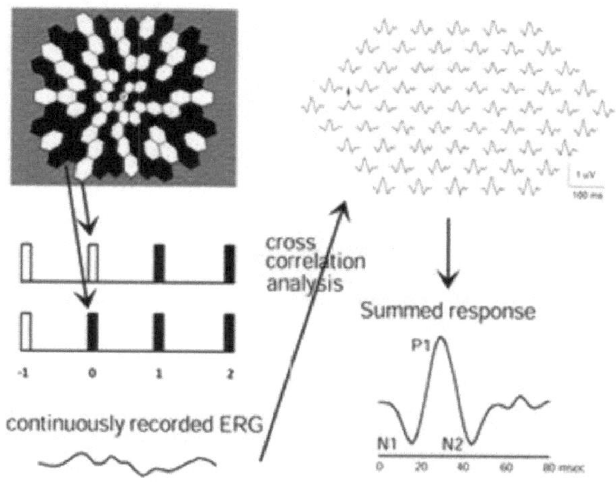

Fig. 5. First-order kernel responses from a normal eye. The mERGs were elicited by an array of black and white hexagons (Upper left). The hexagons go through a pseudo-random sequence of black and white as the frame changes (Middle left). Then a cross-correlation technique produces multiple ERGs (Lower left and upper right). For comparisons to full-field ERGs, 61 focal ERGs are summed (Lower right). Modified and reproduced from (Hood & Greenstein 2003) with permission from Elsevier.

3.2 Waveform of mfERGs

The local response elicited by each hexagon is computed as the cross correlation between the response cycle and the m-sequence. An example of this response is shown in Figure 5 and is called the first-order kernel. The derivation of the first- and second-order kernels as determined by Sutter et al.(Sutter et al., 1999) and Hood(Hood & Greenstein 2003) is shown in Figure 6. The first-order kernel can be thought of as the average response from a particular retinal area unaffected by stimulation of any other area, i.e., a linear approximation of the response from the small retinal area. It is obtained by adding all the records following presentation of a white hexagon and then subtracting all the records following a black hexagon (Fig. 5). The second-order kernel is a non-linear response, and is a measure of how the multifocal response is influenced by the adaptation of the retina to successive flashes. The first slice of the second-order kernel is calculated by comparing the two responses in Figure 6 (arrows). The upper large arrow points to the response to a preceding flash, and the lower large arrow points to the response to a flash of a preceding dark hexagon. If these two responses are not identical, the first slice of the second-order kernel appears, and it is calculated by subtracting one response from the other. The first slice of the second-order kernel represents the effect of an immediately preceding flash; the second slice of the second-order is a measure of the effect of the flash two frames earlier. A similarity of the implicit times of full-field ERGs and that of mfERGs has been reported, and the two techniques can be compared. The waveforms and implicit times of the mfERGs vary with retinal position; however, individuals with retinal dysfunction can be differentiated from those with normal function.

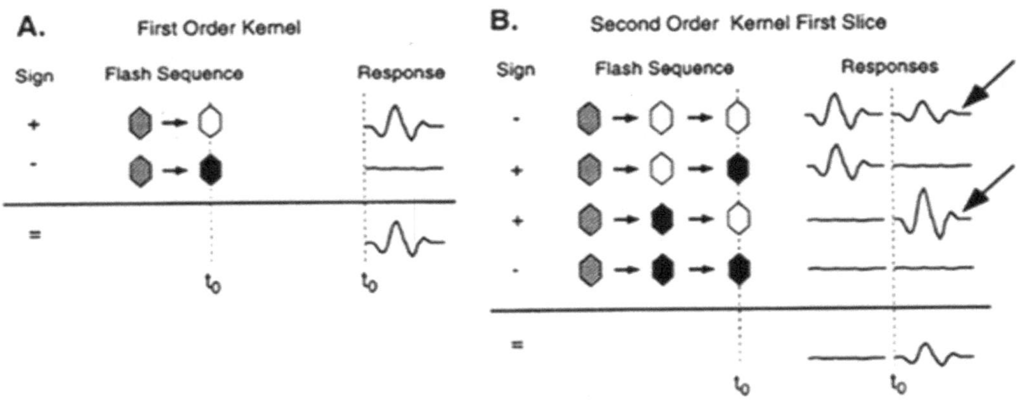

Fig. 6. Deviation of the first- and second-order kernels of mfERGs. White and black hexagons indicate whether the hexagon is bright (white) or when it is dark (black) during the recording. Hexagons with diagonal lines indicate a frame that could have been flash or non-flash. Modified and reproduced from (Hood & Greenstein 2003) with permission from Elsevier.

4. Clinical applications of fmERGs and mfERGs

4.1 Occult retinal lesions

Occult macular dystrophy (OMD) and acute zonal occult outer retinopathy (AZOOR) are representative disorders where the fmERGs and mfERGs findings were key in making a diagnosis.(Miyake et al., 1989b,1996;Miyake 2006;Arai et al., 1998;Piao et al., 2000) OMD was discovered in 1989 by the fmERG findings of the Miyake group. It is a hereditary macular dystrophy characterized by a progressive decrease of the visual acuity, normal fundus, and normal fluorescein angiograms. OMD is an autosomal dominant disease, and the responsible mutation was recently identified as the retinitis pigmentosa 1-like 1 *(RP1L1)* gene.(Akahori et al., 2010) It was demonstrated that *RP1L1* plays important roles in the cone functions in humans, and disruption of *RP1L1* function leads to OMD. The cone and rod components of the full-field ERGs are normal but the fmERGs are reduced. A reduction of the visual acuity without visible fundus abnormalities can lead to a misdiagnosis of amblyopia, optic nerve disease, or a non-organic visual disorder.

The findings from a typical patient with OMD are shown in Figure 7. Although the fundus and fluorescein angiograms are normal, the OCT images show some mild abnormalities such as foveal thinning, irregular and discontinuous photoreceptor inner and outer segment (IS/OS) line, and abnormal cone outer segment tips (COSTs) line.(Park et al., 2010) It is noteworthy that it was Miyake and his co-workers who developed the technique to record fmERGs, who discovered and named patients with these findings as OMD. They determined the clinical characteristics of OMD and identified the responsible gene mutation for OMD. Therefore, OMD has been referred to as Miyake's disease.

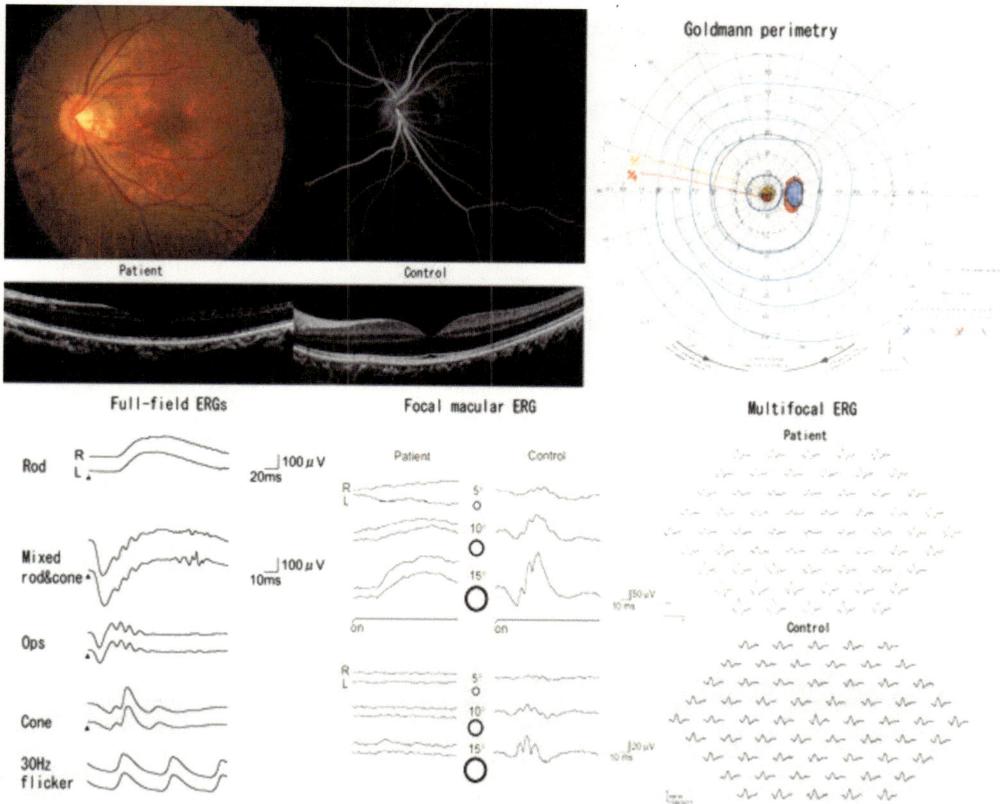

Fig. 7. Fundus photograph, fluorescein angiogram, visual field, full-fielr ERGs, mfERGs, and fmERGs of a typical OMD patient and a control subject. The macular function is selectively depressed. The findings from the fellow eye were almost the same. The fundus appearance, fluorescein fundus angiography, and full-field ERGs were completely normal. The a- and b-waves (upper), and the OPs (lower) of the fmERGs (right column) are reduced. Optical coherence tomographic image showing that the IS/OS line, the middle cone outer segment tip (COST) line between the IS/OS line and the retinal pigment epithelium (RPE) are discernible in the control subject, but the IS/OS line is relative obscure and the COST line is absent in the patient. Modified and reproduced from (Hanazono et al., 2011) with permission from Dove Medical Press Ltd.

Acute idiopathic blind spot enlargement (AIBSE) syndrome is a clinical entity in which the patients report sudden scintillations, and visual field tests show a temporal scotoma enlarging the blind spot. The fundus is otherwise normal, and it was recently reported that AIBSE belongs to the family of AZOOR and associated diseases called the AZOOR-complex. (Fletcher et al., 1988;Gass 2003) The pathological site for the visual field abnormalities is not the optic nerve but the retina, and the diagnosis is made from the mfERG findings (Figure 8).(Sugahara et al., 2011) The spectral domain OCT (SD-OCT) images showed abnormalities in the microstructures of the outer retina, e.g., disruption or loss of the external limiting membrane (ELM), the IS/OS line, and/or an absence of the COST line in the areas of the visual field defects (Figure 9). (Spaide et al., 2008;Sugahara et al., 2011;Tsunoda et al., 2011) It is still under discussion whether fmERGs are better than OCT in detecting the early abnormalities in OMD and in monitoring the changes in the severity or stage of OMD and AZOOR-complex.

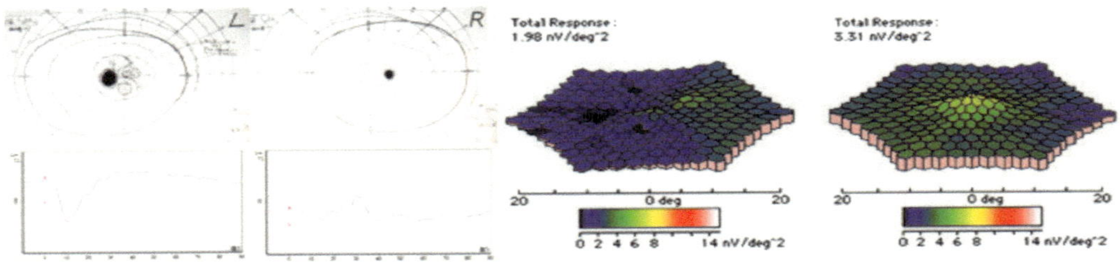

Fig. 8. Findings in a 44-year-old man with acute idiopathic blind spot enlargement (AIBSE) syndrome. (Left) Visual fields (top left) and full-field ERGs (bottom left) from a 44-year-old man who developed an arcuate scotoma connected to the physiological blind spot in the left eye. The amplitudes of the mfERGs (Right) are reduced in the area corresponding to the scotoma indicating that the visual field deficit was retinal in origin. Modified and reproduced from (Sugahara et al., 2011) with permission from S. Karger AG, Basel.

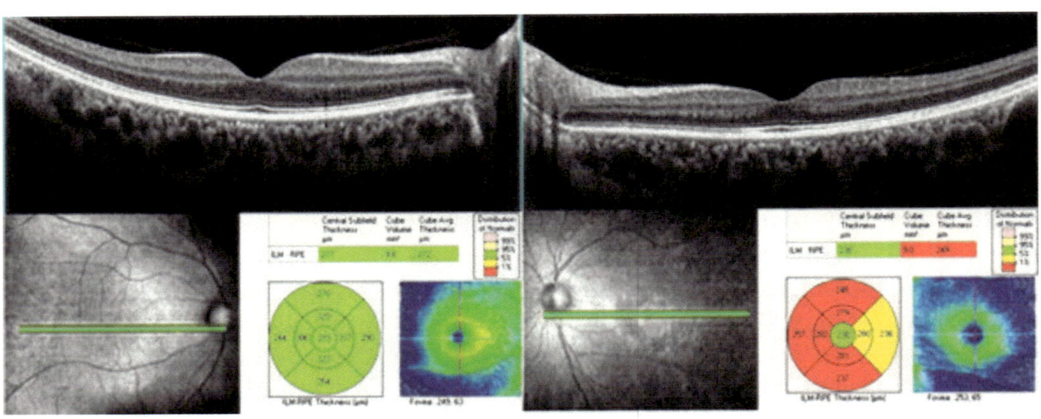

Fig. 9. Findings in the patient shown in Figure 8. (Top) Optical coherence tomographic image showing that both the external limiting membrane (ELM) and the IS/OS line are intact but the middle cone outer segment tip (COST) line between the IS/OS line and the retinal pigment epithelium (RPE) is absent in the nasal macula area of the left eye (top right). The ELM, IS/OS line, COST line, and RPE/Bruch membrane are intact in the right eye (top left).(Bottom) Mean retinal thickness was within normal limits in each of the 9 ETDRS areas in the right macula (bottom left) whereas it was significantly thinner in the corresponding area for thevisual field defect in the left macula (bottom right). Modified and reproduced from (Sugahara et al., 2011) with permission from S. Karger AG, Basel.

4.2 Other retinal dystrophies

Electrophysiological studies have detected macular dysfunction in other retinal dystrophies. In Best vitelliform macular dystrophy (BMD), the full-field ERGs are normal but the fmERGs are reduced.(Falsini et al., 1996) The amplitudes of the central mfERGs are also reduced but the implicit times are relatively well preserved.(Palmowski et al., 2003)
Flicker fmERGs can be used to separate receptoral and postreceptoral activity in BMD and Stargardt macular dystrophy (STD).(Falsini et al., 1996) The fmERGs elicited by 8 and 32 Hz flicker stimuli were reported to have peak amplitudes at the fundamental and 2nd harmonic frequencies. The reduction of the amplitudes at both frequencies was found in both BMD and STD. The fundamental/2nd harmonic ratio is increased in BMD while it is normal in STD suggesting that receptoral and postreceptoral dysfunctions are present in BMD while a receptoral dysfunction appears to be the primary alteration in STD. The amplitude at the fundamental frequency tended to decrease during the follow-up period suggesting a progressive receptoral dysfunction in BMD but not in STD.
mfERGs have been used to compare the patterns of local cone and rod system impairments in patients with progressive cone dystrophy, and the findings clearly showed a pattern of eccentricity-related loss in the cone and rod systems.(Holopigian et al., 2002) Thus, the cone central responses were the most impaired, and the degree of impairment decreased with eccentricity, whereas the rod system was only mildly impaired and the degree of impairment did not change with increasing eccentricities. On the other hand, the peripheral responses were more impaired in patients with retinitis pigmentosa, and a relative sparing of either cone or rod system function was not observed.(Holopigian et al., 2001)
Peripheral cone dystrophy is rare and is an unusual form of cone dystrophy in which the peripheral cone system is more affected than the central cone system. The rod system is relatively normal. To diagnose this type of cone dystrophy accurately and to understand its pathophysiologic features, the findings of fmERGs or mfERGs combined with those of full-field ERGs are necessay.(Kondo et al., 2004)
Studies of the functional anatomy of the macula in albinism showed that the mfERGs were flat in the macular area, and the amplitudes were constant at all retinal eccentricities when the responses were scaled by the stimulated area (Figure 10).(Kelly&Weiss 2006; Nusinowitz & Sarraf, 2008)

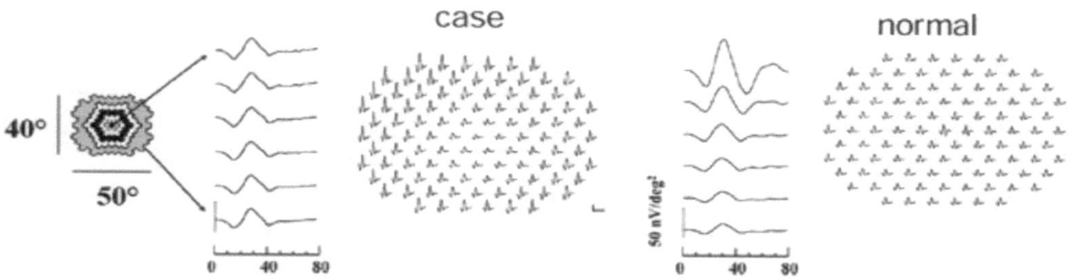

Fig. 10. Topographic map of mfERGs of patient with oculocutaneous albinism (left) compared to that of an adult normal subject (right). The patient has lower amplitude mfERGs at the macula, whereas normal eye has larger amplitude mfERGs at the macula. The mfERGs were averaged across six rings ranging from central retina to 20 degrees peripheral (Left), then scaled for stimulus area. The results show that the amplitude density is constant from the macula to the periphery whereas the normals showed a decrease with increasing eccentricity. Modified and reproduced from (Kelly&Weiss 2006) with permission from Elsevier.

Marmor et al made morphological and functional analyses by Fourier domain OCT (FD-OCT), adaptive optics, and mfERGs in two patients with albinism who lacked a foveal pit.(Marmor et al., 2008) The visual acuities of these two patients ranged from 0.4 to 1.0. They found a thickening of the outer nuclear layer and lengthening of the cone outer segments with normal cone diameters in the central 1° to 2°. Functional analyses showed that the single amplitudes and summed ring-response densities of the main positive peak were within the normal limits, and the response density in the foveal zone was larger, although still low borderline, than that in the peripheral rings. The normal mfERGs from the central macula without a foveal pit suggested that a lack of foveal pit does not always result in retinal dysfunction.

Macular function was assessed in eyes with x-linked retinoschisis by fmERGs (Miyake et al., 1993a) and mfERGs.(Piao et al., 2003) Both tests showed a dysfunction of the retina in the areas corresponding to the foveal schisis. In the early stage of x-linked retinoschisis, the ratio of the b-wave to a-wave (b/a ratio) amplitude of the fmERGs gradually decreased toward the fovea. This suggested that the retinal function in the middle and inner retinal layers were more affected in the central retina, and also that the on-bipolar cells may be more affected than the off-bipolar cells because the a-wave was better preserved than the b-wave. The amplitudes of the first-order kernel of the mfERGs were reduced in the central retina while they varied outside the foveal area. The implicit times were significantly delayed both in the central and extrafoveal regions.(Piao et al., 2003) These findings suggest that the pathology of XLRS affected the implicit times more than the amplitudes of the mfERGs. The amplitudes of the second-order kernels were also more reduced than those of the first-order kernels probably because of a widespread dysfunction of the proximal retina. Alternatively, the delayed implicit time of the first-order kernel may be due to a reduction of the second-order kernel.

Delays in the implicit times of the first-order kernel and reductions in the amplitude of the second-order kernel have been reported in eyes with diabetic retinopathy (Palmowski et al., 1997), retinal vascular disease (Hasegawa et al., 2001), and congenital stationary night blindness (Kondo et al., 2001).

4.3 Retinal vascular diseases

Because the first slice of the second order kernel represents the degree to which the retinal response is affected by an immediately preceding stimulus, this component represents the effects of the fast adaptive mechanisms of the retina. Analysis of this component showed that the recovery of sensitivity following a flash was abnormal in eyes of diabetic patients even before the development of diabetic retinopathy.(Palmowsli et al., 1997) Shimada et al (Shimada et al., 2001) recorded mfERGs using a periodic "global" flash inserted between the multifocal stimuli that enhanced the fast adaptive mechanisms. Then, the periodic global flashes produced a greater reduction in the mfERGs in diabetic eyes without retinopathy than in age-matched normal subjects. This indicated an impairment of recovery from the bright preceding flash. The multifocal OPs were also reported to have prolonged latencies in the eyes of diabetic patients without retinopathy.(Kurtenbach et al., 2000)

The fmERGs can also be a sensitive indicator of macular function in eyes with diabetic maculopathy. In some eyes at the early stage of diabetic maculopathy, the macular OPs were selectively reduced leaving the a- and b-waves intact.(Yoon et al., 1990) This is in good agreement with early studies(Yonemura et al., 1962) with full-field ERGs that showed that the full-field OPs were reduced with delayed implicit times during the early stage of diabetes mellitus.

mfERGs have been used to assess macular function in eyes with age-related macular degeneration (AMD).(Feigl et al., 2005) The mfERGs were used to monitor the changes in the function of parafoveal locations after photodynamic therapy (PDT). In the future, mfERGs can be used to document the effects of different treatments for AMD, e.g., PDT, anti-vascular endothelial growth factor therapies, and retinal pigment epithelial transplantation, and combination of some of these therapies.

The fmERGs have been used to differentiate macular dysfunction from optic nerve disease in cases of acute central scotoma. For example, we studied a 75-year-old man who presented with a unilateral acute decrease of vision and central scotoma (Figure 11).

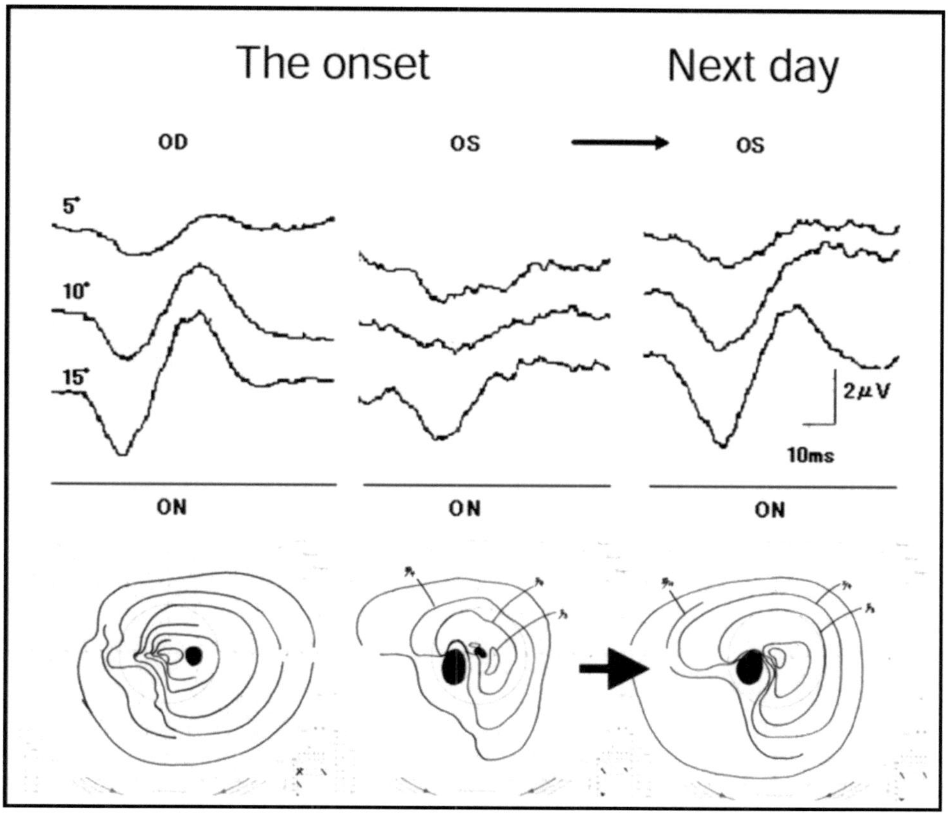

Fig. 11. Visual fields showing ipsilateral hemianopsia in both eyes due to an earlier cerebral infarction and central scotoma in the left eye coupled with an acute visual decrease to 0.01. The optic discs were normal except for enlarged optic disc cups due to glaucoma. Fluorescein angiograms were normal except for a relative prolonged arm-to-retina time of 20 seconds. These findings together with a relative afferent pupillary defect required a differential diagnosis between optic nerve disease and local retinal disease. The reduced fmERGs together with the rapid improvement led to a diagnosis of transient ischemia. Modified and reproduced from (Terauchi et al., 2007) with permission from BMJ Publishing Group Ltd.

A left relative afferent pupillary defect was present. His visual acuity was 0.01 in the left affected eye. The fundus was normal except for an enlarged optic disc cup in both eyes. Fluorescein angiography showed a delayed arm-to-retina circulation time of 20.0 seconds in the left eye. The fmERGs were decreased in the left eye suggesting that the visual dysfunction was of retinal origin. The following day, the visual acuity in the left eye improved to 0.7. The results of full-field ERGs and VEPs were within normal limits. We concluded that the acute decrease in the visual acuity resulted from a macular dysfunction due to a transient macular ischemia.(Terauchi et al., 2007)

Wide-field (WF)-mfERGs are used to assess focal areas of the retina in the far (out to 90°) periphery that might be dysfunctional. The WF-mfERGs have been compared to the full-field flicker ERGs in patients with central retinal vein occlusion (CRVO).(Dolan et al., 2003) In the affected eye, 98% of the central P1 implicit times and 91% of the peripheral P1 implicit times fell outside the normal limits as opposed to 35% of the 30-Hz flicker implicit times in the same eyes. The investigators suggested that this was because the WF-mfERGs were more sensitive than the standard full-field ERGs to detect the changes in the nonlinear dynamics of the eye because the stimulus used for the recordings of the WF-mfERG consisted of many frequencies (Dolan et al., 2003).

In the management of CRVO, it is important to determine whether the CRVO is the ischemic or non-ischemic type, and whether iris neovascularization (NVI) will develop. An earlier study showed that the b/a ratio of the full-field mixed rod and cone ERGs of the affected eyes were significantly lower in patients who developed NVI than that in individuals who did not develop NVI.(Sabates et al., 1983) More recently, it was reported that both the implicit times and amplitudes of the 30-Hz flicker, reflecting predominantly cone photoreceptor function, were good predictors of neovascular complications. (Lasson&Andreasson 2001) However, more useful parameters of the mfERGs are needed to predict neovascular complications in patients with CRVO.

The usefulness of fmERGs in evaluating macular function in eyes with a CRVO has recently been reported.(Ogino et al., 2011) The relative amplitudes (affected eye/fellow eye) of the a- and b-waves and the PhNR of the fmERGs were significantly correlated with the visual acuity. The relative amplitude of the PhNR was most strongly correlated with the central foveal thickness. The relative amplitudes were reduced more severely in eyes with ischemic CRVO than in eyes with nonischemic CRVO.

4.4 Optic nerve diseases

The photpic negative response (PhNR) is a negative-going wave of photopic full-field ERGs that appears immediately after the b-wave. This component is also present in the fmERGs, and intensive investigations on this component by Frishman and colleagues(Frishman 2006) have demonstrated its clinical value. Because all evidence indicated that this component arises from activity of the inner retinal neurons, viz., RGCs, IPL and NFL, the findings have stimulated investigators to find new applications of PhNRs.

Thus, the PhNRs of the fmERGs were significantly reduced in patients with open-angle glaucoma (Machida et al., 2011), optic neuritis(Nakamura et al., 2011), and macular edema associated with CRVO.(Ogino et al., 2011) The threshold for eliciting a focal PhNR was significantly higher than that for the full-field PhNR in eyes at early and intermediate stages of glaucoma. (Machida et al., 2011) The authors recorded from the macular area, and from the supero-temporal and infero-temporal areas of the macula to study regional functions and were able to do a layer-by-layer analyses as well as topographical analyses. In patients with acute optic neuritis, (Nakamura et al., 2011) the focal PhNRs were reduced at the onset of symptoms of optic neuritis, but the full-field PhNRs were unchanged. With time, the PhNRs decreased as the retinal nerve fiber layer became thinner.(Gotoh et al., 2004) Interestingly, the a- and b-waves were also attenuated, and both recovered significantly at 6 months after the onset, but the PhNRs did not improve significantly.

4.5 Surgical or medical intervention

The PhNR of the fmERGs has been reported to be useful in evaluating new medical and surgical treatments for different retinal diseases.(Terasaki et al., 2001) In the evaluation of the effects of macular hole surgery, a selective delay in the recovery of the fmERG b-waves 6 months after surgery was reported. This suggested an alteration of retinal physiology in the macular region. The authors also reported a selective reduction in the amplitude of the PhNR of the full-field ERG after macular hole surgery. This suggested that the ganglion cells were damaged by the indocyanine green dye-assisted internal limiting membrane peeling and gas tamponade.(Ueno et al., 2006)

New treatments have been recently introduced for retinal diseases, e.g., macular edema, neovascular maculopathy, whose pathogenesis is related to the activation of VEGF. In these treatments, fmERGs and/or mfERGs can be used to evaluate the outcomes. Thus, intraocular triamcinolone acetonide (TA), (Moschos et al., 2007) intraocular bevacizumab, (Moschos et al., 2008), and PDT for exudative AMD (Palmowski et al., 2002;Mackay et al., 2007) have been studied by fmERGs and mfERGs. In most studies, the changes in the mfERGs were compared to that of the visual acuity, OCT images, and retinal sensitivities. One of the uses of mfERGs is to monitor the improvements of paramacular function. Consequently, mfERGs can play significant roles in the assessment of retinal function after many treatment trials.

4.6 Miscellaneous

A selective reduction of the OP amplitudes of the fmERGs was reported (Miyake 2006) in the early stage of macular edema, (Miyake et al., 1993b) epiretinal membrane (ERM), (Tanikawa et al., 1999; Niwa et al., 2003), and at the convalescent stage of central serous chorioretinopathy (CSC). (Miyake et al., 1988) The amplitudes of the OPs of the fmERGs were reduced and the implicit times delayed regardless of the visual acuity in aphakic eyes or pseudophakic cystoid macular edema (CME). (Salzman et al., 1986) A layer-by-layer analysis of the components of the fmERGs showed that the a- and b-waves and OPs were reduced in these eyes with CME. (Miyake et al., 1993b; Miyake 2006) With increasing severity of the CME, the OPs, the b-waves, and then the a-waves were reduced. Interestingly, the amplitudes of OPs of the full-field ERGs were significantly smaller in the affected eye than in the normal fellow eye although the a- and b-waves were not significantly different. (Terasaki et al., 2003) In addition, the degree of the reduction was significantly correlated with the visual acuity. These findings suggested that the abnormality was not limited to the macula although ophthalmoscopy and fluorescein angiography did not show any abnormalities of the retina. For the OPs, the contribution of the electrical signals from the macular area may be relative higher than that to the a- or b-waves, and fmERGs may be more sensitive than full-field ERGs in assessing the retinal function in eyes with a CME.

fmERGs were used to assess eyes with ERM before and after surgery, and the properties of the fmERGs were similar to that in eyes with CME.(Tanikawa et al., 1999;Niwa et al., 2003) The results of these studies showed that the relative amplitudes (affected eye/fellow eye) of the a- and b-waves and the OPs before surgery were 75%, 69%, and 45%, respectively. The OPs were most affected and the b-wave was more affected than the a-wave, and a significant reduction of the b/a ratio was found in eyes with a relatively preserved a-wave. In contrast, the b/a ratio in the eyes with a greater reduction of the a-wave were not significantly different from that in the normal fellow eyes. Therefore, it was suggested that the reduction of the b-wave occurred first and was followed by the reduction of the a-wave as the disease progressed. The greater functional impairment of the inner retinal layers shown by fmERGs was correlated with the OCT-determined morphological changes. After surgery, the a-wave recovered first followed by the recovery of the b-waves as in eyes with aphakic CME(Miyake et al., 1993b) and CSC.(Miyake et al., 1988) The postoperative visual acuity was significantly correlated with the preoperative relative a-wave amplitude.

The fmERGs findings indicated that there would be pathophysiological changes in eyes with CSC. It is possible that there was functional damage to the photoreceptors in the macular area. Actually, all of the components of the fmERGs were reduced with delayed implicit times indicating that the expectations were correct.(Miyake et al., 1988) However, fmERG analyses revealed that the inner retinal layers were also damaged, and the recovery was delayed even after the serous retinal detachment (SRD) was resolved. Concomitant analyses with fmERGs and OCT provided good evidence for the cause of these changes. Thus, the sensory retina was thickened not only in the acute phase but also after the SRD was resolved and the only the macular OPs were abnormal. These findings suggest that the functional changes in eyes with CSC may result from the SRD and by the macular edema.

5. Multifocal VEP and its clinical applications

The visual evoked potential (VEP) has traditionally been an important method for assessing the state of visual pathways. However, the conventional VEP has limited ability to reflect field loss in non-central areas since the pattern limited ability to reflect field loss in non-central areas since the pattern VEP is predominantly generated by cortical elements receiving projections from the central retina and it has been estimated that the central 2°of visual field contributes 65% of the response.(Gray et al., 1997) The multifocal stimulation techniques (Figure 12) have enabled assessment of multiple sites in the field out to 30° eccentricity. (Baseler et al., 1994;Klistorner et al., 1998;Betsuin et al., 2001)

It was reported that the topographic map of the amplitudes of the mfVEPs showed good agreement or concordance with the results of conventional visual field tests if occipital bipolar electrodes are used. Scotomas can be identified, and field defects in glaucomatous optic neuropathy and optic neuritis have been well defined.(Klistorner et al., 2000; Hood et al., 2000, 2003, 2004; Goldberg et al., 2002;Graham et al., 2005)

The mfERGs and multifocal visual evoked potentials (mfVEPs) recorded from a patient who developed an acute visual field loss after vitrectomy are shown in Figure 13. (Shinoda et al., 2000) The patient had undergone uncomplicated vitrectomy for a long-lasting vitreous hemorrhage associated with proliferative diabetic retinopathy. The patient complained of superior visual field defects on the following day. Visual field testing, mfERGs, and mfVEPs revealed that the visual field defect was not retinal but of optic nerve origin. A diagnosis of ischemic optic neuropathy was made.

Interestingly, the alterations of the topographic map of the mfVEPs may show discordance with the subjectively determined visual fields in some cases with hemianopic field defects.

(**Figure 14**) (Watanabe et al., 2007) In some patients with occipital lesions, the subjective (Goldmann's perimetry etc) and objective (mfVEP) visual field results are discordant, and some of them will show a recovery of the visual field deficits.

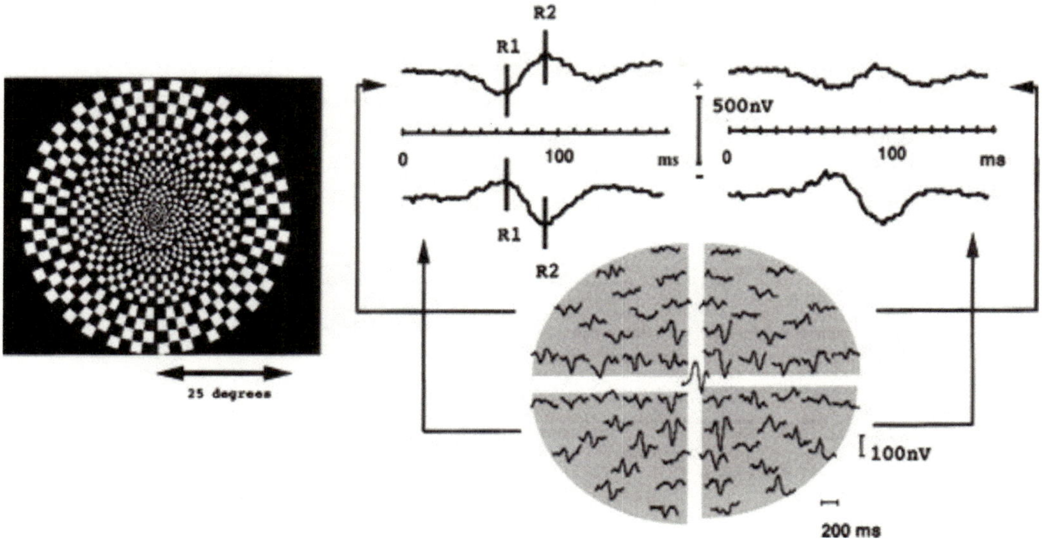

Fig. 12. Stimulus for multifocal visual-evoked potentials. (Left) Stimulus was a dartboard pattern consisting of 61 sectors. (Right) Individual second-order kernels of the multifocal visual evoked potentials (mfVEPs) are plotted retinotopically in the lower half. The sums of the responses in each of the four quadrants are plotted in the sectors in the upper half except for the response from the very central sector. Modified and reproduced from (Watanabe et al., 2007) with permission with permission from Elsevier.

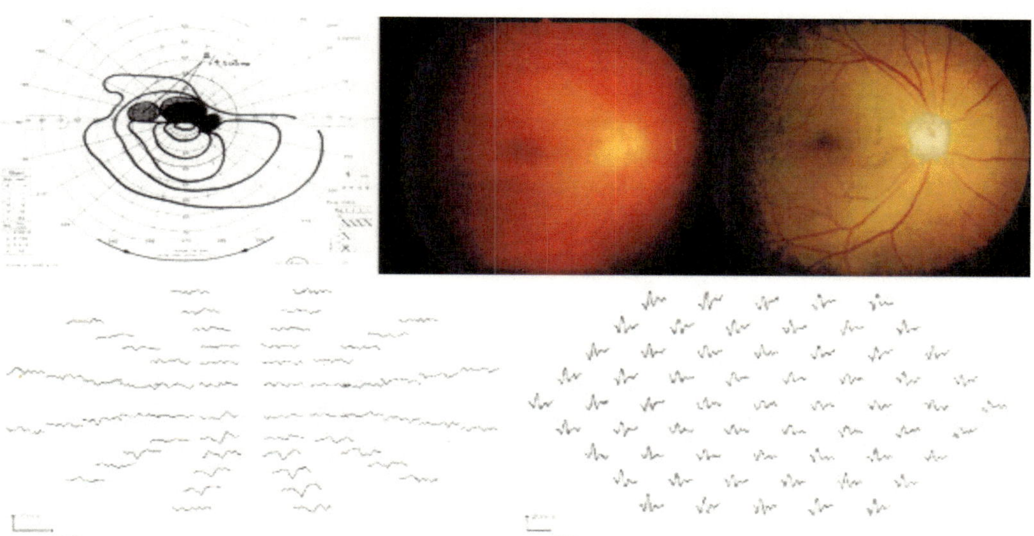

Fig. 13. Visual field, mfERGs, and mfVEPs from an eye with a superior hemianopsia which developed one day after vitrectomy. The pupil was dilated by the atropine instilled before

the surgery and residual mild vitreous hemorrhage hampered the light reflex and detailed fundus view (fundus picture taken on the next day: upper middle). A superior horizontal hemianopsia is present (upper left). The amplitudes of the mfERGs (lower left) were relatively reduced and the delayed implicit times in all retinal areas whereas the amplitudes of the mfVEPs (lower right) were reduced and delayed especially from the area corresponding to the visual field defect. With the resolution of the vitreous hemorrhage, the visual acuity improved to 0.7 but the visual field defects remained. Six months later the inferior margin of the optic disc appeared pale (upper right), supporting that the visual field defect had been optic nerve origin. Modified and reproduced from (Shinoda et al., 2000) with permission.

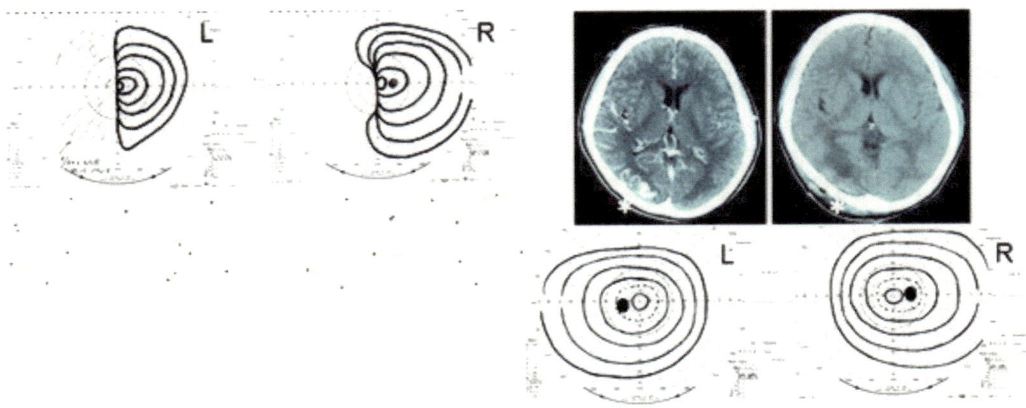

Fig. 14. Findings in a 28-year-old man who underwent neurosurgery for an arteriovenous malformation in the right occipital lobe. (Top left) Goldmann visual fields showing a left homonymous hemianopsia. (Bottom left) The multifocal visual evoked potentials (mfVEPs) are presented so that the average waveforms are seen in each of the quadrants where in the visual field each waveform originates. The mfVEPs were not extinguished in the temporal fields of the left eye and the nasal fields of the right eye. (Top right, left) Computed tomographic (CT) image showing an arteriovenous malformation in the right occipital lobe. (Top right, right) CT image showing a low-density area indicating postoperative edema in the right occipital region. (Bottom right) Goldmann perimetric fields showing complete recovery of visual fields three months later. Modified and reproduced from (Watanabe et al., 2007) with permission with permission from Elsevier.

6. Conclusion

Although evaluations of the macula of the retina by electrophysiological methods have been available for less than a quarter-of-a-century, their uses in clinical and research studies have been expanding with great enthusiasm. The techniques continue to advance for the diagnosis of macular diseases, and in determining the underlying pathology of macular diseases. In addition, focal ERGs have been used and will continue to be used to monitor the course of a disease process, to assess the favorable and adverse effects of therapy, and to discover new retinal and optic nerve diseases. Coupled with the development of imaging technology, advances in surgical techniques, psychophysical tests, circulatory evaluations, and enthusiasm of clinical and laboratory electrophysiologists, fmERG and mfERG will certainly produce much more advances in ophthalmology.

7. Acknowledgements

We express our deepest appreciation to Professor Yozo Miyake for his critical and valuable advices concerning the interpretation and clinical importance of electrophysiological results throughout the chapter. We acknowledge Professor Duco Hamasaki for sharing his great knowledge in electrophysiology and English correction. Support of this chapter was provided by Researches on Sensory and Communicative Disorders from the Ministry of Health, Labor, and Welfare, Japan.

8. References

Akahori M, Tsunoda K, Miyake Y, Fukuda Y, Ishiura H, Tsuji S, Usui T, Hatase T, Nakamura M, Ohde H, Itabashi T, Okamoto H, Takada Y, Iwata T. (2010). Dominant mutations in RP1L1 are responsible for occult macular dystrophy. *Am J Hum Genet.* Vol. 87, No.3pp.(424-9).

Arai M, Nao-i N, Sawada A, Hayashida T. (1998).Multifocal electroretinogram indicates visual field loss in acute zonal occult outer retinopathy. *Am J Ophthalmol,* Vol.126, No.3, pp.(466-9).

Baseler HA, Sutter EE, Klein SA, Carney T. (1994). The topography of visual evoked response properties across the visual field. *Electroencephal Clin Neurophysiol,* Vol.90, No.1, pp.(65–81).

Betsuin Y, Mashima Y, Ohde H, Inoue R, Oguchi Y. (2001). Clinical application of the multifocal VEPs. *Curr Eye Res,* Vol.22, No.1, pp(54–63).

Choshi T, Matsumoto CS, Nakatsuka K. (2003). Rod-driven focal macular electroretinogram. *Jpn J Ophthalmol,* Vol.47, No.4, pp.(356-61).

Curcio CA, Sloan KR, Kalina RE, Hendrickson AE. (1990). Human photoreceptor topography. *J Comp Neurol,* Vol. 292, No.4, pp.(497-523).

Dolan FM, Parks S, Keating D, Dutton GN, Evans AL. (2003). Multifocal electroretinographic features of central retinal vein occlusion. *Invest Ophthalmol Vis Sci,* Vol.44, No.11, pp.(4954-9).

Falsini B, Porciatti V, Porrello G, Merendino E, Minnella A, Cermola S, Buzzonetti L. (1996). Macular flicker electroretinograms in Best vitelliform dystrophy. *Curr Eye Res,* Vol.15, No.6, PP.(638-46).

Feigl B, Lovie-Kitchin J, Brown B. (2005). Objective functional assessment of age-related maculopathy: a special application for the multifocal electroretinogram.*Clin Exp Optom,* Vol.88, No.5, pp.(304-12).

Fletcher WA, Imes RK, Goodman D, Hoyt WF. (1988). Acute idiopathic blind spot enlargement. A big blind spot syndrome without optic disc edema. *Arch Ophthalmol,* Vol.106, No.1, pp.(44-49).

Frishman LJ. (2006). Origins of the Electroretinogram, In : *2nd eds Principle and practice of clinical electrophysiology of vision,* Heckenlively JR & Arden GB, pp.(139-183), The mit press Cambridge, Massachusetts, London, England.

Gass JD. (2003) Are acute zonal occult outer retinopathy and the white spot syndromes (AZOOR complex) specific autoimmune diseases? *Am J Ophthalmol,* Vol.135, No.3, pp.(380-381).

Goldberg I, Graham SL, Klistorner AI. (2002). Multifocal objective perimetry in the detection of glaucomatous field loss. *Am J Ophthalmol,* Vol.133, No.1, pp.(29 -39).

Gotoh Y, Machida S, Tazawa Y. (2004). Selective loss of the photopic negative response in patients with optic nerve atrophy. *Arch Ophthalmol,* Vol.122, No.3, pp.(341-6).

Graham SL, Klistorner AI, Goldberg I. (2005). Clinical application of objective perimetry using multifocal visual evoked potentials in glaucoma practice. *Arch Ophthalmol,* Vol.123, No.6, , pp.(729–39).

Gray LG, Galetta SL, Siegal T, Schatz NJ. (1997) The central visual field in homonymous hemianopia. Evidence for unilateral foveal representation. *Arch Neurol,* Vol.54, No.3, pp.(312–7).

Hanazono G, Ohde H, Shinoda K, Tsunoda K, Tsubota K, Miyake Y. (2010). Pattern-reversal visual evoked potential in patients with occult macular dystrophy. *Clin Ophthalmol,* Vol.4, pp.(1515-20).

Hasegawa S, Ohshima A, Hayakawa Y, Takagi M, Abe H. (2001). Multifocal electroretinograms in patients with branch retinal artery occlusion. *Invest Ophthalmol Vis Sci,* Vol.42, No.1, pp.(298–304).

Hirose T, Miyake Y, Hara A. (1977). Simultaneous recording of electroretinogram and visual evoked response. Focal stimulation under direct observation. *Arch Ophthalmol,* Vol.95, No.7, pp.(1205-8).

Holopigian K, Seiple W, Greenstein VC, Hood DC, Carr RE. (2001). Local cone and rod system function in patients with retinitis pigmentosa. *Invest Ophthalmol Vis Sci,* Vol.42, No.3pp.(779-88).

Holopigian K, Seiple W, Greenstein VC, Hood DC, Carr RE. (2002). Local cone and rod system function in progressive cone dystrophy. *Invest Ophthalmol Vis Sci,* Vol.43, No.7, pp.(2364-73).

Hood DC, Odel JG, Zhang X. (2000).Tracking the recovery of local optic nerve function after optic neuritis:a multifocal VEP study. *Invest Ophthalmol Vis Sci,* Vol.41, No.12, pp.(4032–8).

Hood DC, Greenstein VC. (2003). Multifocal VEP and ganglion cell damage: applications and limitations for the study of glaucoma. *Prog Retin Eye Res,* Vol.22, No.2, pp.(201-51).

Hood DC, Thienprasiddhi P, Greenstein VC, Greenstein VC, Winn BJ, Ohri N, Liebmann JM, Ritch R. (2004). Detecting early to mild glaucomatous damage: a comparison of the multifocal VEP and automated perimetry. *Invest Ophthalmol Vis Sci,* Vol.45, No.2, pp.(492- 498).

Hood DC, Bach M, Brigell M, Keating D, Kondo M, Lyons JS, Palmowski-Wolfe AM. (2008). ISCEV guidelines for clinical multifocal electroretinography (2007 edition). *Doc Ophthalmol,* Vol.116, No.1, pp.(1-11).

Kelly JP, Weiss AH. (2006). Topographical retinal function in oculocutaneous albinism. *Am J Ophthalmol,* Vol.141, No.6, pp.(1156-8).

Klistorner AI, Graham SL, Grigg JR, Billson FA.(1998). Multifocal topographic visual evoked potential: improving objective detection of local visual field defects. *Invest Ophthalmol Vis Sci*. Vol.39, No.6, pp.(937–50).

Klistorner A, Graham SL. (2000). Objective perimetry in glaucoma. Ophthalmology, Vol.107, No.12, pp.(2283–99).

Kondo M, Miyake Y, Kondo N, Tanikawa A, Suzuki S, Horiguchi M, Terasaki H. (2001). Multifocal ERG findings in complete type congenital stationary night blindness. *Invest Ophthalmol Vis Sci*. Vol.42, No.6, pp.(1342–1348).

Kondo M, Miyake Y, Kondo N, Ueno S, Takakuwa H, Terasaki H. (2004). Peripheral cone dystrophy: a variant of cone dystrophy with predominant dysfunction in the peripheral cone system. *Ophthalmology,* Vol.111, No.4, pp.(732-9).Kurtenbach A, Langrova H, Zrenner E. (2000). Multifocal oscillatory potentials in type 1 diabetes without retinopathy. *Invest Ophthalmol Vis Sci,* Vol.41, No.10, pp.(3234-41).

Larsson J, Andreasson S. (2001).Photopic 30 Hz flicker ERG as a predictor for rubeosis in central retinal vein occlusion. *Br J Ophthalmol,* Vol.85, No.6, pp.(683–685).

Machida S, Tamada K, Oikawa T, Gotoh Y, Nishimura T, Kaneko M, Kurosaka D. (2011). Comparison of photopic negative response of full-field and focal electroretinograms in detecting glaucomatous eyes. *J Ophthalmol,* in press..

Mackay AM, Brown MC, Hagan RP, Fisher AC, Grierson I, Harding SP. (2007). Deficits in the electroretinogram in neovascular age-related macular degeneration and changes during photodynamic therapy. *Doc Ophthalmol,* Vol.115, No.2, pp.(69-76).

Marmor MF, Choi SS, Zawadzki RJ, Werner JS. (2008) Visual insignificance of the foveal pit: reassessment of foveal hypoplasia as fovea plana. *Arch Ophthalmol,* Vol.126, No.7, pp.(907-13).

Miyake Y, Shiroyama N, Ota I, Horiguchi M. (1988). Local macular electroretinographic responses in idiopathic central serous chorioretinopathy. *Am J Ophthalmol,* Vol.106, No.5, pp.(546-50).

Miyake Y. (1998). Focal macular electroretinography. *Nagoya J Med Sci,* Vol.61, No.3-4, pp.(79-84).

Miyake Y, Shiroyama N, Horiguchi M, Ota I. (1989a). Asymmetry of focal ERG in human macular region. *Invest Ophthalmol Vis Sci,* Vol.30, No.8, pp.(1743-9).

Miyake Y, Ichikawa K, Shiose Y, Kawase Y. (1989b). Hereditary macular dystrophy without visible fundus abnormality. *Am J Ophthalmol,* Vol.108, No.3, pp.(292-9).

Miyake Y, Shiroyama N, Ota I, Horiguchi M. (1993a). Focal macular electroretinogram in X-linked congenital retinoschisis. *Invest Ophthalmol Vis Sci,* Vol.34, No.3, pp.(512-5).

Miyake Y, Miyake K, Shiroyama N. (1993b). Classification of aphakic cystoid macular edema with focal macular electroretinograms. *Am J Ophthalmol,* Vol.116, No.5, pp.(576-83).

Miyake Y, Horiguchi M, Tomita N, Kondo M, Tanikawa A, Takahashi H, Suzuki S, Terasaki H. (1996). Occult macular dystrophy. *Am J Ophthalmol,* Vol.122, No.5, pp.(644-53).

Miyake Y, (2006). Electrodiagnosis of Retinal Disease. pp.(1-234), Springer-Verlag Tokyo, Tokyo

Moschos MM, Brouzas D, Loukianou E, Apostolopoulos M, Moschos M. (2007). Intraocular triamcinolone acetonide for macular edema due to CRVO. A multifocal-ERG and OCT study.*Doc Ophthalmol,* Vol.114, No.1, pp.(1-7).

Moschos MM, Moschos M. (2008). Intraocular bevacizumab for macular edema due to CRVO. A multifocal-ERG and OCT study. *Doc Ophthalmol,* Vol.116, No.2, pp.(147-52).

Nakamura H, Miyamoto K, Yokota S, Ogino K, Yoshimura N. (2011). Focal macular photopic negative response in patients with optic neuritis. *Eye (Lond),* Vol.25, No.3, pp.(358-64).

Niwa T, Terasaki H, Kondo M, Piao CH, Suzuki T, Miyake Y. (2003). Function and morphology of macula before and after removal of idiopathic epiretinal membrane. *Invest Ophthalmol Vis Sci,* Vol.44, No.4, pp.(1652-6).

Nusinowitz S, Hood DC, Birch DG. (1995). Rod transduction parameters from the a wave of local receptor populations. *J Opt Soc Am A Opt Image Sci Vis,* Vol.12, No.10, pp.(2259-66).

Nusinowitz S, Sarraf D. (2008). Retinal function in X-linked ocular albinism (OA1). *Curr Eye Res,* Vol.33, No.9, pp.(789-803).

Ogino K, Tsujikawa A, Nakamura H, Miyamoto K, Murakami T, Muraoka Y, Kurashige Y, Yoshimura N. (2011). Focal Macular Electroretinogram in Macular Edema Secondary to Central Retinal Vein Occlusion. *Invest Ophthalmol Vis Sci,* in press.

Palmowski AM, Sutter EE, Bearse MA Jr., Fung W. (1997). Mapping of retinal function in diabetic retinopathy using the multifocal electroretinogram. *Invest Ophthalmol Vis Sci,* Vol.38, No.12, pp.(2586–2596).

Palmowski AM, Allgayer R, Heinemann-Vernaleken B, Ruprecht KW. (2002). Influence of photodynamic therapy in choroidal neovascularization on focal retinal function assessed with the multifocal electroretinogram and perimetry. *Ophthalmology,* Vol.109, No.10, pp.(1788-92).

Palmowski AM, Allgayer R, Heinemann-Vernaleken B, Scherer V, Ruprecht KW. (2003).Detection of retinal dysfunction in vitelliform macular dystrophy using the multifocal ERG (MF-ERG). *Doc Ophthalmol,* Vol.106, No.2, pp.(145-52).

Park SJ, Woo SJ, Park KH, Hwang JM, Chung H. (2010). Morphologic photoreceptor abnormality in occult macular dystrophy on spectral-domain optical coherence tomography. *Invest Ophthalmol Vis Sci,* Vol.51, No.7, pp.(3673-3679).

Piao CH, Kondo M, Tanikawa A, Terasaki H, Miyake Y. (2000). Multifocal electroretinogram in occult macular dystrophy. *Invest Ophthalmol Vis Sci,* Vol.41, No.2, pp.(513-7).

Piao CH, Kondo M, Nakamura M, Terasaki H, Miyake Y. (2003). Multifocal electroretinograms in X-linked retinoschisis. *Invest Ophthalmol Vis Sci,* Vol.44, No.11, pp.(4920-30).

Sabates R, Hirose T, McMeel JW. (1983). Electroretinography in the prognosis and classification of central retinal vein occlusion. *Arch Ophthalmol,* Vol.101, No.2, pp.(232-5).

Salzman J, Seiple W, Carr R, Yannuzzi L. (1986). Electrophysiological assessment of aphakic cystoid macular oedema. *Br J Ophthalmol,* Vol.70, No.11, pp.(819-24).

Sandberg MA, Pawlyk BS, Berson EL.(1996). Isolation of focal rod electroretinograms from the dark-adapted human eye. *Invest Ophthalmol Vis Sci,* Vol.37, No.5, pp.(930-4).

Shimada Y, Li Y, Bearse MA Jr, Sutter EE, Fung W. (2001). Assessment of early retinal changes in diabetes using a new multifocal ERG protocol. *Br J Ophthalmol,* Vol.85, No.4, pp.(414-9).

Shinoda K, Ohde H, Ishida S, Kawashima S, Kitamura S, Mita S, Inoue M, Katsura H. (2000). A case of proliferative diabetic retinopathy with development of ischemic optic neuropathy after pars plana vitrectomy. *Folia Ophthalmol Jpn,* Vol.51, pp.(925-929). Japanese.

Spaide RF, Koizumi H, Freund KB. (2008). Photoreceptor outer segment abnormalities as a cause of blind spot enlargement in acute zonal occult outer retinopathy-complex diseases. *Am J Ophthalmol,* Vol.146, No.1, pp.(111-120).

Sutter EE, Tran D. (1992). The field topography of ERG components in man--I. The photopic luminance response. *Vision Res,* Vol.32, No.3, pp.(433-46).

Sutter EE, Shimada Y, Li Y, Bearse MA. (1999). Mappig inner retinal function through enhancement of adaptive components in the m-ERG, In: *Vision science and its applications. OSA Technical Digest Series,* Pp.(52-55), Optical Society of America, Washington, DC.

Sugahara M, Shinoda K, Matsumoto CS, Satofuka S, Hanazono G, Imamura Y, Mizota A. (2011). Outer Retinal Microstructure in Case of Acute Idiopathic Blind Spot Enlargement Syndrome. *Case Reports in Ophthalmol,* Vol.2, No.1, pp.(116-22).

Tanikawa A, Horiguchi M, Kondo M, Suzuki S, Terasaki H, Miyake Y. (1999). Abnormal focal macular electroretinograms in eyes with idiopathic epimacular membrane. *Am J Ophthalmol,* Vol.127, No.5, pp.(559-64).

Terasaki H, Miyake Y, Nomura R, Piao CH, Hori K, Niwa T, Kondo M. (2001). Focal macular ERGs in eyes after removal of macular ILM during macular hole surgery. *Invest Ophthalmol Vis Sci,* Vol.42, No.1, pp.(229-34).

Terasaki H, Miyake K, Miyake Y. (2003). Reduced oscillatory potentials of the full-field electroretinogram of eyes with aphakic or pseudophakic cystoid macular edema. *Am J Ophthalmol,* Vol.135, No.4, pp.(477-82).

Terauchi N, Fujinami K, Shinoda K, Tsunoda K, Hanazono G, Miyake Y, Inomata K. (2007). Transient macular dysfunction determined by focal macular electroretinogram. *Br J Ophthalmol,* Vol.91, No.12, pp.(1709-10).

Tsunoda K, Fujinami K, Miyake Y. (2011). Selective abnormality of cone outer segment tip line in acute zonal occult outer retinopathy as observed by Fourier domain optical coherence tomography. *Arch Ophthalmol,* in press.

Ueno S, Kondo M, Piao CH, Ikenoya K, Miyake Y, Terasaki H.(2006). Selective amplitude reduction of the PhNR after macular hole surgery: ganglion cell damage related to ICG-assisted ILM peeling and gas tamponade. *Invest Ophthalmol Vis Sci,* Vol.47, No.8, pp.(3545-9).

Watanabe K, Shinoda K, Kimura I, Mashima Y, Oguchi Y, Ohde H. (2007). Discordance between subjective perimetric visual fields and objective multifocal visual evoked potential-determined visual fields in patients with hemianopsia. *Am J Ophthalmol,* Vol.143, No.2, pp.(295-304).

Yamada K., Matsumoto CS, Nakatsuka, K. (2006). Effect of spatial frequency of simulus on focal macular ERGs in monkeys. *Doc Ophthalmol,* Vol. 113, pp.(83-91).

Yonemura D, Aoki T, Tsuzuki K. (1962). Electroretinogram in diabetic retinopathy. *Arch Ophthalmol,* Vol.68, No.68, pp.(19-24).

Yoon IH, Shiroyama N, Miyake Y, Awaya S. (1990). Oscillatory potentials of local macular ERG in diabetic retinopathy. *Korean J Ophthalmol,* Vol.4, No.1, pp.(40-5).

4

Signal Pathways in the Electroretinogram

Jan Kremers
University of Erlangen-Nürnberg
Germany

1. Introduction

The electroretinogram (ERG) is an electrical potential of retinal origin elicited by a visual stimulus. The basis of the ERG is the same photochemical process that leads to the neural response of the retina and the visual system[1]: photon absorptions in the photoreceptoral opsin pigments[2]. In addition, it is a purely retinal response that reflects the retinal physiology. It is not surprising that the ERG received substantial attention because it is a potentially useful way to study the function of the retina and its disease-related changes. Indeed, it still is a very important tool in the clinic. In addition, there was hope that the ERG might be related to the visual responses of retinal neurones whose signals are transmitted to the brain for visual perception and motor responses. However, even though the ERG is known for nearly 150 years now, the similarities with visually relevant neuronal signals and with visual perception were disappointingly small. In the 1970s, Armington (1974) wrote in his book "The Electroretinogram" when discussing the link between ERGs and psychophysics (chapter 7): "The electroretinogram is unique because its components allow the experimenter to follow several separate retinal activities, while recording is performed with a minimum of discomfort to the subject. Furthermore, the subject may make verbal reports or judgements regarding the same stimulus, which was used to elicit the electroretinogram. It is thus possible to relate the visual appearance of a stimulus to the underlying physiological processes. The full potential for doing this in a sophisticated manner, however, has not been yet realized." As a result, ERGs were mainly used in studies that had a clinical interest. It was treated as an epiphenomenon of the responses of the visual pathways without showing a direct relationship with them. In this chapter, I will argue that under well chosen circumstances, which can be created owing to modern stimulus and recording techniques, a correlation with the physiological properties of the major pathways projecting to the brain and the related visual performances can be obtained.

---

[1] in this chapter I will mainly confine myself to the situation in mammals and more specifically primates, but the basic mechanism is probably similar in all vertebrates; in invertebrates the differences are possibly larger.

[2] I neglect for the time being that light absorption in the melanopsin containing retinal ganglion cells may also elicit a detectable ERG signal see: FUKUDA, Y., TSUJIMURA, S., HIGUCHI, S., YASUKOUCHI, A. & MORITA, T. (2010): The ERG responses to light stimuli of melanopsin-expressing retinal ganglion cells that are independent of rods and cones. *Neurosci Lett* 479, 282-286..

2. Historical overview of the ERG and stimulus types

The electroretinogram was discovered twice independently by Holmgren and by Dewar and McKendrick around 1870 (for a historical overview see de Rouck (2006)). The stimuli that initially were most often used, were high intensity flashes, probably because they were relatively easy to deliver with the early techniques and a single stimulus elicited a response that was large enough to be measured. Improvements in the electrodes and amplifiers and the advent of averaging techniques enabled recording of smaller response components. At a later stage, other stimulus techniques (such as trains of flashes to elicit a flicker ERG or long flash ERGs, pattern ERGs etc) became available so that other features of the ERG could be studied. This chapter is not meant to give a complete overview of all ERG types and their properties. Instead, a short description of the flash and the conventional flicker ERGs is given, because it provides a context for comparison the results of the work performed in my lab.

The responses elicited by flashes have a complex waveform with different components. The responses to a flash stimulus contain a-, b- and c-waves that each have different cellular origins (Frishman, 2006). With flashes that last long enough, the responses to stimulus onset and offset can be separated and compared and it was shown that the two responses are quite different. Whereas the response to stimulus onset is similar in appearance (but certainly not identical) to the response to the short flash the response to stimulus offset displays a cornea positive peak called the d-wave. Systems that are linear or that contain simple contrast dependent nonlinearities have mirror imaged responses to stimulus on- and offset. Obviously, this is not the case in the flash ERG indicating that its signal pathway contains substantial nonlinearities, which makes interpretation of the signals difficult.

As an alternative to the flash ERG, the response to a repetition of pulses (called the flicker ERG) can be measured. The response waveform with pulse trains at about 30 Hz is much simpler than the flash ERG and therefore might also be easier to interpret. The flicker ERG can have certain properties that are comparable to perceptual properties. Already in the 70s of the 20th century, it was found that the spectral sensitivities of the flicker ERGs at relatively high temporal frequencies were similar to the spectral luminosity function (Padmos & van Norren). After refining this method, the correlation was so strong that inter-species and inter-individual differences in the spectral luminosity function could be retraced in the flicker ERG. This technique has been employed extremely successfully by Gerald Jacobs and his colleagues (Neitz & Jacobs, 1984; Jacobs *et al.*, 1987; Neitz *et al.*, 1991; Jacobs & Deegan Ii, 1993b, a; Jacobs *et al.*, 1993a; Jacobs & Neitz, 1993; Jacobs *et al.*, 1996a; Jacobs *et al.*, 1996b; Jacobs *et al.*, 1996c; Jacobs & Deegan Ii, 1997; Jacobs, 1998; Jacobs & Deegan Ii, 1999; Jacobs *et al.*, 2004).

Through the development of light emitting diodes (LEDs) and their use in creating stimuli, recordings and interpretation of the flicker ERG could be further improved. First, the stimulus waveform can be chosen because the LEDs can be controlled at a high temporal resolution. For instance, pure sine-wave modulation can be generated at all relevant temporal frequencies. A sine-wave contains only one frequency component whereas a pulse train has considerable higher harmonics. This can make the interpretation of the ERG responses elicited by sine-waves easier. A second possibility that can be achieved with LEDs is that sine-waves and other periodic waveforms can be modulated around a mean luminance. Stimulus strength can be varied by changing the modulation depth without changing the mean luminance and chromaticity of the stimulus and therefore without changing the state of adaptation. The stimulus strength can be quantified by Michelson contrast C:

$$C = \frac{(L_{max} - L_{min})}{(L_{max} + L_{min})} \tag{1}$$

L_{max} is the maximal and L_{min} is the minimal intensity of the output. In contrast, flash trains are mostly delivered upon a steady background. Changing the stimulus strength is achieved by changing the pulse intensity and therefore is confounded with changes in the state of adaptation. In that case the stimulus strength is quantified by Weber fraction:

$$F = \frac{\Delta L}{L_{back}} \tag{2}$$

ΔL is the flash intensity and L_{back} is the intensity of the background. A third advantage of the use of LEDs is that many differently coloured diodes are available, with which a multidimensional stimulus space can be created with according flexibility enabling, for instance, the stimulation of single photoreceptor types. Thus, the retinal signal flow originating in the different photoreceptor types can be studied. To be able to do this optimally, at least four differently coloured light sources are necessary to study the human retina. In the next section, a description is given of how photoreceptor isolating stimuli can be made and how this method can be extended to conditions in which the stimulus strength in each photoreceptor type can be quantified and how more than one photoreceptor types can be stimulated simultaneously.

3. Cone isolating stimuli

In the early days, isolation of photoreceptor responses was achieved by using a selective adaptation paradigm. A background light was chosen that adapted the photoreceptor systems that were not of interest and a flashed stimulus was delivered having a wavelength at which the photoreceptor of interest was sensitive. This method was used before by Stiles to describe psychophysically the photoreceptor spectral sensitivities of π mechanisms (Stiles, 1939, 1953, 1959, 1978). However, although the response will be strongly dominated by one photoreceptor type, isolation is never complete. In addition, this method has the disadvantage that strongly varying adapting fields have to be used to isolate the responses of different photoreceptor types. As a result, the state of adaptation is also variable. The state of adaptation can have a strong influence upon the cone driven signals (see below), indicating that measurements that are performed at different states of adaptation cannot be compared quantitatively.

A new stimulation method that does not have the above-described disadvantages is the silent substitution method. After more data became available on photopigments and photoreceptor physiology, Donner and Rushton (1959) described a new method of isolating single photoreceptor mechanisms which they called the 'spectral compensation' method. This method is based upon the principle of univariance (Naka & Rushton, 1966), stating that each photoisomerization leads to an identical response of the photoreceptor independent of the wavelength of the photon that was absorbed by the photopigment. As a result, the replacement of one stimulus by another will not lead to a change in photoreceptor excitation if the number of isomerizations is not altered (for a review see Kremers, 2003). This method was later renamed into 'silent substitution' and has been developed further by Estévez and Spekreijse (Estévez & Spekreijse, 1974, 1982) and by Smith and Pokorny and colleagues (e.g.

Shapiro *et al.*, 1996). It was used to create stimuli for psychophysical experiments (Zele *et al.*, 2006) and for single cell recordings (e.g. Yeh *et al.*, 1995). In the 1990s it was introduced in ERG measurements (Usui *et al.*, 1998a; Kremers *et al.*, 1999). Briefly, when using silent substitution, the number of photoisomerizations is in one or more photoreceptor types is not altered. Consider a monochromatic light of 535 nm that is replaced by another monochromatic light of 600 nm. When the two lights have equal energy than, according to the cone fundamentals (DeMarco *et al.*, 1992; Stockman *et al.*, 1993) the M-cones are about 3 times more sensitive to the 535 nm than to the 600 nm light. However, if the radiance of the 600 nm light is three times the radiance of the 535 nm light then the number of isomerizations in the M-cones is not changed by the replacement. Therefore this condition would be a silent substitution for the M-cones. The L-cones, however, are about as sensitive to the 535 nm as to the 600 nm light. Taking into account that the intensity of 600 nm is three times that of the 535 nm light, then the number of isomerizations increases by a factor of about three when the 600 nm light replaces the 535 nm light. If the radiances of the two lights are equal, then we would have a reversed situation with a silent substitution of L-cone and a threefold larger number of isomerizations in the M-cones when the 535 nm light replaces the 600 nm stimulus. Of course, the situation is normally more complicated because broadband sources are generally used instead of monochromatic lights. Nevertheless, the numbers of isomerizations can be calculated by multiplying the rod and cone fundamentals with the emission spectra of the light sources and integrating over wavelength. Furthermore, the human retina contains four receptor types and not just two. The latter problem can be solved when more light sources are used. Theoretically, four light sources are sufficient to be able to stimulate each photoreceptor type independently. For a more extensive explanation of the silent substitution technique I refer to Kremers (2003).

The silent substitution method can be more generalized because it is based upon the fact that the method actually allows to calculate the number of photoisomerizations in each photoreceptor type. The stimulus strength of photoreceptor can be calculated for each stimulus (and similar to the above-mentioned Michelson contrast expressed as cone contrast or rod contrast defined as:

$$PC = \frac{(PI_{max} - PI_{min})}{(PI_{max} + PI_{min})} \tag{3}$$

in which PC is photoreceptor contrast and PI are the numbers of photoisomerizations in the concerning photoreceptor. As mentioned above, the number of photoisomerizations is calculated by the integral of the multiplication of emission spectra of the stimuli and the absorption spectra of the photoreceptor types. With four differently coloured stimuli, this process of calculating stimulus strength in a particular photoreceptor type is a linear and one to one process. "Linear" means that if the stimulus contrasts are multiplied by a certain factor, the resulting photoreceptor contrasts are multiplied by the same factor. "One to one" means that each combination of stimulus contrasts gives a unique combination of photoreceptor contrasts. With a sufficient number independently coloured light stimuli it is also possible to calculate what stimulus condition has to be used to obtain a particular set photoreceptor contrasts. In the human retina, there are normally four photoreceptor types (one rod and three cone types). That means that theoretically four differently and independently coloured stimuli (independent means that the emission spectrum of one stimulus cannot be obtained by a combination of the other stimuli) are sufficient to obtain every combination of photoreceptor stimulus strengths (in practise this dynamic range is limited because stimulus contrasts cannot be smaller than zero and larger than one). Silent substitution is a special case in which the contrast in one or more photoreceptor types is zero. Thus, using the silent substitution method it is possible to study the response pathway starting in one photoreceptor type. The method is, however, more powerful, because in principle every wanted combination can be obtained, so that the interactions between photoreceptor driven responses can be studied. I would like to stress once more that the different stimulus strengths are obtained by changing the stimulus contrasts. The mean outputs of the stimuli are not altered. In the next section, I will give an overview about the results of cone and rod driven ERG responses.

4. Cone and rod driven flicker-ERG responses

In collaboration with Tomoaki Usui I started to measure ERG response to L- and M-cone isolating stimuli (Usui *et al.*, 1998a, b; Kremers *et al.*, 1999). For a more complete review of the data with cone isolating stimuli I refer to Kremers (2003). We first explored the influence of stimulus strength of a 30 Hz modulation on the response. A response was defined as the fundamental component (the component at the stimulus frequency) out of the Fourier analysis on the recordings. At this temporal frequency, the complete response was mainly determined by the fundamental component (to which I also refer as the first harmonic component). We found that the response amplitude depended linearly on contrast (Usui *et al.*, 1998a). This was surprising because often ERG components in responses to flash stimuli have a more complex dependency on stimulus strength. In my opinion, this has two important consequences. First, it shows that the flicker ERG displays fundamental properties of the visual system without distortion by nonlinear processes. Second, the data imply that cone and rod contrast are an adequate measure to quantify stimulus strength. With a linear relationship between response amplitude and stimulus strength, the contrast gain (which is the increase in response amplitude per increase in cone contrast) is identical to the slope of the linear regression through the data. Furthermore, the results of the response properties at a pre-defined threshold do not depend on the threshold criterion.
We further found that the response phase increased (i.e. the time delay decreased) with increasing contrast. However, the phase relationship could be different when a retinal disorder is present (Usui *et al.*, 1998b). These data show that the response phases might be a sensitive indicator of retinal diseases. Indeed in subsequent experiments on e.g. patients with retinitis pigmentosa, Stargardt's disease, Morbus Best it turned out that the response phases were altered (Scholl & Kremers, 2000; Scholl *et al.*, 2000; Scholl *et al.*, 2001). Because the phases of L- and M-cone driven responses were often differently altered, this could lead to changed responses when the two were simultaneously stimulated.
When the L- and M-cones were simultaneously stimulated, the responses could be described by a vector addition of the L- and M-cone driven signals. As mentioned above, it is possible to construct such stimuli and the stimulus strength in each photoreceptor type can be theoretically chosen. In addition, all stimuli are presented at the same state of adaptation so that the results of the different measurements (L-cone isolation; M-cone isolation; simultaneous L- and M-cone modulation) can be directly compared. A vector addition means that the signals driven by the two cone types are linearly added at each time instant. Thus, any delay difference between the two cone driven signals is accounted for.
In conclusion, the flicker ERG, measured with high temporal frequency stimuli, display characteristics that can be related to L- and M-cone driven retinal pathways. However, the

question is, if these pathways only reflect photoreceptor properties or if post-receptoral pathways also play a role. For instance, the above-mentioned vector addition can be the result of an interaction of independent signals at the electrode. Alternatively, they may also reflect the properties of post-receptoral pathways. In the next section, I will argue that the flicker ERG does indeed reflect the properties of post-receptoral mechanisms. In addition, I will argue that these post-receptoral mechanisms are probably pathways of the retino-geniculate system that are important for different aspects of visual perception.

5. Post-receptoral responses in retino-geniculate pathways

The stimuli used for measuring ERG responses to isolated and combined photoreceptor stimulations were used before to describe the responses of cells belonging to different retino-geniculate pathways. Because the signals in the retino-geniculate pathways are transmitted to the visual cortex, where they are further processed for visual perception and motor reactions, a correlation of ERG signals with those of the retino-geniculate pathways would indicate that the ERGs can be discussed in a perceptual context.

In primates, three major retino-geniculate pathways are well described and the photoreceptor inputs to these post-receptoral mechanisms are known (Dacey & Lee, 1999; Silveira *et al.*, 2005; Lee, 2011). In the retina, the magnocellular pathway contains diffuse bipolar cells and parasol ganglion cells that project to the magnocellular layers of the lateral geniculate nucleus (LGN). Physiologically, these cells are characterized by a high sensitivity to luminance stimuli, a high temporal resolution and large receptive fields. The magnocelular pathway receives additive input from the L- and M-cones. The L- and M-cone input weights are most probably determined by the numbers of L- and M-cones, which, in humans, varies between individuals. S-cone inputs are either absent or very small. At low illuminances, they receive rod input. The magnocellular pathway is most probably responsible for luminance vision, motion perception, vernier acuity and probably also other psychophyical tasks.

The parvocellular pathway also only receives input from L- and M-cones but not from S-cones. There are contradictory results concerning rod inputs. In contrast to the magnocellular pathway, the L- and M-cone interact subtractively (i.e. antagonistically) at low temporal frequencies. This is caused by the antagonistic input to receptive field centres and surrounds which receive differently weighted L- and M-cone inputs[3]. It is not clear whether the receptive field centres and surrounds are cone selective or receive a mixture of L- and M-cone input (Buzas *et al.*, 2006; Jusuf *et al.*, 2006). Another difference compared to the magnocellular pathway is that there is psychophysical evidence that L- and M-cones have about equal input independent of their densities in the retina (Krauskopf, 2000; Kremers *et al.*, 2000) and state of adaptation (Kremers *et al.*, 2003). Midget bipolar and midget ganglion cells are the anatomical retinal substrate of the parvocellular pathway. Physiologically, the retinal ganglion cells are characterized by cone opponency and thus by red-green colour sensitivity, small receptive fields and low temporal resolution. These cells are most probably involved in red-green colour vision, form perception and others.

The koniocellular pathway is a heterogeneous pathway containing cells with different physiological properties. One important sub-type are the blue-on cells. These cells receive

---

[3] Owing to a latency difference between receptive field centres and surrounds there may be an additive interaction at high temporal frequencies.

strong excitatory S-cone input and inhibitory signals from L- and M-cones. Anatomically the blue cone bipolar cells are responsible for transmitting S-cone signals. Diffuse bipolar cells transmit the inhibitory L- and M-cone signals (Martin *et al.*, 1997). Retinal ganglion cells belonging to this pathway are anatomically described as small-field bistratified cells (Dacey & Lee, 1994). The blue-on pathway is responsible for blue-yellow colour vision. Probably there are many other cell types that receive S-cone input, although these cell types probably belong to minor pathways.

When correlating ERG signals with properties of post-receptoral retino-geniculate pathways it is important to keep the above mentioned properties in mind.

6. Flicker-ERG signals reflecting retino-geniculate pathways

As mentioned, many measurements showed that the responses of the flicker ERG at high temporal frequencies are correlated with activity of the luminance pathway. Both have identical spectral sensitivities and the same inter-individual variability can be found in the two. It is not clear if this correlation reflects a causal relationship between the two (Fig. 1, left). The alternative explanation could be that, if all L- and M-cones contribute to the flicker ERG and if the latencies between their signals are not too large, then their signals are summed just as in the luminance channel. The correlation between the ERG and the luminance pathway would then merely be the result of analogous cone signal processing without sharing the same signal pathways (Fig. 1, middle).

However, we found that cone signal weights both in the flicker ERG and in psychophysical luminance pathway strongly depend on the state of adaptation (Kremers *et al.*, 2003). In conclusion, adaptation has the same effect in both pathways. Since adaptation probably involves post-receptoral processing, it is also probable that the luminance pathway and the pathway leading to an ERG signal really share these post-receptoral mechanisms.

The question whether there is a causal relationship between the signal flow in the flicker ERG and in the retino-geniculate pathways is very important because, if the ERG indeed directly reflects the activity of the retino-geniculate pathways, it then can possibly be used for non-invasive studies of the electrophysiological properties of the retino-geniculate pathways in human subjects. This would increase the value of the flicker ERG tremendously beyond its pure clinical application.

If the flicker ERG can reflect activity of the magnocellular luminance pathway then possibly, under other stimulus conditions, it may also reflect activity of the parvocellular red-green chromatic pathway (Fig. 1 right). In 2006, my colleagues and I began to explore the possibility if the responses of the red-green chromatic (parvocellular) pathway can be detected in the ERG. In the next sections, I will describe the results of two experiments showing that indeed there are stimulus conditions at which the flicker ERG is directly related to activity in the red-green chromatic system.

7. Flicker ERGs and the red-green chromatic system

7.1 Methods

ERGs were measured in human observers using full field modulation at different temporal frequencies. For details in recording conditions, I refer to the original publications (Usui *et al.*, 1998a, b; Kremers *et al.*, 1999; Kremers *et al.*, 2003; Kremers & Link, 2008; Kremers *et al.*, 2010). Briefly, ERGs were recording using DTL electrodes with skin electrodes on the ipsilateral temple as reference and on the forehead as ground. The signals were amplified, band-pass filtered (generally between 1 and 300 Hz) and digitized at a frequency of at least 1 KHz. Within the two described experiments, the mean luminance and chromaticity was constant in all stimulus conditions so that the retina was always in the same state of adaptation and the results could be compared with each other. The states of adaptation were differed between the experiments. In these experiments, luminance and chromatic modulations were varied in the different stimulus conditions.

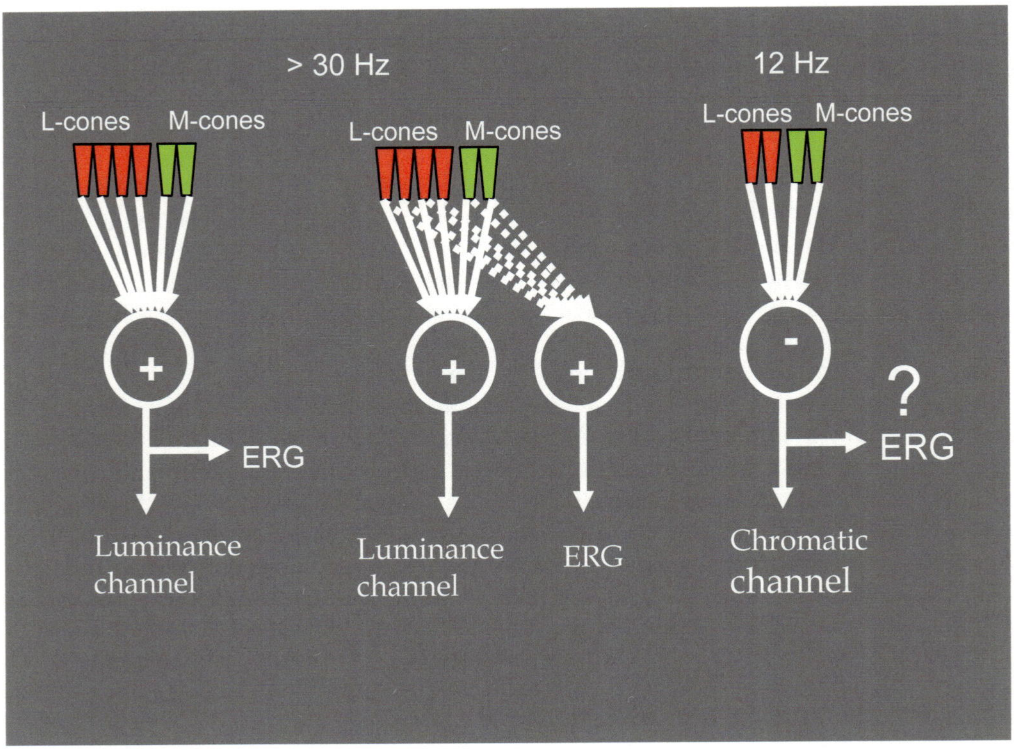

Fig. 1. Possible ideas concerning the relationship between the origins of the flicker ERG and the activity in major retino-geniculate pathways that are responsible for different aspects of visual perception. A correlation between the magnocellularly based luminance channel and the flicker ERGs using high temporal frequency stimuli is well established. The question is if this correlation is the result of the two pathways sharing common mechanisms (left graph) or of two separated pathways that more or less by accident process cone driven signals in an analogous manner (middle graph). If there is a direct causal relationship between the two, it could be expected that under certain stimulus conditions, the flicker ERG also reflects the activity of the parvocellular pathway, which is the physiological basis for red-green chromatic vision but, until recently, there was not much evidence for that proposal (right graph). Observe, that the L-/M-ration is about unity in the red-green chromatic channel whereas the L-/M- ratio is, on average, larger than one in the luminance channel.

Healthy subjects with normal colour vision participated in the experiments. In some experiments, as indicated, deuteranopic subjects and glaucoma patients participated. The glaucoma patients had no or only minor visual field defects and were basically diagnosed on the appearance of the optic nerve heads.

7.2 Experiment 1

7.2.1 Stimuli

On a CRT screen, L- and M-cone isolating stimuli were created. In addition, L- and M-cone excitations were modulated simultaneously at different relative strengths (expressed in cone contrast). In all conditions, the L- and the M-cones were modulated in counter-phase. The stimulus conditions are displayed in Fig 2 (Kremers & Link, 2008). An L-/M-cone modulation ratio of 1 indicates equal modulation strength for the L- and M-cones. A ratio of 2 indicates that the L-cones were modulated at twice the strength at which the M-cones were modulated; with a ratio of 0.5 the M-cone modulation strength was twice the L-cone modulation strength, etc. The rods were not modulated using the above-described silent substitution method. Because a CRT monitor contains three light sources (the red, green and blue phosphors), the excitation of only three photoreceptors can be controlled. Thus, S-cones were modulated at various contrasts at the different stimulus conditions. We repeated the measurements under conditions at which the S-cones were not modulated (S-cone silent substitution) and rods were modulated at various contrasts. The results of the S-cone silent measurements were basically similar and are not shown here. At each relative strength of L- and M-cone modulation, responses were measured at stimulus strengths for which

$$L_C^2 + M_C^2 = const \tag{4}$$

in which *Lc* and *Mc* are the L- and M-cone contrasts. When depicted in a coordinate system with M-cone contrast on the abscissa and L-cone contrast on the ordinate (as in Fig. 2), these stimuli had equal distances to the origin. In pre-experiments it was found that for all conditions, the ERG amplitude depended approximately linearly on the stimulus strength. For additional information I refer to the original publication (Kremers & Link, 2008). The measurements were repeated at four different temporal frequencies (12, 18, 24 and 30 Hz).

7.2.2 Results

For the different stimulus conditions (selective L- and M-cone stimulation and different counter-phase combinations of the two), the ERG amplitudes and phases (defined as the amplitudes and phases of the first harmonic components, which dominated most responses, indicating that the responses were mainly sinusoidal in shape) were determined. The mean amplitudes and phases for measurements performed at 12 and 30 Hz in one observer are displayed in Figure 3. It is obvious that the response data at the two temporal frequencies were quite different. At 30 Hz, the response amplitude to selective M-cone stimulation (L-fraction 0) was substantially smaller than the L-cone response (L-fraction 1). In addition, the phase changed relatively strongly as a function of L-fraction. At 12 Hz, the responses to L- and M-cone selective stimuli had similar amplitudes and phases. Because the stimuli were constructed to modulate L- and M-cones in counterphase, this means that the L- and M-cone driven ERG responses in fact differed by about 180 deg.

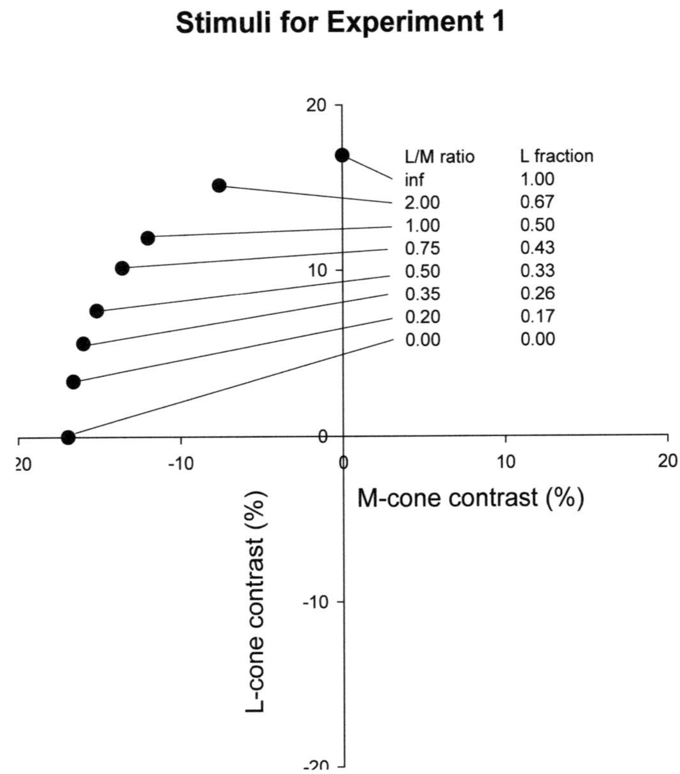

Fig. 2. Schematic description of the stimuli used in experiment 1. A modulating stimulus is produced on a CRT screen. Eight stimuli were constructed. The rods were not stimulated by any of the stimuli. The stimulus strength for the M- and L-cones (in terms of cone contrast) are given by the X- and Y-values respectively. When the two were modulated simultaneously, they modulated in counter-phase.

The curves are fits of a linear model to the data. The model is identical to the vector summation model mentioned above and assumes that the L- and M-cone driven responses have different delays and weightings before they are added; this model assumes that L- and M-cone driven responses are added at each time. With sine wave responses, as is basically the case here, responses with an amplitude and a time delay, can be expressed by a vector, the length of which depicts the response amplitude. The phase of the response is reflected by the angle of the vector with the X-axis. In the vector addition model, the vector reflecting the response to a simultaneous L- and M-cone stimulation, is equal to the addition of the vectors reflecting the response to the selective L- and M-cone stimulation. For a more detailed description of a vector addition, see Kremers (2003). In the fits, amplitudes and phases were simultaneously considered. There were four free parameters: weights (amplitudes) and phases of the L- and M-cone driven ERG signals. Therefore, from the fits L-/M- amplitude ratios in the ERGs and their relative phases can be estimated. These were estimated for all subjects and all four temporal frequencies. Figure 4 shows the average L-/M-ratios and phase differences for six different observers measured at the different temporal frequencies. The phase difference increases with decreasing temporal frequency. At 12 Hz, the phase difference between the cone inputs is approximately 180° indicating cone opponent inputs. Observe also that the inter-individual variability is substantially smaller at 12 Hz. The L-/M-ratio decreases with decreasing temporal frequency and is about unity at 12 Hz.

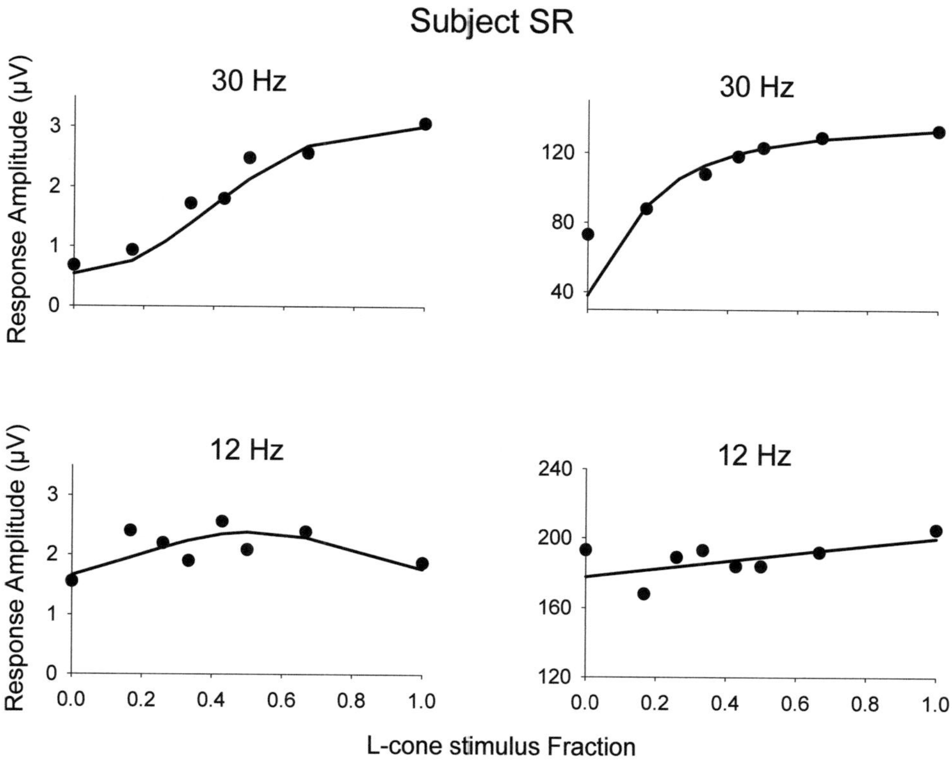

Fig. 3. Response amplitudes (left plots) and phases (right plots) displayed as a function of L-cone stimulation fraction (see Fig. 2 for explanation of stimulus conditions) in one subject measured at 30 Hz (upper plots) and 12 Hz (lower plots). The data are representative for the results obtained in all subjects with normal colour vision. At 30 Hz, the response amplitude to L-cone isolating stimuli (L-cone stimulus fraction equals 1) is larger than the response amplitude to M-cone isolating stimuli (L-cone stimulus fraction equals 0). At 12 Hz stimulation, the response amplitudes are all similar. In addition, the response phases at these two conditions are more similar at 12 Hz. Owing to the counter-phase stimulation of L- and M-cones this means that the L- and M-cone driven signals are about 180 degrees apart at 12 Hz.

The stimuli used in these experiments are combinations of chromatic and luminance modulations. Previous psychophysical data suggest that flicker detection of these types of stimuli is mediated by the (parvocellularly based) red-green chromatic channel at low temporal frequencies and by the (magnocellularly based) luminance channel at high temporal frequencies (Kelly & van Norren, 1977; Kremers *et al.*, 1992). More importantly, the L-/M-sensitivity ratio for flicker detection is about unity (i.e. the sensitivity to L- and M-cone stimuli are equal) when the red-green chromatic channel mediates flicker detection. The L-/M-sensitivity ratio is on average larger than one (but with substantial inter-individual variability) when the luminance channel mediates flicker detection (Miyahara *et al.*, 1998; Krauskopf, 2000; Kremers *et al.*, 2000; Kremers *et al.*, 2003).

The cone opponent input and the amplitude ratio of about one (with smaller inter-individual variability) in the 12 Hz flicker ERGs suggest that these responses reflect activity of the parvocellularly based red-green chromatic channel. At 30 Hz, the phases between L- and M-cone driven signals are smaller than 180° [see also Usui *et al.* (1998a) and Kremers *et al.*(1999)]. In addition, the individual L-/M-ratios can be correlated with the psychophysically determined L-/M-ratios for luminance mediated flicker detection (Jacobs & Neitz, 1993; Jacobs *et al.*, 1996c; Kremers *et al.*, 2000). Both probably find their origin in the ratio of L- to M-cone numbers in the retina (Brainard *et al.*, 2000; Kremers *et al.*, 2000). There is a large inter-individual variability in the L- to M-cone numbers but with a general bias towards L-/M-ratios larger than unity (Hofer *et al.*, 2005). This is reflected in the L-/M-ratio in the high temporal frequency ERG and in the psychophysical luminance channel. In conclusion, the 30 Hz flicker ERG seems to reflect magnocellularly based activity of the luminance pathway. In the described experiments rods were not stimulated indicating that rod intrusion cannot explain the results. To confirm this interpretation of the data, an additional experiment was conducted (experiment 2).

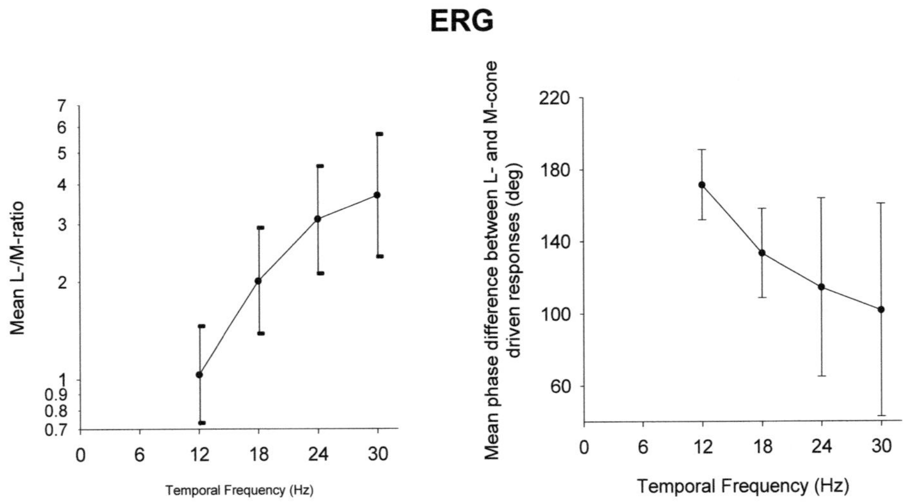

Fig. 4. L-/M-ratio (left) and L-M phase difference plotted versus temporal frequency. The L-M/-ratio decreases with decreasing temporal frequency and is about unity at 12 Hz. The L-M phase difference increases with decreasing temporal frequency and is about 180 degrees at 12 Hz.

7.3 Experiment 2

7.3.1 Stimuli

In a Ganzfeld bowl with differently coloured light emitting diodes (LEDs), the red and green LEDs were modulated in counter-phase at varying different ratios while leaving the overall modulation unchanged (Kremers *et al.*, 2010). The stimulus condition is expressed as the fraction of red LED (R) contrast of the total red and green modulation contrast (R+G). A red fraction of zero (R/(R+G)=0) means that only the green LEDs were modulated while the red LEDs were steady at its mean luminance. A red fraction of one (R/(R+G)=1) means that only the red LEDs were modulated while the green LEDs were steady at its mean luminance. A red fraction of 0.5 (R/(R+G) = 0.5) indicates that the red and the green LEDs were modulated at equal contrast. The upper panel in Fig. 5 displays the calculated response amplitudes (defined as a contrast in excitation analogous to rod and cone contrasts as a definition for the responses in the rods and cones respectively) of the luminance and red-green chromatic systems as a function of R/(R+G). In addition, the response phases of the luminance and chromatic channels are displayed in the lower graph. The luminance modulation in the stimulus strongly depends on the stimulus condition whereas chromatic modulation is the same for all conditions. For the luminance system we assumed here a V_λ-like spectral sensitivity. As a result, the minimum is at an R/(R+G) of 0.5. Inter-individual variability in the spectral luminosity function (related to the above-mentioned individual differences of L-/M-ratios) results in a variability of this minimum. Dichromats are expected to have a spectral luminosity functions that are identical with the L- (deuteranopes) or M-cone (protanope) fundamentals. The minima of the luminance based responses therefore coincide with the silent substitution points of the L- and M-cone (i.e. those points where the L- and M-cone contrasts equal 0) in deuteranopes and protanopes respectively.

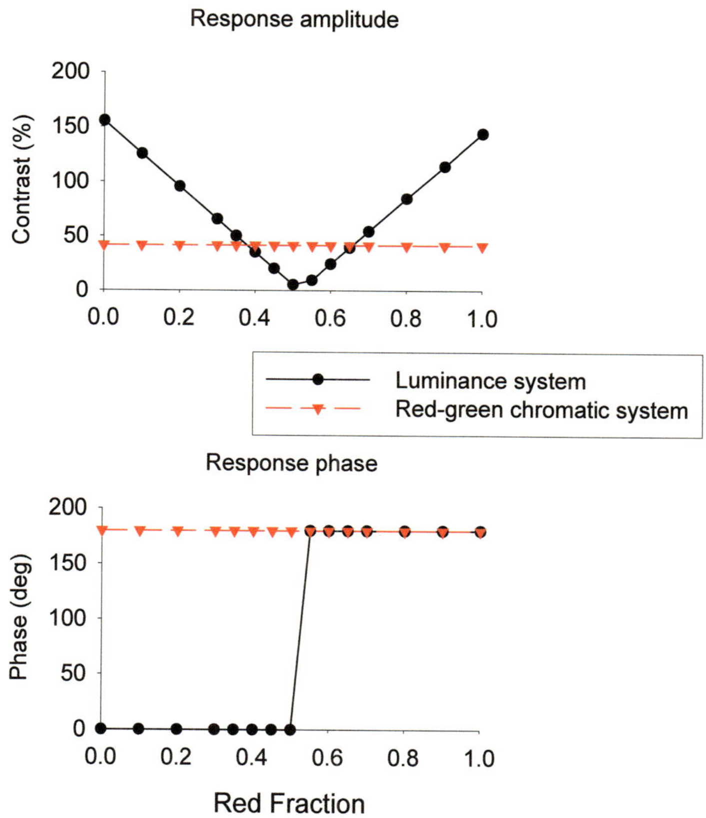

Fig. 5. Theoretical response amplitudes (upper plot) and phases (lower) of the luminance and red-green chromatic pathways given as a function of the stimulus conditions used in experiment 2.

7.3.2 Results

In Fig. 6, the 36 Hz and 12 Hz responses are displayed for three different trichromatic subjects. Obviously, the 36 Hz ERG responses closely correspond to the (magnocellularly based) activity of the luminance channel whereas the 12 Hz ERGs is more reminiscent of the response of the (parvocellularly based) red-green chromatic system (cf. Fig. 5). This experiment confirms the results of experiment 1 that the 36 Hz ERGs reflect magnocellular activity whereas the 12 Hz ERGs mainly reflect parvocellular activity. The results at intermediate temporal frequencies (data not shown) could be described as a linear vector addition of the magno- and parvocellular activity. The advantage of this experiment in comparison with experiment 1 was that larger stimulus contrasts and thus also larger ERG

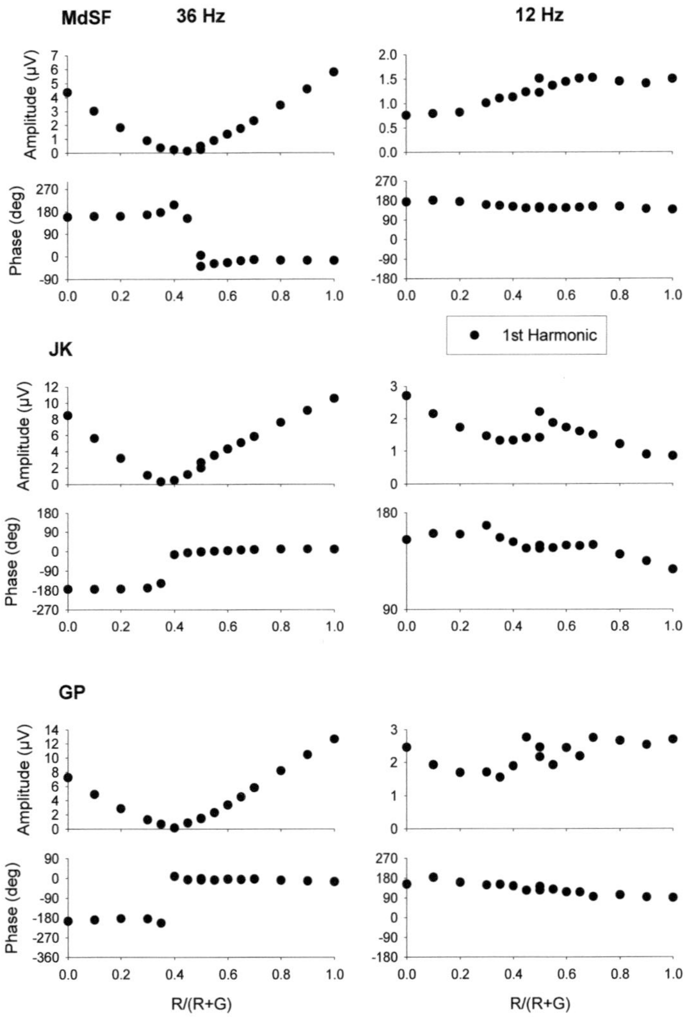

Fig. 6. Measured response amplitudes and phase in flicker ERGs at 36 Hz (left plots) and 12 Hz (right plots) for three different colour normal subjects obtained in experiment 2. Observe the resemblance of the response properties at 36 Hz with those of the luminance pathway and at 12 Hz with those of the red-green chromatic pathway (see fig. 5).

signals could be obtained. This was possible because the narrow band emission spectra of the LEDs allow larger contrasts than the phosphors of a CRT screen. However, in contrast to experiment 1 rods and S-cones responded to the stimuli as well. In principle, rod or S-cone intrusion could lead to similar results. To exclude this explanation of the data, the experiment was repeated in a deuteranope who has normal rods and S-cones but no L-cones and no functional parvocellularly based red-green colour system. If the above described effects were caused by rod and S-cone intrusion then the same results would be obtained in the measurements with the deuteranope. If the ERGs indeed reflected activity of the magno- and parvocellular pathways then it could be expected that the 12 Hz responses would depend on the different stimulus conditions in a similar manner as the 36 Hz responses. The later case was confirmed experimentally (see Figure 7). Therefore, we can conclude that the data in the trichromats were dominated by activity of the red-green chromatic pathway at 12 Hz. In addition, as expected (see above), the minima at 36 Hz and 12 Hz coincided with the silent substitution condition of the L-cones confirming that this subject had no functional M-cones.

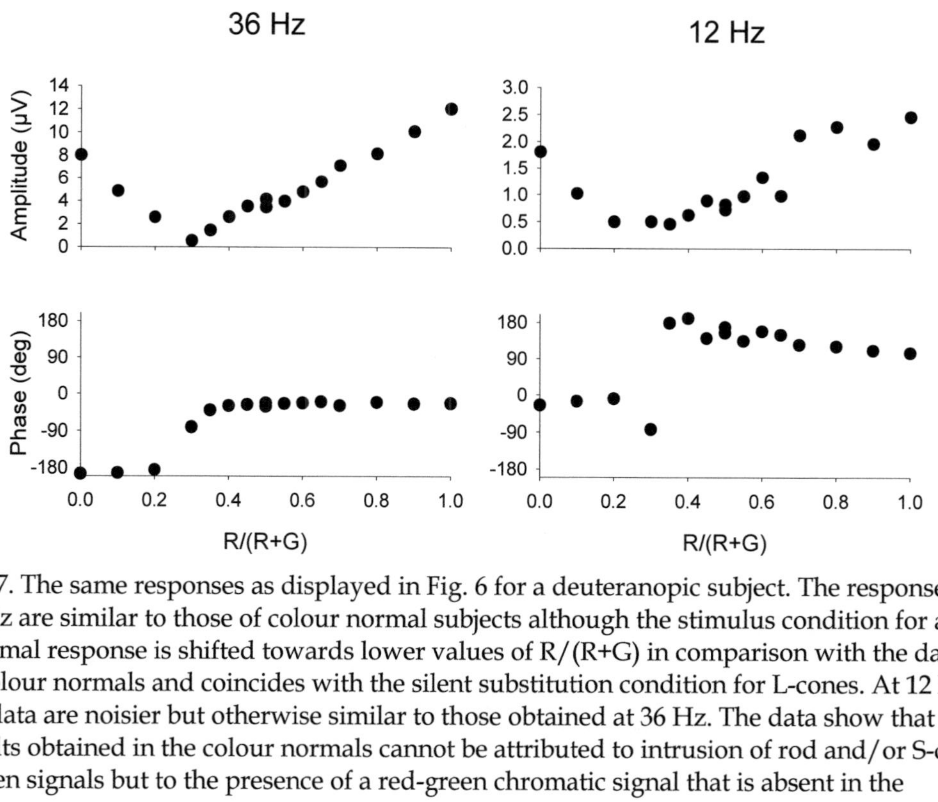

Fig. 7. The same responses as displayed in Fig. 6 for a deuteranopic subject. The responses at 36 Hz are similar to those of colour normal subjects although the stimulus condition for a minimal response is shifted towards lower values of R/(R+G) in comparison with the data of colour normals and coincides with the silent substitution condition for L-cones. At 12 Hz, the data are noisier but otherwise similar to those obtained at 36 Hz. The data show that the results obtained in the colour normals cannot be attributed to intrusion of rod and/or S-cone driven signals but to the presence of a red-green chromatic signal that is absent in the deuteranope.

These experiments were also performed in patients with mild glaucoma. These patients either had no or mild visual field defects. In these experiments, only a subset of the above described stimuli was employed on a larger population of participants. The results of these measurements, shown in Fig. 8, with the healthy subjects were in agreement with the results of the more extended measurements, described above. The response amplitudes measured with the patients were very similar to those of the normal subjects. However, the response phases differed significantly. Although the differences were not large, the small inter-individual variability in phase data made the phase parameter very useful for detecting differences between groups.

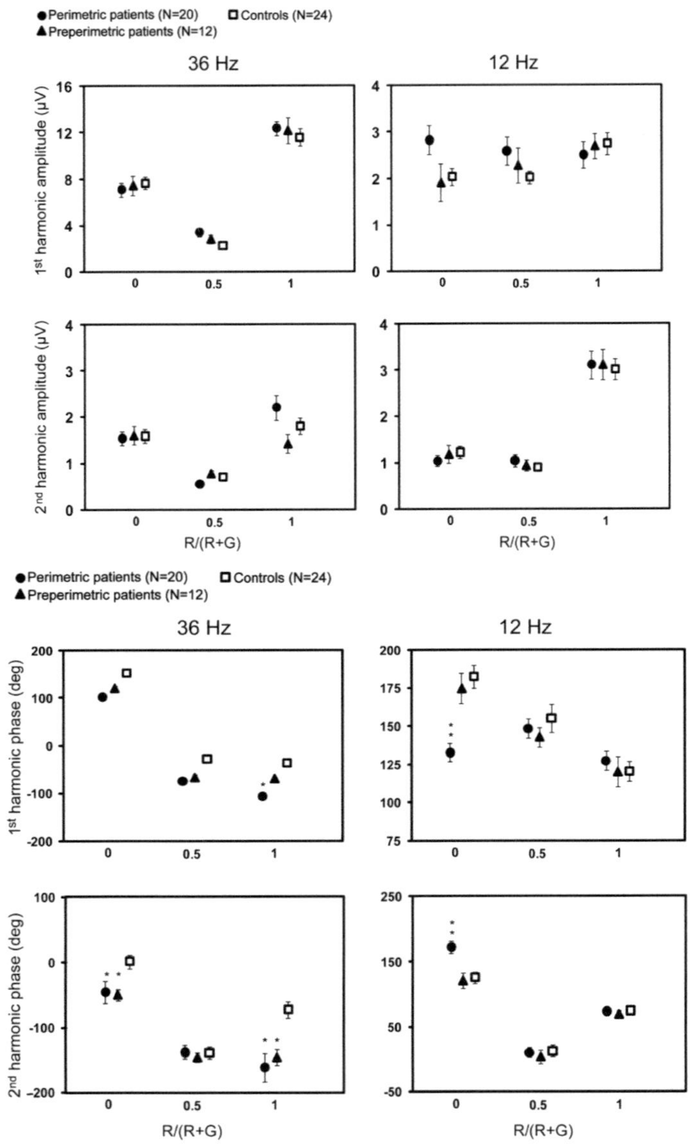

Fig. 8. Responses to a subset of stimuli displayed in Figs. 6 and 7 in larger group of normal subjects, preperimetric and perimetric glaucoma patients (i.e. glaucoma patients without and with visual field losses respectively). The largest differences between the perimetric patients and normals were found in the response phases rather than in the response amplitudes.

In conclusion, in two independent experiments we have shown that it is possible to record ERGs that reflect magnocellularly based luminance activity at high temporal frequency and parvocellularly based red-green chromatic activity at 12 Hz. As I will discuss below, these data may have important implications for our understanding of the visual information processing in the retina. However, the ERG is an important clinical tool. The results with the glaucoma patients may be a starting point for studying the disease related functional changes in distinct retino-geniculate pathways.

8. Discussion

The individual L-/M-ratio in the ERGs with 30 Hz stimuli was measured in previous experiments by us and by others (Jacobs & Harwerth, 1989; Jacobs & Neitz, 1993; Jacobs *et al.*, 1996b; Jacobs *et al.*, 1996c; Brainard *et al.*, 1999; Kremers *et al.*, 1999; Brainard *et al.*, 2000; Kremers *et al.*, 2000; Kremers, 2003; Kremers *et al.*, 2003) and it was found that they correlated well with the individual L-/M-ratios in the psychophysical luminance channel. In addition, the spectral sensitivity of the high temporal frequency ERG corresponds well with the luminous efficiency function in different human individuals (Jacobs & Neitz, 1993; Kremers *et al.*, 2000) and in different primate species (Jacobs *et al.*, 1987; Jacobs & Harwerth, 1989; Jacobs, 1991; Jacobs & Deegan Ii, 1993b, a; Jacobs *et al.*, 1993a; Jacobs *et al.*, 1993b; Jacobs, 1996; Jacobs *et al.*, 1996a; Jacobs *et al.*, 1996b; Jacobs *et al.*, 1996d; Jacobs, 1997; Jacobs & Deegan Ii, 1997; Banin *et al.*, 1999; Jacobs *et al.*, 2002). It was further found that the L-/M-ratio was correlated with the ratio of L- to M-cone pigment content in the retina (Kremers *et al.*, 2000) and with the ratio of L- to M-cone numbers (Brainard *et al.*, 2000). Therefore, it seems that the high frequency ERG and the luminance channel share a similar type of post-receptoral processing by summing the information of all available L- and M-cones. However, does this mean that the two are intimately related or is the correlation between the two merely the result of an analogous processing in the two signal pathways without a closer relationship (see Fig. 1 for the alternative explanations)? This question was raised in part 6 of this chapter. The data of the two described experiments strongly suggest high temporal flicker ERG is indeed causally related to activity of the luminance channel. This is consistent with our previous finding that selective cone adaptation had similar effects on flicker detection thresholds mediated by the luminance channel and the high temporal frequency flicker ERG (Kremers *et al.*, 2003). The most parsimonious explanation for this observation is that the pathway leading to a high frequency flicker ERG and the magnocellular pathway share substantially parts of visual information processing mechanisms (Fig. 9 left graph). Furthermore, the flicker ERG, measured at a temporal frequency of about 12 Hz, is directly related to activity of the parvocellularly based red-green chromatic pathway (see Fig. 9 where the question mark in the right graph of fig. 1 has been replaced by an exclamation mark).

Based on these data, we conclude that the flicker ERG can reflect activity in the parvocellular and magnocellular retino-geniculate pathways and shares signal processing mechanisms with them. It has been previously proposed that flicker ERGs probably originate in bipolar cell activity (Bush & Sieving, 1996). Possibly, the flicker ERGs reflect activity of diffuse and midget bipolar cells rather than of retinal ganglion cells. That would implicate that the bipolar cells already have response properties that resemble those of the retinal ganglion cells. This is in agreement with the results of intracellular measurements from primate bipolar cells in which it was shown that the bipolar cells have centre-surround structures (Dacey *et al.*, 2000). These findings may have important implications for basic and clinical science. It may now be possible to study some physiological properties of the two major retino-geniculate pathways objectively in human observers.

A clinical application was introduced above with glaucoma patients. I want to give two examples of basic vision science issues to which the ERG data may contribute. As mentioned above, the 12 Hz ERG data are consistent with psychophysical data showing that the L-/M-ratio in the red-green chromatic channel is about unity despite the generally larger L-/M-ratios and the large inter-individual differences in the luminance channel and in the cone numbers. Moreover, the L-/M-ratio remains at unity in different adaptation conditions although the same adaptation conditions have a large influence upon the responses in the luminance channel (Kremers *et al.*, 2003). This strongly suggests the presence of a sophisticated compensatory mechanism in the retina. I propose that this compensatory mechanism needs to develop in early lifetime of an individual through experience-based weighting and recalibrating of the cone input to the red-green chromatic system. The consequence of this viewpoint is that the cone signal inputs are transformed continuously. This proposal of a dynamic system is in contrast with ideas of a static and hard random wiring in the parvocellular pathway which suggests that the presence of two photoreceptor types with distinct absorption spectra, that are both connected to the midget bipolar cells, is sufficient for the existence of red-green colour vision. In a recent experiment it was found that dichromatic monkeys transfected with an extra opsin gene, express this gene and that the extra photopigment is used behaviourally (Mancuso *et al.*, 2009). It has been suggested that this behaviour is caused by colour vision. This would not be in line with my suggestion that colour vision is experience based. However, an alternative explanation of the monkey data is that the extra pigment has introduced retinal areas that are intrinsically dichromatic (so do not have extra colour vision) but have different spectral sensitivities. This proposal could also explain the behavioural data.

What would the functional and evolutionary advantage of such compensatory mechanism be? This is highly speculative but the answer may be found if we consider the fundamental difference between luminance and chromatic perception. Luminance perception is relative: we are able to see differences in luminances, meaning that we are able to recognize whether one structure is more luminant or brighter than the other, but it is not possible to state what the absolute luminance or brightness is. In contrast, colour perception can be given in absolute terms: we can recognize the colour of a structure directly without a comparison with another structure. We are able to see and identify whether a flower is red or some other colour. It is not necessary to say whether it is more reddish or more greenish than another structure. In addition, we are able to communicate this colour to another person without confusion (provided the two persons have normal colour vision). If somebody asks colour normal persons to pick the red flower in bouquet with a blue, a green, a yellow and an orange, all persons will pick the same flower without any dissent and they will pick correctly the requested flower. Thus, colour vision is absolute and very similar in different individuals despite the large variability in L- and M-cone numbers in their retinae and despite the variability in lighting conditions. That means that the colour system continuously is recalibrated. The proposed compensatory mechanism could be the basis for this. The ERG data may now contribute to these contemplations on basic questions.

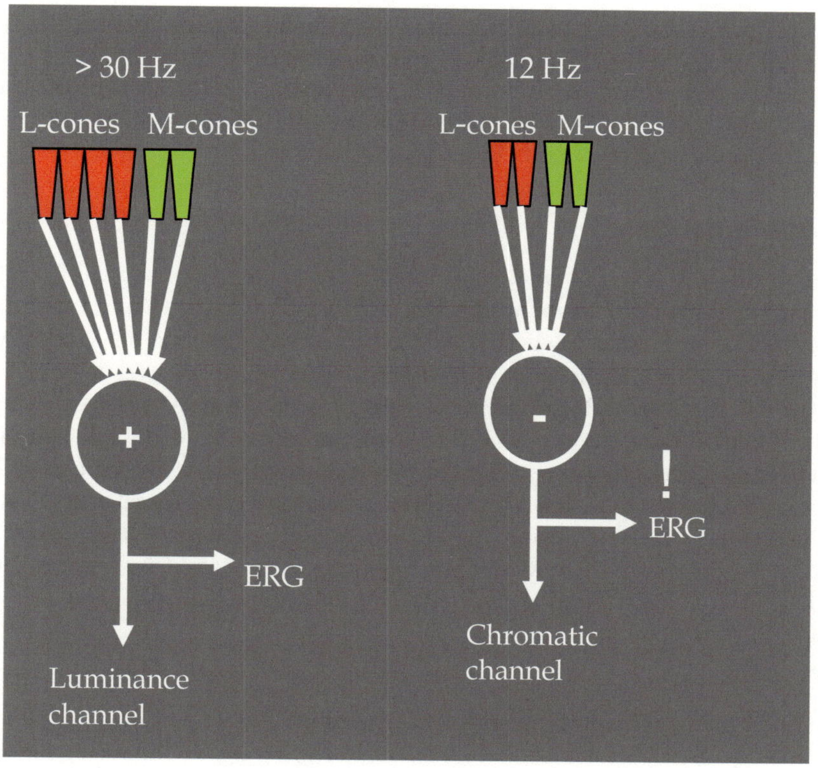

Fig. 9. The proposal based on the results of experiments 1 - 3. The activity of the flicker ERG directly reflects the activity of the luminance channel when high temporal frequency stimuli are used. It reflects the activity of the red-green chromatic pathway when stimulated at 12 Hz.

A second basic issue is that the ERG data can also be used to obtain information about dynamics of photoreceptor driven signals in the human retina. The ERG data can be compared with psychophysical data, but they provide additional information about response delays which can not easily be obtained from psychophysical experiments. The ERG data can be used to explain interesting observations. For instance, it was found that the phase differences between L- and M-cone driven ERG responses at high temporal frequency stimuli (and therefore reflecting luminance activity) were particularly large (1) in subjects with high L-/M-ratios (Kremers *et al.*, 2011), (2) in the periphery of the retina (Challa *et al.*, 2010) and (3) in retinitis pigmentosa patients (Scholl & Kremers, 2000). In all of these cases, the large phase differences were accompanied by a change in M-cone driven phases. The phases of the L-cone driven responses were much more stable and there was less inter-individual variability. Do the phase changes in the M-cone driven ERGs have the same causes in these three cases? If so, what could this cause be? The factor that these cases possibly have in common is a low number of M-cones. Normal subjects with high L-/M-ratios have lower numbers of M-cones. The number of cones decreases with increasing retinal eccentricity. Finally, the numbers of cones also decrease in RP patients. Possibly, if the M-cone numbers fall below a threshold the response phases change. This proposition implies that a reasonable number of cones of one type should be present so that their responses can be synchronized amongst each other and with the other cone types. Although this idea is quite speculative, it provides a testable working hypothesis for future experiments. In addition, it provides a common solution for the three puzzling results given above. Finally, it may explain why L- and M-cone driven signals have different properties even though the L- and M-cones, and the postreceptoral pathways connected to them, are biochemically and structurally nearly identical.

9. Acknowledgment

The work presented in this chapter was performed over a period of about 15 years in which I was lucky to collaborate with many great scientists and friends. I would therefore like to thank Tomoaki Usui, Hendrik Scholl, Neil Parry, Ian Murray, Declan McKeefry, Naveen Challa, Barbara Link, Luiz Carlos Silveira, Anderson Rodrigues, Manoel da Silva Filho, Dora Ventura, Mirella Barboni, Maciej Stepien, Cezar Saito, Lindsay Sharpe, Folkert Horn, Anselm Jünemann for their contributions and discussions. The work has been financially supported through several grants from the German Research Council (through a Heisenberg Fellowship), the Hertie Foundation (a Fellowship in the Hertie Excellence Program), the German Academic Exchange Council, the Ministry of Education and Research, CNPq (Brazil) and CAPES (Brazil) for collaborative grants with Brazil. Finally, I would like to thank the Head of the Department, Prof. Kruse, for his general support.

10. References

Armington, J. C. (1974). *The Electroretinogram*. Academic Press, New York.

Banin, E., Cideciyan, A. V., Aleman, T. S., Petters, R. M., Wong, F., Milam, A. H. & Jacobson, S. G. (1999). Retinal rod photoreceptor-specific gene mutation perturbs cone pathway development. *Neuron* 23, 549-557.

Barboni, M.T.S., Pangeni, G., Vetura, D.F., Horn, F.K., Kremers, J. (2011). Hetreochromatic flicker electroretinograms reflecting luminance and cone opponent activity in glaucoma patients. *Investigative Ophthalmology & Visual Science,* in press.

Brainard, D. H., Calderone, J. B., Nugent, A. K. & Jacobs, G. H. (1999). Flicker ERG responses to stimuli parametrically modulated in color space. *Investigative Ophthalmology & Visual Science* 40, 2840-2847.

Brainard, D. H., Roorda, A., Yamauchi, Y., Calderone, J. B., Metha, A. B., Neitz, M., Neitz, J., Williams, D. R. & Jacobs, G. H. (2000). Functional consequences of the relative numbers of L and M cones. *Journal of the Optical Society of America A* 17, 607-614.

Bush, R. A. & Sieving, P. A. (1996). Inner retinal contributions to the primate photopic fast flicker electroretinogram. *Journal of the Optical Society of America A* 13, 557-565.

Buzas, P., Blessing, E. M., Szmajda, B. A. & Martin, P. R. (2006). Specificity of M and L cone inputs to receptive fields in the parvocellular pathway: random wiring with functional bias. *J Neurosci* 26, 11148-11161.

Challa, N. K., McKeefry, D., Parry, N. R. A., Kremers, J., Murray, I. J. & Panorgias, A. (2010). L- and M-cone input to 12Hz and 30Hz flicker ERGs across the human retina. *Ophthalmic and Physiological Optics* 30, 503-510.

Dacey, D. M. & Lee, B. B. (1994). The 'blue-on' opponent pathway in primate retina originates from a distinct bistratified ganglion cell type. *Nature* 367, 731-735.

Dacey, D. M. & Lee, B. B. (1999). Functional architecture of cone signal pathways in the primate retina. In *Color Vision; From genes to perception*, vol. first. ed. Gegenfurtner, K. R. & Sharpe, L. T., pp. 181-202. Cambridge University Press, Cambridge.

Dacey, D. M., Packer, O. S., Diller, L., Brainard, D. H., Peterson, B. & Lee, B. B. (2000). Center surround receptive field structure of cone bipolar cells in primate retina. *Vision Research* 40, 1801-1811.

de Rouck, A. F. (2006). History of the electroretinogram. In *Principles and Practice of Clinical Electrophysiology of Vision*. ed. Heckenlively, J. R. & Arden, G. B., pp. 3-10. The MIT Press, Cambridge, USA, London, UK.

DeMarco, P., Pokorny, J. & Smith, V. C. (1992). Full-spectrum cone sensitivity functions for X-chromosome-linked anomalous trichromats. *Journal of the Optical Society of America A* 9, 1465-1476.

Donner, K. O. & Rushton, W. A. H. (1959). Retinal stimulation by light substitution. *Journal of Physiology* 149, 288-302.

Estévez, O. & Spekreijse, H. (1974). A spectral compensation method for determining the flicker characteristics of the human colour mechanisms. *Vision Research* 14, 823-830.

Estévez, O. & Spekreijse, H. (1982). The "silent substitution" method in visual research. *Vision Research* 22, 681-691.

Frishman, L. J. (2006). Origins of the electroretinogram. In *Principles and Practice of Clinical Electrophysiology of Vision.*, vol. 2nd. ed. Heckenlively, J. R. & Arden, G. B., pp. 139-183. The MIT Press, Cambridge, London.

Fukuda, Y., Tsujimura, S., Higuchi, S., Yasukouchi, A. & Morita, T. (2010). The ERG responses to light stimuli of melanopsin-expressing retinal ganglion cells that are independent of rods and cones. *Neurosci Lett* 479, 282-286.

Hofer, H., Carroll, J., Neitz, J., Neitz, M. & Williams, D. R. (2005). Organization of the Human Trichromatic Cone Mosaic. *Journal of Neuroscience* 25, 9669-9679.

Jacobs, G. H. (1991). Variations in colour vision in non-human primates. *Inherited and Acquired Colour Vision Deficiencies, D.H.Foster (ed)*, 199-214.

Jacobs, G. H. (1996). Primate photopigments and primate color vision. *Proceedings National Academy of Sciences USA* 93, 577-581.

Jacobs, G. H. (1997). Color vision polymorphisms in New World monkeys: Implications for the evolution of primate trichromacy. In *New World Primates; Ecology, evolution and behavior*. ed. Kinzey, W. G., pp. 45-74. Aldine de Gruyter, New York.

Jacobs, G. H. (1998). A perspective on color vision in platyrrhine monkeys. *Vision Research* 38, 3307-3313.

Jacobs, G. H. & Deegan Ii, J. F. (1993a). Photopigments underlying color vision in ringtail lemurs (Lemur catta) and brown lemurs (Eulemur fulvus). *American Journal of Primatology* 30, 243-256.

Jacobs, G. H. & Deegan Ii, J. F. (1993b). Polymorphism of cone photopigments in new world monkeys: is the spider monkey unique? *Investigative Ophthalmology and Visual Science (SUPPL)* 34, 749.

Jacobs, G. H. & Deegan Ii, J. F. (1997). Spectral sensitivity of macaque monkeys measured with ERG flicker photometry. *Visual Neuroscience* 14, 921-928.

Jacobs, G. H. & Deegan Ii, J. F. (1999). Five distinct M/L photopigments in a New World monkey. *Investigative Ophthalmology and Visual Science (SUPPL)* 40, 981.

Jacobs, G. H., Deegan Ii, J. F., Neitz, J., Crognale, M. A. & Neitz, M. (1993a). Photopigments and color vision in the nocturnal monkey, Aotus *Vision Research* 33, 1773-1783.

Jacobs, G. H., Deegan Ii, J. F., Neitz, M. & Neitz, J. (1996a). Presence of routine trichromatic color vision in new world monkeys. *Investigative Ophthalmology and Visual Science (SUPPL)* 37, 346.

Jacobs, G. H., Deegan Ii, J. F., Tan, Y. & Li, W. H. (2002). Opsin gene and photopigment polymorphism in a prosimian primate. *Vision Research* 42, 11-18.

Jacobs, G. H., Deegan, I. J. S. & Moran, J. L. (1996b). ERG measurements of the spectral sensitivity of common chimpanzee (Pan troglodytes). *Vision Research* 36, 2587-2594.

Jacobs, G. H. & Harwerth, R. S. (1989). Color vision variations in Old and New World primates. *American Journal of Primatology* 18, 35-44.

Jacobs, G. H. & Neitz, J. (1993). Electrophysiological estimates of individual variation in the L/M cone ratio. In *colour vision deficiencies XI*. ed. Drum, B., pp. 107-112. Kluwer Academic publishers.

Jacobs, G. H., Neitz, J. & Crognale, M. (1987). Color vision polymorphism and its photopigment basis in a callitrichid monkey (saguinus fuscicollis). *Vision Research* 27, 2089-2100.

Jacobs, G. H., Neitz, J. & Krogh, K. (1996c). Electroretinogram flicker photometry and its applications. *Journal of the Optical Society of America A* 13, 641-648.

Jacobs, G. H., Neitz, J. & Neitz, M. (1993b). Genetic basis of polymorphism in the color vision of platyrrhine monkeys. *Vision Research* 33, 269-274.

Jacobs, G. H., Neitz, M., Deegan, J. F. & Neitz, J. (1996d). Trichromatic colour vision in New World monkeys. *Nature* 382, 156-158.

Jacobs, G. H., Wiliams, G. A. & Fenwick, J. A. (2004). Influence of cone pigment coexpression on spectral sensitivity and color vision in the mouse. *Vision Research* 44, 1615-1622.

Jusuf, P. R., Martin, P. R. & Grünert, U. (2006). Random wiring in the midget pathway of primate retina. *Journal of Neuroscience* 26, 3908-3917.

Kelly, D. H. & van Norren, D. (1977). Two-band model of heterochromatic flicker. *Journal of the Optical Society of America* 67, 1081-1091.

Krauskopf, J. (2000). Relative number of long- and middle-wavelength-sensitive cones in the human fovea. *Journal of the Optical Society of America A* 17, 510-516.

Kremers, J. (2003). The assessment of L- and M-cone specific electroretinographical signals in the normal and abnormal retina. *Progress in Retinal and Eye Research* 22, 579-605.

Kremers, J., Lee, B. B. & Kaiser, P. K. (1992). Sensitivity of macaque retinal ganglion cells and human observers to combined luminance and chromatic modulation. *Journal of the Optical Society of America A* 9, 1477-1485.

Kremers, J. & Link, B. (2008). Electroretinographic responses that may reflect activity of parvo- and magnocellular post-receptoral visual pathways. *Journal of Vision* 8, 1-14.

Kremers, J., Parry, N. R., Panorgias, A. & Murray, I. J. (2011). The influence of retinal illuminance on L- and M-cone driven electroretinograms. *Vis Neurosci*, 1-7.

Kremers, J., Rodrigues, A. R., Silveira, L. C. L. & da Silva-Filho, M. (2010). Flicker ERGs Representing Chromaticity and Luminance Signals. *Investigative Ophthalmology & Visual Science* 51.

Kremers, J., Scholl, H. P. N., Knau, H., Berendschot, T. T. J. M., Usui, T. & Sharpe, L. T. (2000). L/M cone ratios in human trichromats assesed by psychophysics, electroretinograpy , and retinal densitometry. *J.Opt.Soc.Am.* 17, 517-526.

Kremers, J., Stepien, M. W., Scholl, H. P. N. & Saito, C. A. (2003). Cone selective adaptation influences L- and M-cone driven signals in electroretinography and psychophysics. *Journal of Vision* 3, 146-160.

Kremers, J., Usui, T., Scholl, H. P. N. & Sharpe, L. T. (1999). Cone signal contributions to electroretinograms in dichromats and trichromats. *Investigative Ophthalmology & Visual Science* 40, 920-930.

Lee, B. B. (2011). Visual pathways and psychophysical channels in the primate. *J Physiol* 589, 41-47.

Mancuso, K., Hauswirth, W. W., Li, Q., Connor, T. B., Kuchenbecker, J. A., Mauck, M. C., Neitz, J. & Neitz, M. (2009). Gene therapy for red-green colour blindness in adult primates. *Nature* 461, 784-787.

Martin, P. R., White, A. J. R., Goodchild, A. K., Wilder, H. D. & Sefton, A. E. (1997). Evidence that blue-on cells are part of the third genicolocortical pathway in primates. *European Journal of Neuroscience* 9, 1536-1541.

Miyahara, E., Pokorny, J., Smith, V. C., Baron, R. & Baron, E. (1998). Color vision in two observers with highly biased LWS/MWS cone ratios. *Vision Research* 38, 601-612.

Naka, K. I. & Rushton, W. A. (1966). S-potentials from colour units in the retina of fish (Cyprinidae). *Journal of Physiology (London)* 185, 536-555.

Neitz, J. & Jacobs, G. H. (1984). Electroretinogram measurements of cone spectral sensitivity in dichromatic monkeys. *Journal of the Optical Society of America A* 1, 1175-1180.

Neitz, M., Neitz, J. & Jacobs, G. H. (1991). Spectral tuning of pigments underlying red-green color vision. *Science* 252, 971-974.

Scholl, H. P. N. & Kremers, J. (2000). Large phase differences between L-cone and M-cone driven electroretinograms in retinitis pigmentosa. *Investigative Ophthalmology & Visual Science* 41, 3225-3233.

Scholl, H. P. N., Kremers, J., Apfelstedt-Sylla, E. & Zrenner, E. (2000). L- and M-cone driven ERGs are differently altered in Best's macular dystrophy. *Vision Research* 40, 3159-3168.

Scholl, H. P. N., Kremers, J., Vonthein, R., White, K. & Weber, B. H. (2001). L- and M-cone driven electroretinograms in Stargardt's macular dystrophy-Fundus flavimaculatus. *Investigative Ophthalmology & Visual Science* 42, 1380-1389.

Shapiro, A. G., Pokorny, J. & Smith, V. C. (1996). Cone-rod receptor spaces with illustrations that use the CRT phosphor and light-emitting-diode spectra. *Journal of the Optical Society of America A* 13, 2319-2328.

Silveira, L. C. L., Grünert, U., Kremers, J., Lee, B. B. & Martin, P. R. (2005). Comparative anatomy and physiology of the primate retina. In *The Primate Visual System; a comparative approach*, vol. 1. ed. Kremers, J., pp. 127-160. Johnn Wiley and sons, Chichester.

Stiles, W. S. (1939). The directional sensitivity of the retina and the spectral sensitivities of the rods and cones. *Proceedings of the Royal Society (London)* 127, 64-105.

Stiles, W. S. (1953). Further studies of visual mechanisms by the two-colour threshold method. In *Cologuio Sobre Problemas Opticas de la Vision*. Union Int Phys Pure Appl, Madrid.

Stiles, W. S. (1959). Color vision: The approach through increment threshold sensitivity. *Proceedings National Academy of Sciences USA* 45, 100-114.

Stiles, W. S. (1978). *Mechanisms of Colour Vision*. Academic Press, London.

Stockman, A., MacLeod, D. I. A. & Johnson, N. E. (1993). Spectral sensitivities of the human cones. *Journal of the Optical Society of America A* 10, 2491-2521.

Usui, T., Kremers, J., Sharpe, L. T. & Zrenner, E. (1998a). Flicker cone electroretinogram in dichromats and trichromats. *Vision Research* 38, 3391-3396.

Usui, T., Kremers, J., Sharpe, L. T. & Zrenner, E. (1998b). Response phase of the flicker electroretinogram (ERG) is influenced by cone excitation strength. *Vision Research* 38, 3247-3251.

Yeh, T., Lee, B. B. & Kremers, J. (1995). Temporal response of ganglion cells of the macaque retina to cone-specific modulation. *Journal of the Optical Society of America A* 12, 456-464.

Zele, A. J., Smith, V. C. & Pokorny, J. (2006). Spatial and temporal chromatic contrast: effects on chromatic discrimination for stimuli varying in L- and M-cone excitation. *Visual Neuroscience* 23, 495-501.

5

Method to Indentify Nonsignificant Responses at Multifocal Electroretinogram Recordings: Technical Note

Aline Corrêa de Carvalho[1], Givago da Silva Souza[1,2], Bruno Duarte Gomes[2], Anderson Raiol Rodrigues[1], Dora Fix Ventura[3] and Luiz Carlos de Lima Silveira[1,2]

[1]*Universidade Federal do Pará, Núcleo de Medicina Tropical*
[2]*Universidade Federal do Pará, Instituto de Ciências Biológicas*
[3]*Universidade de São Paulo, Instituto de Psicologia*
Brazil

1. Introduction

Multifocal electroretinography (mfERG) was developed by Erich Sutter and colleagues (Sutter & Tran, 1992) and since the beginning was an important non invasive method to record simultaneously evoked electrical activity from several retinal areas in a relative short time. This method may reveal the presence or absence of electrical activity in a number of retinal locations, mapping the functional state of a large retinal area.

The stimulus is composed by multiple patches. Usually, each patch has a command to show flashes according to a pseudorandom sequence called binary m-sequence. The decision to show or not a flash in the patch is programmed in periodic intervals, the base period (Sutter, 2000). The evoked responses, called kernels, are derived from a cross-correlation technique (Sutter, 2001).

Usually, the stimulus is scaled in order to elicit similar waveforms across the visual field. The results of an mfERG session is presented in an array of traces or in a three dimensional plot showing the response density to the different sectors of the stimulus. The response density plot may lead the clinician to misinterpretation, because the plot generates a central peak, even when no responses are recorded from the patient (Kretschmann et al., 2000; Hood et al., 2003). Waveform array is safer than response density to decide about an outcome of the mfERG test. It is relatively easy for clinicians to recognize true responses (large signal plus noise) in the mfERG trace array. However, it is very difficult to decide between decreased responses (small signal plus noise), and pure noise.

Some analysis methods have suggested different ways to discriminate signal from noise in recorded data that can be applied to a variety of electrophysiological techniques. It was shown that the dot product between the responses and an artificial signal template could increase the signal-to-noise ratio (SNR) of the data (Sutter & Tran, 1992). Few studies have suggested objective methods to evaluate the reliability of the mfERG (Hood et al., 1998, Seeliger et al., 1998). Hood et al. (1998) proposed the comparison of the signal RMS amplitude of the recording with the RMS amplitude of a template in different time intervals. The closer in time was the equivalence between both RMS amplitudes, the better was the SNR. Seeliger et al. (1998) measured mfERG implicit times to determine their distribution across the retina. They found a low intersubject variability and higher implicit times in the blind spot, upper and lower retina, and macula. They calculated the median of implicit time of each sector of normal subjects and subtracted this value from the implicit times of patients. The larger the difference, the higher the chance to find a functionally decreased area. Other work compared human scores and automated methods to distinguish signal information of mfERG from noise. The authors concluded that automated routines can be used to increase the sensitivity of signal detection of the mfERG compared to human scoring (Wright et al., 2006).

Here, we describe a method to identify an optimal SNR that can be used to classify waveforms with normal amplitude, low amplitude and without signal.

2. Subjects

We recorded mfERGs from 10 healthy subjects (25.4 ± 3.5 years old). Their pupils were dilated and their eyes were anesthetised before electrode placement (Mydriatics. Tropicamide 1%, Alcon; Phenylephrine chloridrate 10%, Allergan. Anesthetic. Proximetacaine chloridrate 0.5%, Alcon). All procedures were in agreement with the tenets of the Declaration of Helsinki and approved by the Research Ethics Committee of the Tropical Medicine Nucleus, Federal University of Pará, Report 57/2008 of 26th November 2008, following the Resolution 196/96 of the National Health Council of Brazil.

3. Visual stimulation

VERIS Science v6.0.5d (Electro-Diagnostic Imaging, EDI, San Mateo, California) was used to generate a black-and-white stimulus comprising a 103 hexagons array covering 45° x 45° of visual field. The stimulus was generated in a colour microdisplay (FMS II, EDI) at 60 Hz frame rate and 1280 x 1024 pixels of spatial resolution. The microdisplay was positioned in front of subject's eye and the optical distance from the eye to the stimulus was adjusted until the best focus was achieved.

The hexagons were scaled with eccentricity to equalize response amplitude across the visual field following ISCEV recommendations (Hood et al., 2008). The luminance of each hexagon was modulated in time by a complete cycle of an m-sequence of 2^{14} -1 elements (Sutter & Tran, 1992). The same m-sequence was used for all hexagons but its starting point was displaced in time from one hexagon to the other. States 1 and -1 of the m-sequence represented the flash and non flash period, respectively. The base period was 16.667 ms (the duration of 1 frame). The stimulation session lasted 4 min and 33 s divided in eight segments of 34.13 s each. A red cross of 1° of visual angle was used as fixation mark. The eye fixation was continuously monitored during visual stimulation by an infrared camera located inside the microdisplay.

4. Recordings

Continuous recordings were obtained by using a Burian-Allen corneal electrode, housing both the recording and reference electrodes, and a ground consisting of a gold-cup surface electrode placed on the subject's ear lobe. Electrode impedance was monitored between stimulus segments and kept below 2 kΩ. The bioelectrical signals were x 50,000 amplified, sampled at 16 times per frame (about 960 Hz), and on-line band-filtered at 10-300 Hz using a 15LT differential amplifier (Grass, Quincy, Massachusetts). An acquisition board (PCI ESeries, National Instruments, Austin, Texas) was used to digitize the analog signal.

5. Description of the method

5.1 RMS amplitude ratio calculus

The VERIS Science v6.0.5d (EDI) software was used to extract the first order kernel. The first order kernel waveform data for the 0-200 ms interval was exported to be analysed by a homemade routine written for MATLAB environment (The Mathworks, Natick, Massachusetts).

We calculated a RMS amplitude ratio for each local mfERG response for all subjects (Zhang et al., 2002). First, we calculated the RMS amplitude of the first order kernel for the signal time interval, located between 0-80 ms, and the RMS amplitude for a time interval comprising only noise uncorrelated with visual stimulation, located between 120-200 ms (Equations 1 and 2, respectively) (Figure 1 shows the noise and signal time intervals for an mfERG recording).

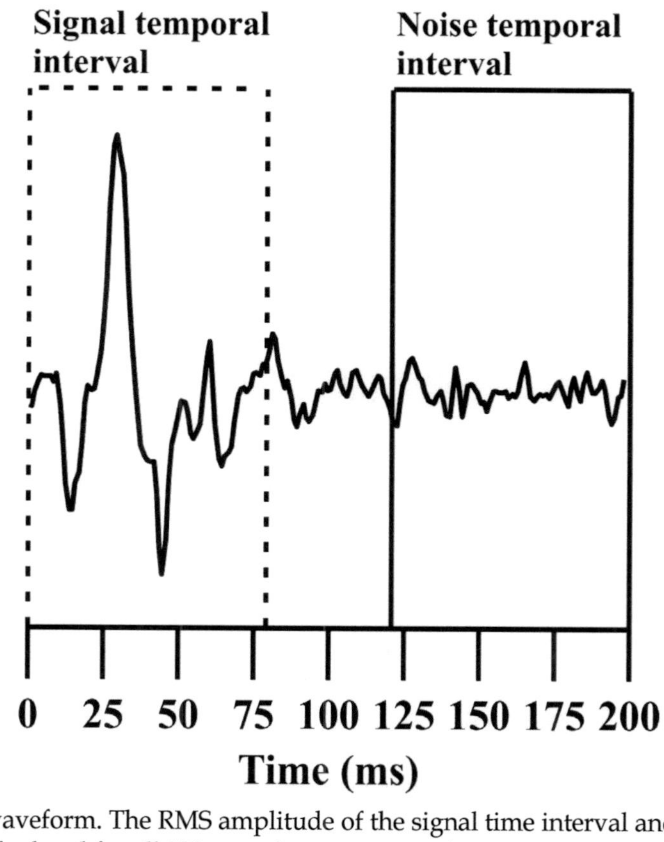

Fig. 1. mfERG waveform. The RMS amplitude of the signal time interval and noise time interval were calculated for all 103 waveforms to quantify a RMS amplitude ratio associated to the signal and noise information of each waveform.

Then, we estimated the ratio between the signal RMS amplitude of the jth hexagon to the mean noise RMS amplitude of the 103 mfERG waveforms obtained from the same subject (Signal Ratio, Equation 3). To obtain an equivalent value for the noise interval, we divided the noise RMS amplitude of the jth hexagon by the mean noise RMS amplitude (Noise Ratio, Equation 4).

$$\text{Signal amplitude} = \sqrt{\frac{\sum_{t=0}^{80} (Rt - \mu_{0 \text{ to } 80})^2}{N}} \tag{1}$$

Signal amplitude of a waveform is the RMS amplitude calculated over the signal time interval of the jth hexagon recording, Rt is the absolute amplitude at time t, μ0 to 80 is the mean amplitude during the signal time interval, and N is number of samples in the signal time interval.

$$\text{Noise amplitude} = \sqrt{\frac{\sum_{t=120}^{200} (Rt - \mu_{120 \text{ to } 200})^2}{N}} \tag{2}$$

Noise amplitude of a waveform is the RMS amplitude calculated over the noise time interval of the jth hexagon recording, Rt is the absolute amplitude at time t, μ0 to 200 is the mean amplitude during the noise time interval.

$$\text{Signal ratio} = \frac{\text{Signal amplitude}}{\text{Mean Noise amplitude}_{\text{hexagon (1 to 103)}}} - 1 \tag{3}$$

Signal Ratio of a waveform is the signal to noise ratio (SNR) to the signal time interval for the jth hexagon recording. Mean Noise amplitude is the average of the noise RMS amplitude for the 103 hexagon waveforms for the same subject.

$$\text{Noise ratio} = \frac{\text{Noise amplitude}}{\text{Mean Noise amplitude}_{\text{hexagon (1 to 103)}}} - 1 \tag{4}$$

Noise Ratio of a waveform is the equivalent to the SNR to the noise time interval for the jth hexagon recording.

5.2 Looking for an optimal RMS amplitude ratio to discriminate normal waveforms from waveforms without signal

For this first analysis, our data were composed of 1030 signal ratios and 1030 noise ratios. We estimated the distribution of frequency of RMS amplitude ratio (Signal ratio and Noise ratio). We then estimated the associated cumulative distribution function for the noise and the signal data distribution (Figure 2A-B). We proceeded to perform a Receiver Operating Characteristic (ROC) analysis using as false positive rate the values of 1 - noise cumulative distribution function and using the signal cumulative distribution function as true positive rate (Figure 2C-D). We obtained the optimal RMS amplitude ratio to distinguish the signal data from noise data as being the one which corresponds to a higher associated trade-off in the ROC space. The trade-off was calculated as the difference between each pair of true positive rate and false positive rate in the ROC space (Figure 2C-D). The optimal RMS amplitude ratio was 0.47.

5.3 Looking for an optimal RMS amplitude ratio to discriminate normal waveforms from waveforms with attenuated signal

In the previous section, we calculated an optimal RMS amplitude ratio to distinguish normal waveforms from those with no signal. But in clinical research we need to know how to distinguish the normal response from responses with different levels of decreased signal amplitude. In order to find an optimal RMS amplitude ratio for this purpose, we first artificially attenuated the original waveforms in a way that the signal could be decreased while keeping the noise level constant. This attenuation method was described by Wright et al. (2006).

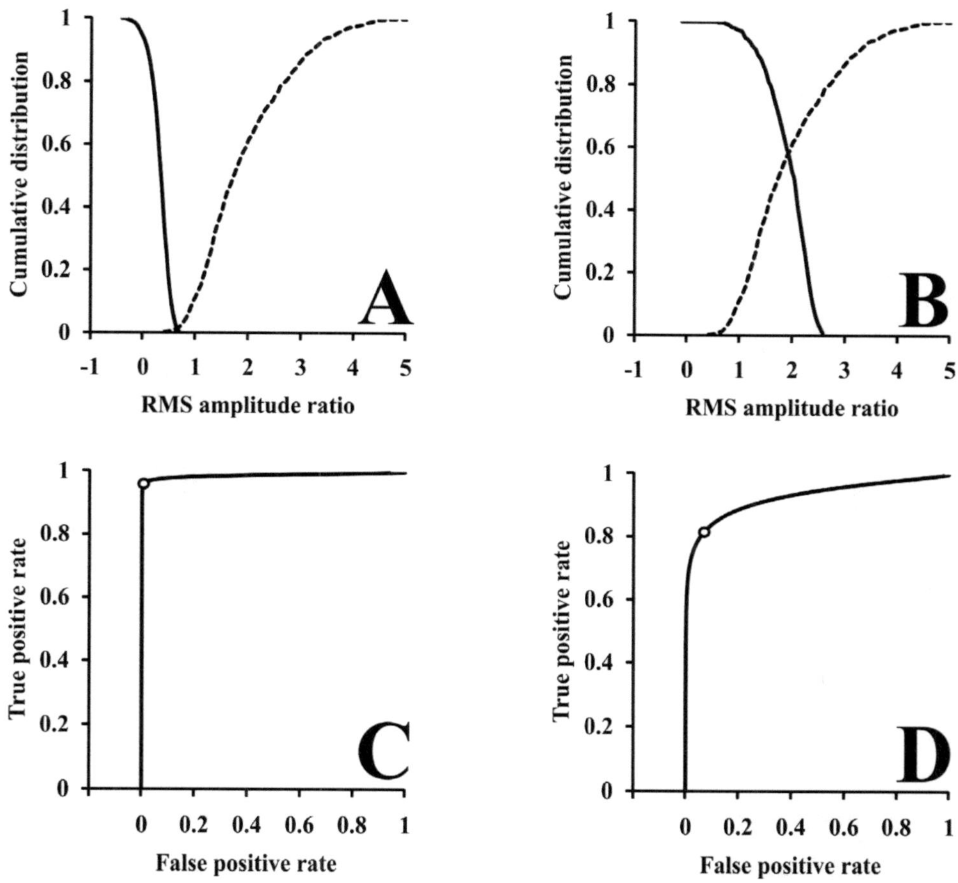

Fig. 2. Analysis implemented to obtain optimal values to distinguish between original waveforms and attenuated waveforms. (A) Cumulative distribution functions (CDF) of noise information (continuous line) and original signal information (dotted line). (B) CDF of attenuated signal information at level 1 (continuous lines) and signal information (dotted line). (C) ROC analysis correlating the CDF from signal and CDF from noise. (D) ROC analysis correlating attenuated signal at level 1 and original signal. The circles at the ROC curves, in C and D, are the higher trade-off between true positive rate and false positive rate. The RMS amplitude ratios associated to the higher trade-off in the ROC space were considered as the optimal values to distinguish two data groups. Functions using data of other attenuation levels are intermediate between the functions showed in this figure.

To attenuate the amplitude of the signal from each waveform, the noise data was added to the signal. The attenuation level corresponded to the number of times the noise data was added to the signal (number of summations between signal and noise). The result was then divided by the attenuation level plus one to keep constant the RMS amplitude of the noise (Equation 5).

$$\text{jth AttenuateWave} = \frac{\text{jth Wave}_{0\text{ to }80} + (\text{attenuation level} \times \text{jth Wave}_{120\text{ to }200})}{\text{attenuation level} + 1} \tag{5}$$

The jth AttenuateWave 0 to 80 is the attenuated signal time interval data, jth Wave 0 to 80 is the original signal time interval data, attenuation level is the number of times that the noise data will be added to the signal data, and the jth Wave120 to 200 is the noise time interval data.

We used 5 attenuation levels, from 1 to 5, in order to simulate different visual loss conditions. Figure 3 shows a scheme representing the different artificial attenuation levels over the same signal in an original waveform.

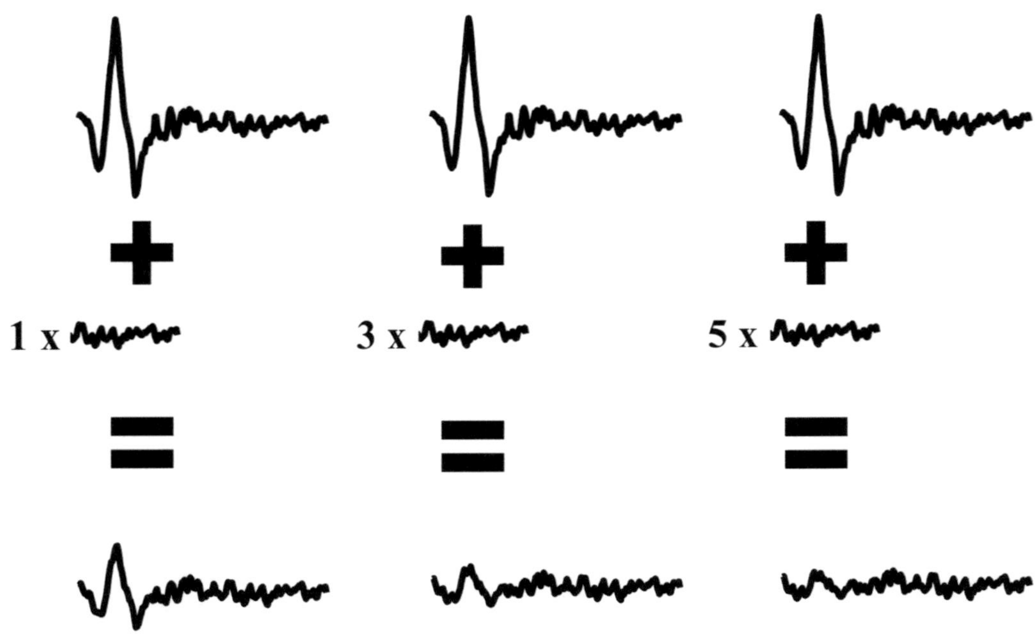

Fig. 3. Diagram representing the artificial attenuation applied over the signal from original waveforms. From left to right, the attenuation level is increasing. Consequently, the signal of the waveform is decreasing. Noise level was kept constant (similar RMS amplitude) across the attenuation levels because the denominator of equation 5 used to normalise the waveforms was dependent how much noise was added in the signal.

Then, the procedure of the previous section was repeated, but now we replaced the noise information by the attenuated signal information. The optimal values found to distinguish the original signal information from attenuated waveforms are indicated in the Table 1.

5.4 Testing the reliability of the optimal RMS amplitude ratios to different waveform attenuation conditions

We quantified the amount of errors that a classifier can present when using each optimal RMS amplitude ratio to distinguish normal waveforms from noisy or attenuated waveforms in different levels. The role of the classifier was to compare the signal ratio of waveforms to each optimal value obtained previously for the different attenuation levels.

Attenuation level	Optimal value
Noise	0.47
5	0.44
4	0.48
3	0.57
2	0.78
1	1.21

Table 1. Optimal value of differentiation from signal waveforms to attenuated waveforms. The optimal value was the RMS amplitude ratio with highest trade-off between hit and errors.

Before the attenuation process, the classifier considered that all waveforms should have signal ratio above the optimal SNR to distinguish normal from any attenuated waveform. We considered as error of classification when after the attenuation process the attenuated signal RMS amplitude ratio was higher than the optimal value. Correct identification was considered when the signal ratio of a waveform was lower than the optimal value.

The hit rate (HR) of the automated classifier was calculated by Equation 6. Table 2 shows the HR obtained by the classifier using each optimal RMS amplitude ratio to distinguish normal waveforms from the different attenuation levels.

$$HR = \frac{\text{correct responses}}{(\text{correct responses} + \text{errors})} \tag{6}$$

The best performance of the classifier in identifying highly attenuated waveforms (attenuation levels 4 and 5) occurred when the optimal value was 0.57. For moderately attenuated waveforms (attenuation levels 2 and 3) the best performance occurred when the optimal value was 0.78, and for slightly attenuated waveforms (attenuation level 1) it occurred with an optimal value of 1.21.

Our analysis seemed to be able to delimit a range of RMS amplitude ratios to classify any mfERG waveform obtained from 103 hexagons array (Table 3). It can be argued if the attenuated waveforms at the level 1 already correspond to a true visual loss or is within the variability of an electrophysiological amplitude recording, but the moderately and highly attenuated waveforms have a considerable decrease of the signal amplitude and their clinical importance must be considered.

For an application to a real situation, we applied the evaluation protocol to recordings obtained from a patient affected by ocular toxoplasmosis. Figure 4 shows the mfERG array of this patient after the analysis, showing the retinal waveforms associated with the retinal scar marked in different colours to indicate Table 3.

We think the same method could be applied for sets of waveforms obtained from other hexagons arrays, in order to find the optimal ranges to classify mfERG waveforms.

	Hit rate (%)				
Optimal value	A.L. 5	A.L. 4	A.L. 3	A.L. 2	A.L. 1
0.47	99 ± 0.8	98.9 ± 0.9	96.4 ± 3.5	84.7 ± 16.7	51.5 ± 30.7
0.44	98.4 ± 1.7	97.5 ± 3.1	94 ± 7.1	81.1 ± 21.3	46.5 ± 32.5
0.48	98.7 ± 1.5	98.3 ± 2.3	95.3 ± 5.8	83.6 ± 18.7	50.4 ± 33
0.57	**99.3 ± 0.7**	**99 ± 1.2**	97.1 ± 4.6	88.6 ± 14.5	57.1 ± 35
0.78	97.6 ± 3	97.6 ± 3	**97.4 ± 2.9**	**94.2 ± 6.1**	68.7 ± 30.4
1.21	81.7 ± 19.3	81.7 ± 19.3	81.7 ± 19.3	81.7 ± 19.2	**73.4 ± 15**

Table 2. Hit rate estimated for the usage of the optimal values in different attenuation levels. The classifier had a better performance in distinguishing normal waveforms from slightly attenuated waveforms (A.L. 1) using the optimal value 1.21, whilst the optimal value of 0.78 was better to differentiate normal waveforms from those with intermediate attenuation (A.L. 2 and 3), and the optimal value of 0.57 was better to distinguish highly attenuated or noisy waveforms (AL. 4 and 5) from the original waves. A.L.: Attenuation level.

6. Discussion

Since the development of the mfERG technology in the 90's, it was immediately applied to different topics of clinical ophthalmology (Huang et al., 1996; Kretschmann et al., 1998; Ventura et al., 2004; Greenstein et al., 2004; Raster et al., 2011), and over 700 articles already discussed the technique. The experience of the ophthalmologist is very important in the functional mapping, but this topographical evaluation is still very subjective (Hood et al., 2003). The method that we are suggesting could be an objective alternative to the conventional subjective evaluation of mfERG.

Classification of mfERG waveform	
Highly attenuated amplitude	SNR < 0.57 (Hit rate > 97%-99%)
Moderately attenuated amplitude	0.78 > SNR ≥ 0.57 (Hit rate ≈ 94 - 97%)
Slightly attenuated amplitude	1.21 > SNR ≥ 0.78 (Hit rate ≈ 73%–94%)
Normal waveforms	SNR ≥ 1.21 (Hit rate ≈ 73%)

Table 3. Classification of mfERG waveforms. Ranges of signal to noise ratio to qualify normal or slightly attenuated waveforms in black, moderately attenuated in yellow, and highly attenuated in red in the Figure 4. In the parenthesis the hit rate of a classifier which use each optimal value.

The application of a SNR evaluation as in the present work in the software that performs mfERG recordings (like Veris system - EDI or Retiscan – Roland Consultant) could help the users to avoid some mistakes in the identification of the waveform as normal response, decreased responses or noise. A color-marked trace array as shown in figure 4 would make the task of the clinician easier.

Another application of the results from SNR analysis would be in the programming of response density plots. It is well established that response density plot can generate a false central peak in conditions of recordings with no signals (Hood et al., 2003, Hood et al., 2008). After the SNR evaluation, it would be possible to identify the patches related to the absence of responses (for the data of the present work, SNR < 0.57), and it would be possible to program the response density plot with this information, setting zero amplitude in the response density of the hexagon with no response. Figure 5 shows a response density plot of the data shown in Figure 4 with and without the SNR evaluation.

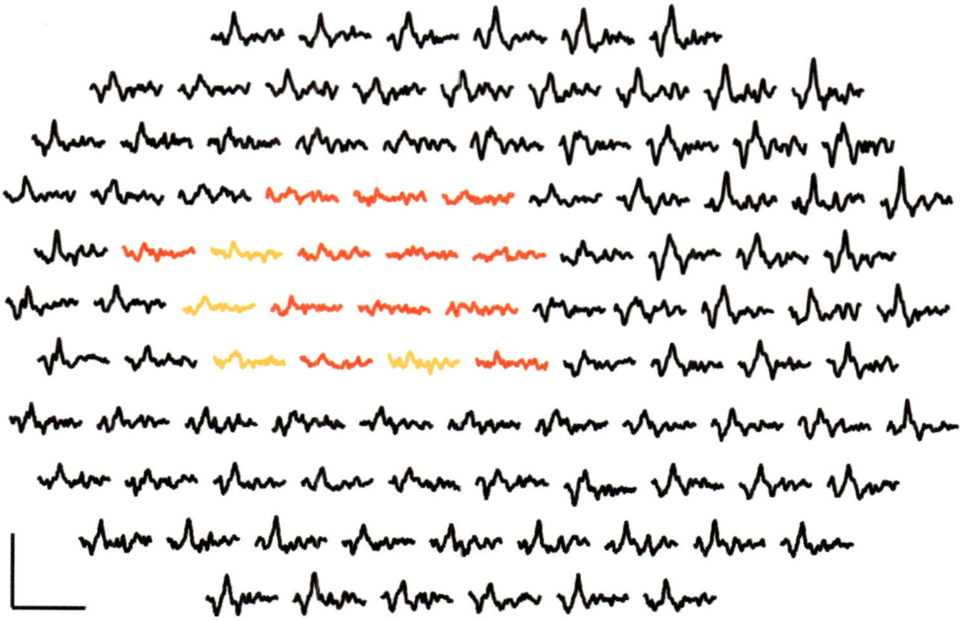

Fig. 4. Evaluation of mfERGs from a patient with visual loss caused by retinal toxoplasmosis. The area of the retinal scar was marked by the protocol in orange (moderately attenuated waveforms) and red (highly attenuated waveforms). Black waveforms indicate normal or slightly attenuated waveforms. Horizontal scale: 100 ms; Vertical scale: 1 μV.

The main contribution of the present technical note is the description of a method to estimate ranges of SNR in order to classify an unknown mfERG waveform. Other methods proposed to measure the difference between mfERG waveform and a template waveform estimated from a control group (Hood & Li, 1997; Wright et al., 2008). The larger the difference between both waveforms, the lower the likelihood that the waveform contained a signal. Seeliger et al. (1998) suggested differences in the implicit time of the P1 component between templates and unknown waveforms. They found high implicit time deviations in recordings obtained from retinitis pigmentosa patients.

The absolute values of SNR can be different when we compare different data settings due different procedures. All data used here was obtained from recordings using Burian-Allen electrodes and 103 hexagons in the stimulus. Other recording and stimulation parameters could change the absolute values of the limit ranges. Other work has described the influence of different experimental conditions in mfERG SNRs (Kretschmann et al., 2000).

The application of our method helps the clinicians to map retinal function and quantify the number of waveforms in each SNR range. It can be of further use as a tool to obtain

parameters of the sequential evaluation of the history of the retinal disease. For the application of our protocol we advise that each laboratory applies it to their own data to obtain the optimal ranges of classification.
In order to facilitate the application of this method by other researchers, in the next section we present the code in MATLAB language of important steps of the method described in the present chapter.

7. Matlab codes for important steps to reproduce the method described in the present technical note

Matlab is a very useful technical programming interpreted language to work with matrix computations. This computational environment has many pre-programmed functions that help a beginner in mathematics or computer science to perform complex numerical calculations in a relative intuitive way. In visual electrophysiology, this language got an important status in the data analysis mainly after multifocal electrophysiology, which requires the researcher to work with multiple vectors simultaneously.

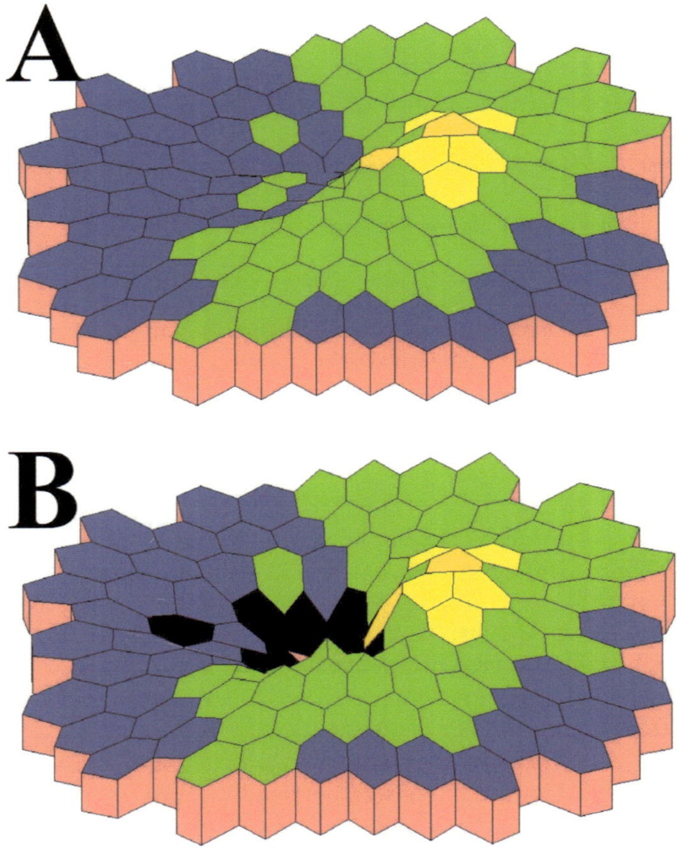

Fig. 5. Response density plots calculated from the same in Figure 4. The plots were programmed without and with SNR evaluation results (A and B, respectively). The hexagons with no responses had zero response density and they are marked in black.

7.1 Code to calculate the Signal ratio and Noise ratio for a subject as described in the equations (3) and (4)

Trace_Array is a matrix with 103 lines and 193 columns. **Trace_Array** represents the waveforms information. Each line represents one of 103 waveforms and each column is each voltage of the recording

```
RMS_Signal = ones(1,103);%RMS_Signal will receive the RMS amplitude of the signal interval
RMS_Noise = ones(1,103);%RMS_Noise will receive the RMS amplitude of the noise interval
SNR_Signal = ones(1,103);%SNR_Signal will receive the Signal ratio
SNR_Noise = ones(1,103);%SNR_Noise will receive the Noise ratio
%Next loop executes the calculus of RMS amplitude of the signal interval
for i = 1:103
   RMS_Signal(1,i) = std(Trace_Array(i,1:78),1);
end
%Next loop executes the calculus of RMS amplitude of the noise interval
for Line= 1:103
   RMS_Noise(1,line) = std(Trace_Array(i,116:193),1);
end
meanRMS_Noise = mean(RMS_Noise);%Calculus of the average of all Noise RMS amplitudes
%Next loop executes the calculus of Signal ratio
for i = 1:103
   SNR_Signal(1,i) = (RMS_Signal(1,i)/meanRMS)-1;
end
%Next loop executes the calculus of Noise ratio
for i = 1:103
   SNR_Noise(1,i) = (RMS_Noise(1,i)/meanRMS_Noise)-1;
end
```

7.2 Code to perform the artificial attenuation in the original waveforms

The code below performs an artificial attenuation in the level 5. To perform other attenuation levels, the user must only change the value of variable **Att_level**

```
Att_Rec = ones(103,193);%Attenuated_recording will receive the attenuated waveforms
Att_level = 5; %Att_level sets the attenuation level to proceed
%Next loop will create build a matrix of attenuated waveforms as indicated in equation (5)
for i = 1:103
Att_Rec(i,:)=[(Trace_Array(i,1:78)+Att_level*Trace_Array(i,116:193))/(F+1),Trace_Array(i,79
:193)];
end
```

7.3 Code to calculate the cumulative distribution of signal information and noise information of the sample

In the next code, **Signal** is the matrix with all Signal ratio values of the sample and **Noise** is the matrix with all Noise ratio values of the sample.

```
interval = 0.05;
max_Signal = max(Signal); % finding maximum value of Signal ratio
min_Noise = min(Noise); %finding minimum value of Noise ratio
x = min_Noise:interval:max_Signal;
data_Signal = histc(Signal,x);%to calculate the number of elements in each Signal ratio of the interval x_Signal
data_Noise = histc(Noise,x); %to calculate the number of elements in each Noise ratio of the interval x_Noise
sum_Signal = sum(data_Signal);
sum_Noise = sum(data_Noise);
percent_sum_Signal = data_Signal ./sum_Signal;
percent_sum_Noise = data_Noise ./sum_Noise;
%Next loop will calculate the cumulative distribution for signal and noise information
for i = 1:1:length(x)
cum_sum_Signal(i)=sum(percent_sum_Signal(1,i:length(percent_sum_Signal)));
cum_sum_Noise(i)=sum(percent_sum_Noise(1,i:length(percent_sum_Signal)));
end
```

7.4 Code to calculate the optimal value to distinguish signal information from noise information

The code below is continuing of the previous code. We kept the name of variables of the previous code in the follow code.

```
x = min_Noise:interval:max_Signal; %Interval including SNR of Noise and Signal information
FA = cum_sum_Noise; %False positive rate
HIT = cum_sum_Signal; %True positive rate
m = length(FA);
trade_off = ones(1,m);
%Next loop will calculate of the trade-off in the ROC space
for i = 1:m
   trade_off(1,i) = abs(FA(1,i)-HIT(1,i));
end
counter = 1;
maximum_trade_off = max(trade_off);%Finding the maximum trade-off between hit and false alarm
```

```
%Next loop will find the position of the maximum_trade_off in the matrix trade_off
for i = 1:m
   if (maximum_trade_off == trade_off(1,t))
      break
   else
      counter = counter + 1;
   end
end
Optimal_SNR = x(1,counter);%Optimal_SNR is the SNR value in the same position in x of maximum_trade_off in trade_off.
```

8. Conclusion

The multifocal electroretinogram is a relatively new method of visual investigation and studies that contribute to the improvement of the effectiveness of the method should be encouraged. The method described in this chapter intended to assist in the neuroophthalmological diagnosis by estimating ranges of SNR as indicators of the quality of the electrophysiological response.

9. Acknowledgements

Supported by FINEP research grant "Rede Instituto Brasileiro de Neurociência (IBN-Net)" #01.06.0842-00, CNPq-PRONEX / FAPESPA #2268, CNPq #486351/2006-8, CNPq #550671/2007-2, CNPq #620037/2008-3, CNPq #476744/2009-1, CNPQ #475860/2010-1. ACC received a CNPq fellowship for graduate students. DFV and LCLS are CNPq research fellows.

10. References

Greenstein, V.C., Holopigian, K., Seiple, W., Carr, RE., & Hood, D.C. (2004). Atypical multifocal ERG responses in patients with diseases affecting the photoreceptors. *Vision Research*, Vol. 44, No. 25, (November 2004), pp. 2867-2874, ISSN 0042-6989

Hood, D.C., Holopigian, K., Greenstein, V., Seiple, W., Li, J., Sutter, E.E., & Carr, R.E. (1998). Assessment of local retinal function in patients with retinitis pigmentosa using the multi-focal ERG technique. *Vision Research*, Vol. 38, No. 1, (January 1998), pp. 163-179, ISSN 0042-6989

Hood, D.C., Odel, J.G., Chen, C.S., & Winn, B.J. (2003). The multifocal electroretinogram. *Journal of Neuro-Ophthalmology*, Vol. 23, No. 3, (September 2003), pp. 225-235, ISSN 1536-5166

Hood, D.C., Bach, M., Brigell, M., Keating, D., Kondo, M., Lyons, J.S. & Palmowski-Wolfe, A.M. (2008). ISCEV guidelines for clinical multifocal electroretinography (2007 edition). *Documenta Ophthalmologica*, Vol. 116, No. 1, (January 2008), pp. 1-11, ISSN 0012-4486

Huang, H.J., Yamazaki, H., Kawabata, H., Ninomiya, T., & Adachi-Usami, E. (1997). Multifocal electroretinogram in multiple evanescent white dot syndrome. *Documenta Ophthalmologica*, Vol. 92, No. 4, (December 1996), pp. 301-309, ISSN 0012-4486

Kretschmann, U., Seeliger, M.W., Ruether, K., Usui, T., Apfelstedt-Sylla, E., & Zrenner, E. (1998). Multifocal electroretinography in patients with Stargardt's macular dystrophy. *British Journal of Ophthalmology*, Vol. 82, No. 3, (March 1998), pp. 267-275, ISSN 0007-1161

Raster, M., Horn, F., Jüneman, A., Rosa, A.A., Souza, G.S., Gomes, B.D., Lima, M.G., Silveira, L.C., & Kremers, J. (2011). Retinal disorders in northern Brazilian patients treated with chloroquine assessed by multifocal ERG. *Documenta Ophthalmologica*, Vol. 122, No. 2, (April 2011), pp. 77:86, ISSN 0012-4486

Seeliger, M.W., Kretschmann, U.H., Apfelstedt-Sylla, E., & Zrenner, E. (1998). Implicit time topography of multifocal electroretinograms. *Investigative Ophthalmology and Visual Science*, Vol. 39, No. 5, (April 1998), pp. 718-723, ISSN

Sutter, E.E., & Tran, D. (1992). The field topography of ERG components in man - I. The photopic luminance response. *Vision Research*, Vol. 32, No. 3, (March 1992), pp. 433-446, ISSN 0042-6989

Sutter, E.E. (2000). The interpretation of multifocal binary kernels. *Documenta Ophthalmologica*, Vol. 100, No. 2-3, (March 2000), pp. 49-75, ISSN 0012-4486

Sutter, E.E. (2001). Imaging visual function with the multifocal m-sequence technique. Vision Research, Vol. 41, No. 10-11, (May 2001), pp. 1241-1255, ISSN 0042-6989

Ventura, D.F., Costa, M.F., Berezowsky, A., Salomão, S.R., Simões, A.L., Lago, M., Pereira, L.H., Faria, M.A., De Souza, J.M., & Silveira, L.C. (2004). Multifocal and full-field electroretinogram changes associated with color-vision loss in mercury vapor exposure. *Visual Neuroscience*, Vol. 21, No. 3, (May 2004), pp. 421-9, ISSN 0952-5238

Wright, T., Nilsson, J., Gerth, C., & Westall, C. (2008). A comparison of signal detection techniques in the multifocal electroretinogram. *Documenta Ophthalmologica*, Vol. 117, No. 2, (September 2008), pp. 163-170, ISSN 0012-4486

Zhang X, Hood DC, Chen CS, Hong JE (2002). A signal-to-noise analysis of multifocal VEP responses: an objective definition for poor records. *Documenta Ophthalmologica*, Vol. 104, No. 3, (May 2002), pp. 287-302, ISSN 0012-448

Part 2

ERG in Human Disease

6

Electroretinogram in Hereditary Retinal Disorders

Fatih Cakir Gundogan[1], Ahmet Tas[2] and Gungor Sobaci[3]
[1]Etimesgut Military Hospital
[2]Ankara Mevki Military Hospital
[3]Gulhane Military Medical Academy
Turkey

1. Introduction

Electroretinogram (ERG) represents the electrical response of retina to a light stimulus. The light stimuli may be either a pattern (spatially structured) stimulus or a flash (unstructured) stimulus, and the retina may be stimulated completely or partially. In this chapter, we will briefly mention about the recording procedures of electroretinographic tests. Electroretinographic testing procedures and findings in hereditary retinal dystrophies will be discussed from a clinical point of view.

1.1 The full-field electroretinogram

Full-field ERG is the diffuse response of both neural and nonneural cells of the retina to a light stimulus. The response recorded after such a stimulus represents the sum of the positive and negative components that originate from different stages of retinal processing overlap in time. The recorded electrical activity is the result of light-induced changes in the transretinal movements of ions, principally sodium and potassium, in the extracellular space (Fishman, 2001). The electrical responses originated in the retina are recorded by active electrodes that contact the cornea or nearby bulbar conjunctiva. These include contact lens electrodes, conductive fibers and foils, conjunctival loop electrodes and corneal wicks. The responses are amplified, averaged and displayed on screens.

The rod and cone responses may be functionally dissected with ERG in the light of International Society for Clinical of Vision (ISCEV) recommendations (Marmor et al., 2009) (Figure 1).

1.1.1 Clinical ERG recording

1.1.1.1 The rod ERG

The patient should be dark-adapted for at least 20 minutes. The recommended stimulus is a dim white flash of strength 2.5 log units below the white standard flash (3.43cd/m^2) on a dark background. Instead, a blue stimulus equivalent to the white standard may be used to stimulate the rod photoreceptors (Figure 1A).

1.1.1.2 The standard combined ERG

After recording rod ERG, a brighter white flash (standard flash) on a dark background is used to stimulate the retina. The standard combined ERG is the combined response of both rod and cone photoreceptors (Figure 1B).

1.1.1.3 The oscillatory potentials

Oscillatory potentials may be recorded from dark-adapted or light-adapted eye (at least 10-min of light adaptation) by using standard flash after standard-combined ERG recording. By adjusting the high-pass and low-pass filters, only the high-frequency responses originated from the amacrine cells are obtained (Figure 1C).

1.1.1.4 The single-flash cone ERG

In order to be able to isolate cone photoreceptor response, the rod photoreceptors must be suppressed by a bright background. The patient should be light-adapted for at least 10-min before the recording. A standard flash is used to obtain cone responses (Figure 1D).

1.1.1.5 Flicker ERG

Flicker ERG is recorded under the same conditions of light-adaptation as the single-flash cone ERG. The standard flashes are presented at a rate of approximately 30 stimuli per second. Rod photoreceptors can not respond to flickering light with a frequency above 20 Hz (Figure 1E).

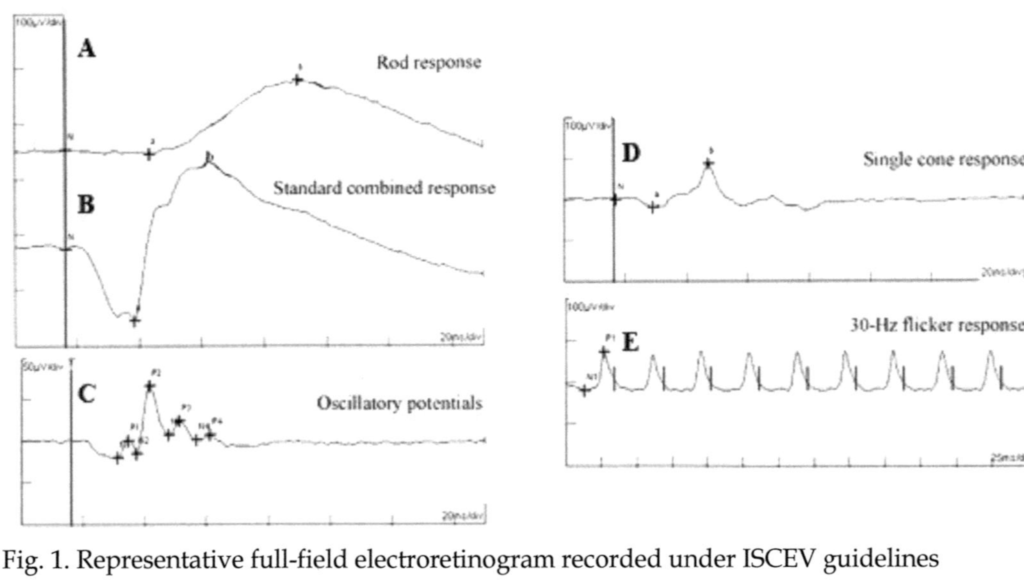

Fig. 1. Representative full-field electroretinogram recorded under ISCEV guidelines

1.1.2 The origins of ERG waves

The ERG generally consists of a negative deflection, called the a-wave, and a positive deflection, called the b-wave (Figure 1B). A-wave is mainly a response of photoreceptors, while the b-wave is mainly associated with on-bipolar cell function. A-wave is generally not recordable in rod ERG responses recorded under ISCEV recommendations (low-intensity flashes). There is a large magnification of electrical activity as signals are transmitted from photoreceptors to inner retinal neurons, for this reason, b-wave may be recorded in lower intensity flashes which does not produce a-wave response (Figure 1A). However, as the intensity of the light stimulus increases, the a-wave begins to be recorded. But, in such intensities, the cone photoreceptors begin to respond to the light flash. This violates the recording of absolute rod photoreceptor function. For this reason, b-wave response in rod ERG shows the on-bipolar cell function originated from the rod photoreceptors. Standard flash stimulates both rod and cone photoreceptor and generates both a- and b-wave deflections (Figure 1B). Oscillatory potentials are a series of wavelets on the ascending limb of the ERG b-wave after stimulation by an intense light flash. These are high-frequency, low-amplitude components of the ERG with a frequency of about 100 to 160 Hz. These responses originate in the circuitry between the amacrine cells and other retinal neurons. By comparison, the a- and b-waves are dominated by frequency components of about 25 Hz (Fishman, 2001). Single-flash cone ERG and 30-Hz flicker ERG have a-and b-wave components representing the cone photoreceptors and cone on-bipolar cell functions, respectively.

1.2 Multifocal electroretinogram

The ERG is the sum activity of the cells of the retina and, small retinal defects may not be detected by standard ERG testing. Pattern electroretinogram (PERG) can provide valuable information about the macular function. However, both of these techniques still lack the topographical information of the retinal response. The multifocal ERG (mfERG) technique was developed by Sutter and Tran to deal with these problems (Sutter & Tran, 1992). The use of mfERG enables topographic mapping of retinal function in the central 40-50 degrees of the retina.

Typically, the multifocal stimulus is displayed on a computer monitor. The display contains an array of hexagons; the most commonly used displays contain either 61 or 103 hexagons (Figure 2). The hexagons may be scaled to produce local cone responses of approximately equal amplitude.

2. Hereditary retinal disorders

Hereditary retinal disorders constitute a heterogenous group of eye disorders. These disorders differ one from another in many aspects, such as the mode of inheritance, the rate of progression, appearance of ophthalmoscopy and the type of visual handicap they cause among affected patients.

In this chapter, we will discuss the electroretinographic findings of hereditary retinal disorders under the main headings of; retinitis pigmentosa and pigmentary retinopathies, cone dystrophies, juvenile X-linked retinoschisis, congenital stationary night blindness, hereditary macular disorders, hereditary vitreoretinal disorders, and hereditary chorioretinal dystrophies.

2.1 Retinitis pigmentosa and pigmentary retinopathies

Retinitis pigmentosa is a significant cause of visual impairment all over the world and belongs to the group of pigmentary retinopathies, a generic name that covers all retinal dystrophies presented with a loss of photoreceptors and retinal pigment deposits. The macular function is generally preserved until adulthood. The primary pathologic mechanism is the degeneration of the rod photoreceptors, and a secondary degeneration of cone photoreceptors. For this reason, classical retinitis pigmentosa may also be described as rod-cone dystrophy, rod photoreceptors being more affected than cones. The sequence of photoreceptor involvement explains why the patients experience night vision impairment in the early stages of the disease, with the visual acuity loss in later stages (Hamel, 2006). In the early stages the patients lose peripheral vision, but eventually central vision deteriorates. In advanced stages, signs include attenuated retinal vessels, intraretinal pigment, and waxy pallor of the optic discs.

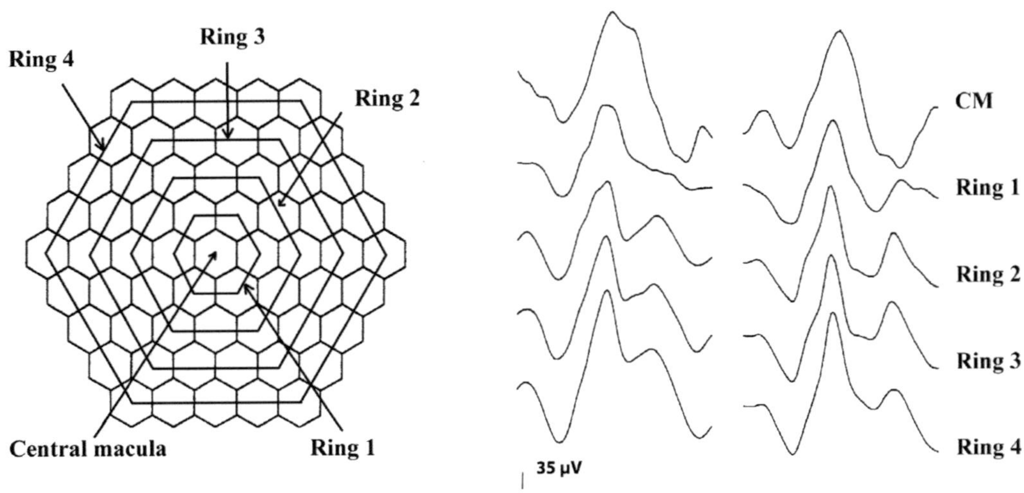

Fig. 2. Multifocal electroretinogram simulus consiting of 61 hexagons (left) and corresponding multifocal electroretinogram responses belonging the five concentric rings from both eyes (right).

The incidence of retinitis pigmentosa has been estimated to be 1 in 3500 to 1 in 3700 births in the United States (Boughman et al, 1980; Bunker et al, 1984) and 1 in 3400 to 1 in 8000 births in Japan (Berson, 1987). Genetic type of retinitis pigmentosa was reported to be 19% dominant, 19% recessive, 8% X-linked, 46% isolates, and 8% undetermined in the United States (Bunker et al, 1984).

Retinitis pigmentosa may be evaluated as syndromic and nonsyndromic from a clinical point of view. Most patients with RP are nonsyndromic; that is they do not have any other associated systemic disease. The syndromic conditions with associated RP are Usher syndrome, Bassen-Kornzweig syndrome (abetalipoproteinemia), Refsum disease, Laurence-Moon-Biedl syndrome, neuronal ceroid lipofuscinosis (Batten disease), Alström disease, and Kearns-Sayre syndrome.

2.1.1 Hereditary types of RP and ERG findings

The most significant factor determining the disease severity of the retinitis pigmentosa is the genetic type. Autosomal dominant retinitis pigmentosa is the mildest form. Some patients with autosomal dominant form experience vision impairment after the age of 50. Autosomal recessive and X-linked recessive types have a more severe course with the typical onset of disease in the first decade (Hamel, 2006). Figure 3 shows classical examples of ERGs recorded from retinitis pigmentosa patients with different hereditary types.

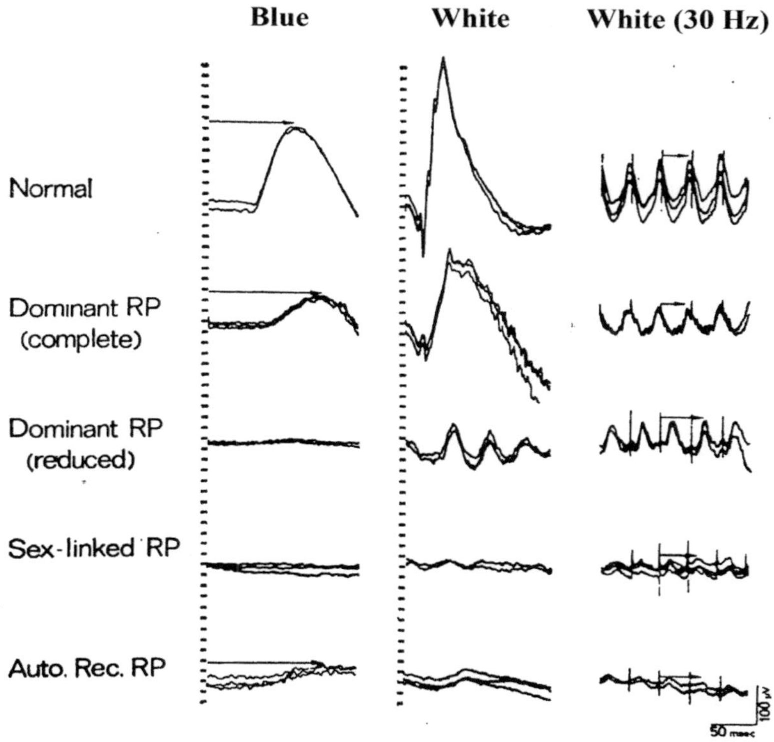

Fig. 3. Full-field electroretinography examples of autosomal dominant, autosomal recessive and, X-linked recessive retinitis pigmentosa. Patients with autosomal recessive and X-linked inheritance patterns have more severe disease course with earlier retinal functional impairment. (Used with permission of American Academy of Ophthalmology and Otolaryngology. From. Retinitis pigmentosa and allied retinal diseases: Electrophysiological findings, Berson,. Transactions - American Academy of Ophthalmology and Otolaryngology, Vol 81, Number 4, pp. OP659-OP666, 1976)

Very small ERG responses may not be recorded under the standardized recording procedures in retinitis pigmentosa patients very with advanced disease. The response may be *nonrecordable* under conditions of ISCEV guidelines. In these circumstances, narrow band filtering method provides the recording of 30-Hz cone response amplitudes below 1 microvolt. In this method, hundreds of 30-Hz cone responses are averaged to reduce the effect of background noise. In addition, a narrow-band electronic filter with bandpass of 29-31 Hz and a center frequency of 30 Hz alters the recorded signal so that only the 30-Hz recorded signals are preserved. (Andreasson et al, 1988).

2.1.2 Implicit time in retinitis pigmentosa

Berson showed that cone b-wave implicit time delay is a consistent finding in generalized retinitis pigmentosa (Berson, 1987). Fishman et al. categorized autosomal dominantly inherited retinitis pigmentosa patients into 4 groups with respect to implicit time of the cone responses (Fishman et al, 1985). Marmor reported that retinitis pigmentosa patients with normal cone b-wave implicit times have a better prognosis (Marmor, 1979). In the presence of *sector* retinitis pigmentosa, cone b-wave implicit time was reported to be normal by the same authors (Berson, Howard, 1971). In normal human eyes, rod-cone interaction mechanism was shown to be responsible for the relation of implicit time of the cone response and the amplitudes of rod response. Birch and Sandberg found that cone response b-wave implicit time seen in patients with retinitis pigmentosa is inversely correlated to the log amplitude of the dark-adapted rod b-wave (Birch & Sandberg, 1987) (Figure 4). Similarly, Iijima et al reported that patients with normal cone b-wave implicit times had better prognosis in terms of the onset of night blindness (Iijima et al, 1993).

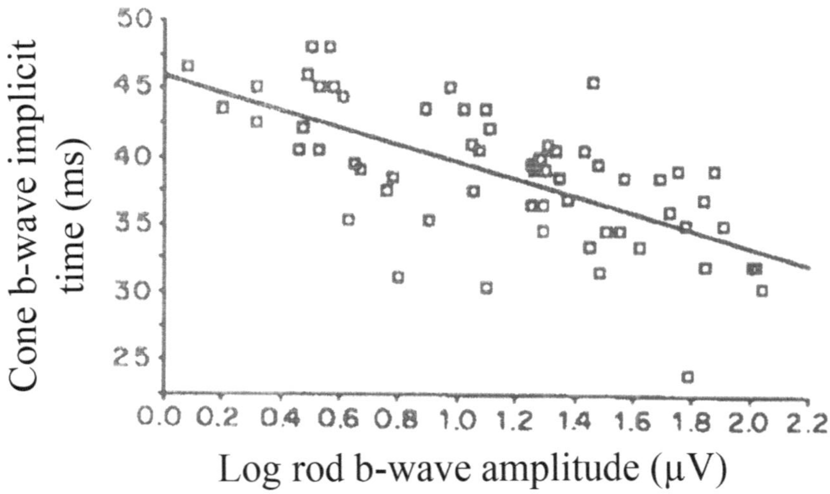

Fig. 4. Scatter plot and linear regression for cone b-wave implict time as a function of log rod b-wave amplitude in retinitis pigmentosa. Regression line is y=46-6.3x and does not control for the nonsignifican effect of cone b-wave amplitude on cone b-wave implicit time (used with permission of Pergamon Journals Ltd. From ,"Dependance of cone b-wave implicit time on rod amplitude in retinitis pigmentosa", Birch et al, Vision Research, Volume 27, Number 7, 1987; permission conveyed through Copyright Clearance Center, Inc)

2.1.3 Electronegative ERG in RP

Electronegative ERG refers to an ERG in which the a-wave is normal and the b-wave is severely subnormal, being smaller in amplitude than the a-wave. This classic description was used for years. However, recently the term electronegative ERG has been used to describe any ERG in which the b-wave amplitude is smaller than the a-wave amplitude whether a-wave amplitude is normal or reduced (Weleber & Francis, 2006). Although the term was initially applied only to the dark-adapted mixed rod-cone ERG, the term has recently been used to describe a similar configuration for the cone ERG (Weleber & Francis, 2006; Kellner & Foerster, 1993; Swain et al, 1997).

There are approximately 120 million rods and 6 million cones in the retina. This difference constitutes the basis of the fact that the ERG is mainly rod-driven. The a-wave in standardized ERG is generated by the rod phototransduction. The b-wave is arises from the

ON bipolar cell depolarization after the signal originated in the outer cell membranes of the photoreceptors. For this reason, electronegative ERG response reflects any pathophysiological process that prevents electrical signals reaching to ON-bipolar cells. This phenomenon is called *postphotoreceptoral transmission defect.*

Cideciyan and Jacobson reported patients with typical clinical features of RP and negative ERG pattern (Cideciyan & Jacobson, 1993) (Figure 5). The authors speculated three mechanisms for this finding. One speculation is that this type of disease expression may be caused by an abnormal gene product at the photoreceptor terminal regions unlike classical retinitis pigmentosa which causes abnormalities in outer segment proteins such as rhodopsin and peripherin (Humphries et al, 1992). This could lead to defective signal transmission between photoreceptors and bipolar cells; the outer segment disease would be ascribed to secondary degenerative processes. Another speculation is that this phonotype of disease may be caused by functional and/or morphological involvement in both the photoreceptor and postphotoreceptoral sites. The third speculation is that the inner retinal dysfunction in this patient group may be caused by a different secondary effect.

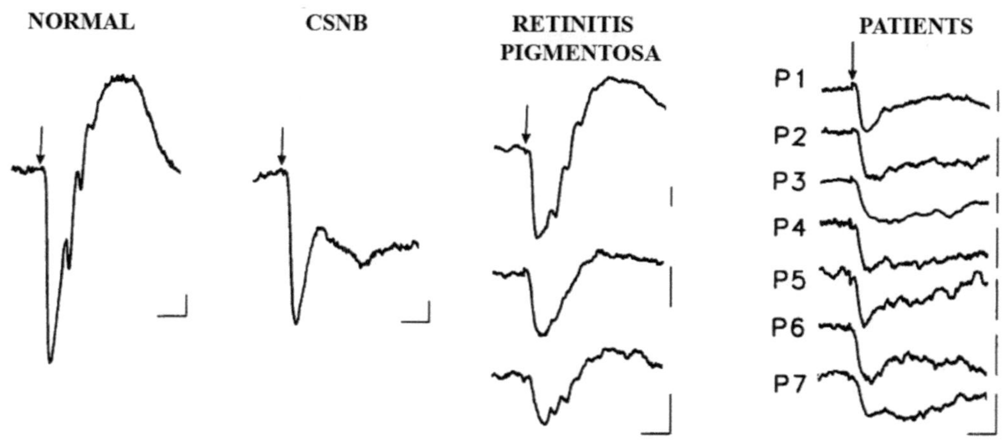

Fig. 5. Full-field electroretinograms in a normal subject, a congenital stationary night blindness (CSNB) patient, representative classical retinitis pigmentosa patients without negative electroretinograms ,and seven patients with negative electroretinograms (Arrow indicates stimulus onset. Horizontal calibration is 20 ms for all traces; vertical calibration is 50 μV) (used with permission of *Association for Research in Vision and Ophthalmology*. From: Negative Electroretinograms in Retinitis Pigmentosa, Cideciyan & Jacobson, Volume 34, Number 12, 1993; permission conveyed through Copyright Clearance Center, Inc)

2.1.4 Multifocal electroretinogram in RP

MfERG assesses local retinal cone functions. The normal mfERG amplitude declines with increasing eccentricity from fixation. MfERG amplitude decline is much more pronounced in patients with retinitis pigmentosa. MfERG may enable the progression of retinitis pigmentosa to be followed more accurately, facilitating a better understanding of the variants of the disease (Keating & Parks, 2006).

Retinitis pigmentosa patients were found to have significant reductions in response amplitudes at all retinal eccentricities and implicit times were generally normal in the central areas but became significantly delayed towards peripheral retina (Chan & Brown,

1998; Felius & Swanson, 1999; Holopigian et al, 2001; Hood et al, 1998; Kondo et al, 1995) (Figure 6). In the advanced stages of retinitis pigmentosa, ERG responses may even be non-detectable in the presence of good visual acuities. In these circumstances, mfERG not only shows the objective function of the fovea, but also the progression of the disease. Hood et al. found that implicit time changes but not amplitude changes in mfERG were correlated with the locations of visual field sensitivity loss (Hood et al, 1998).

2.1.5 The variants of classic RP

The variants of classic RP show diverse patterns both morphologically and electrophysiologically.

2.1.5.1 Unilateral RP

Unilateral retinitis pigmentosa is used to define unilateral retinal pigmentary degeneration with abnormal ERG while the other eye is clinically and functionally normal. In order to diagnose unilateral retinitis pigmentosa, the patient should be followed for a period of time by means of clinical and electroretinographic methods to ensure that retinal function in the unaffected eye does not impair with time. This method may explore asymmetric bilateral retinitis pigmentosa in most cases. ERG recording may document diminished response in the ''normal'' eye with normal fundoscopic appearance. In addition, pigmentary changes in the affected eye should not be due to acquired retinal disorders such as ophthalmic artery occlusion, syphilis, rubeola, diffuse unilateral subacute neuroretinitis and, traumatic retinal injuries (Auerbach et al, 1969). Kolb and Galloway stressed the importance of family history in diagnosing unilateral retinitis pigmentosa. The authors suggested that unilateral retinitis pigmentosa is probably a partial manifestation of a bilateral disease, however, true unilateral retinitis pigmentosa really exists (Kolb & Galloway, 1964). Kandori et al. reported two cases of ophthalmic artery occlusion causing unilateral pigmentary retinopathy mimicking retinitis pigmentosa (Kandori et al, 1968).

2.1.5.2 Sector RP

Sector retinitis pigmentosa defines typical retinitis pigmentosa signs including attenuated retinal vessels, and retinal pigmentary changes when confined to one or two quadrants of the retina. The most frequent inheritance pattern is autosomal dominant, but autosomal recessive and X-linked recessive traits were also reported. Mostly, inferior and nasal retina is involved which causes a superior or superotemporal visual field defect. Sector retinitis pigmentosa is mostly bilateral, and symmmetric. In contrast to classical retinitis pigmentosa types, sector retinitis pigmentosa is considered stationary or only very slowly progressive, and the fovea preserves its normal function at old age (Abraham, 1975).

The ERG changes are generally proportional to the area involved in the retina. However, perimetric and electrophysiologic studies demonstrated that normal-appearing retina may also have functional deficits. Berson et al reported normal rod and cone implicit time in sector retinitis pigmentosa (Berson & Howard, 1971) in contrast to widespread retinitis pigmentosa which causes typical implicit time delays.

2.1.5.3 RP sine pigmento

Retinitis pigmentosa sine pigmento is used to define the condition of normal-appearing retina and diffuse photoreceptor cell dysfunction. However, whether this clinical condition is a distinct entity other than classical retinitis pigmentosa or an early stage or a variant of retinitis pigmentosa remains to be clarified (Fishman, 2001).

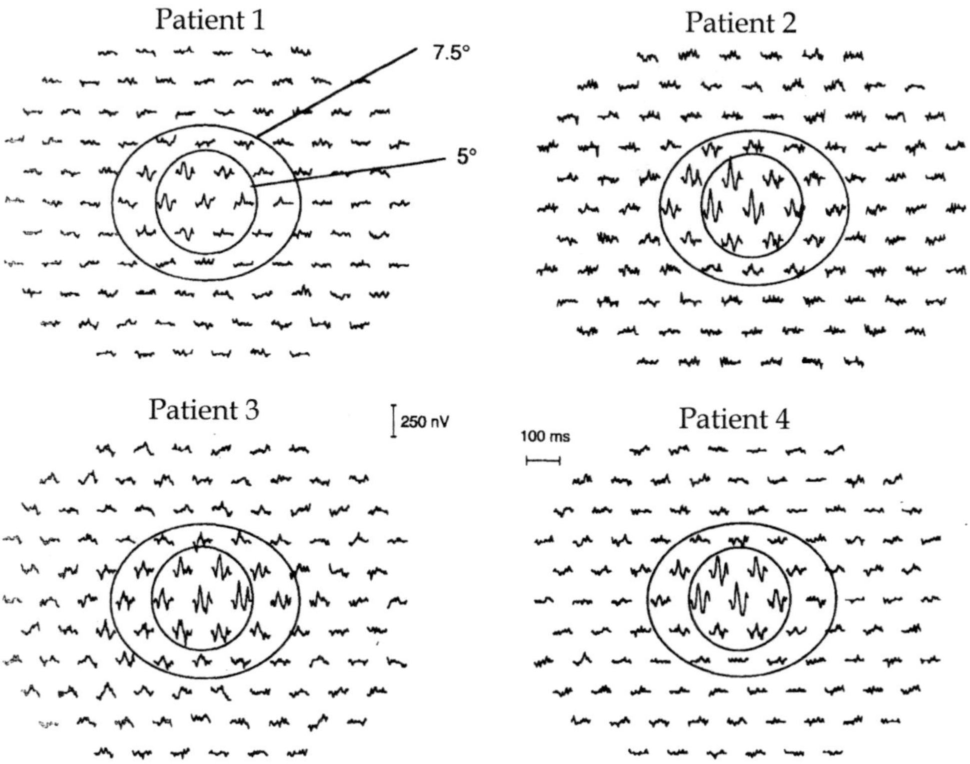

Fig. 6. Multifocal eletroretinography responses from four patients. The circles in each panel indicate the areas with a radius of 5 or 7.5 degree. Multifocal electretinogram responses are diminished in peripheral retina and preserved in the central areas (Used with permission of Elsevier Science Ltd. From: Vision Research, Vol 38, Number 1, Hood et al, Assessment of local retinal function in patients with retinitis pigmentosa using the multi-focal ERG technique, 1997, permission conveyed through Copyright Clearance Center, Inc).

2.1.5.4 Retinitis punctata albescens

Retinitis punctata albescens is a type of retinitis pigmentosa characterized by diffuse white, deep, punctate lesions throughout the retina. The retinal degeneration has a progressive nature with night blindness and peripheral visual field loss.

2.1.5.5 Usher syndrome

Usher syndrome is an autosomal recessive disease characterized by retinitis pigmentosa and bilateral sensorineural hearing loss or deafness. It is the most frequent cause of deaf-blindness. Based on clinical findings, three types of Usher syndrome were described (Van Aarem et al, 1995). The sensorineural hearing loss is profound in type 1, and moderate in type 2 (Fishman et al 1983; Kimberling et al, 1989). A rare third type was also described with progressive hearing loss (Sankila et al, 1995). Seeliger et al. found that type 1 patients and control subjects had almost identical 33-Hz flicker implicit times, and the same was true for type 2 and classical retinitis pigmentosa patients (Seeliger et al, 2001).

2.1.6 Treatable RP types

Classical retinitis pigmentosa is not a treatable disease. However, there are some forms of treatable retinitis pigmentosa associated with systemic involvement.

2.1.6.1 Abetalipoproteinemia

Abetalipoproteinemia or Bassen-Kornzweig syndrome is a hereditary disorder characterized by gastrointestinal symptoms (steatorrhea), haematologic disorders (acanthocytosis), neuromuscular disturbances (ataxia), and retinitis pigmentosa, all appearing in the first decade of life (Bishara et al, 1982). The first case was reported by Bassen and Kornzweig in 1950 in an 18 year-old girl who had generalized retinal degeneration, abnormal red blood cells and Freidreich ataxia (Lam, 2005). The disease is recessively inherited.

The early appearance of the retinal disease differs from the isolated retinitis pigmentosa, which usually appears during the second or third decade. The pathologic process is caused by a rare inborn error of lipoprotein metabolism (Runge et al, 1986). The primary defect appears to be an inability to secrete apolipoprotein B-100 which is a major protein of very low density lipoproteins and low density lipoproteins and an inability to secrete apolipoprotein B-48 which is a major protein of intestinal chylomicrons (Berson, 1987). Thus, the impairment in the production of chylomicrons causes the impairment in the fat absorption which in turn causes the impairment in the absorption of fat soluble vitamins, such as vitamin A, vitamin E, and vitamin K. Serum levels of cholesterol and triglyceride in abetalipoproteinemia are extremely low. The treatment consists of low-fat diet and oral vitamin A and vitamin E supplementation.

Studies showed that vitamin A supplementation results in a return of dark adaptation thresholds and ERG responses to normal in the early stages (Gouras et al, 1971). Bishara et al. reported that vitamin E also should be administered concomitantly with vitamin A (Bishara et al, 1982).

2.1.6.2 Refsum disease

Refsum disease was first described by Refsum in two consanguineous families. This syndrome was originally termed as *heredopathia ataxia polyneuritiformis,* and more recently *phytanic acid storage disease.* It is an autosomal recessive disorder characterized by peripheral neuropathy, ataxia and, retinitis pigmentosa (Refsum, 1981). Some of the patients have anosmia and neurogenic hearing loss. The metabolic defect is an inability in the conversion of phytanic acid to alpha-hydroxy-phytanic acid. Exogenous phytanic acid accumulates in a variety of tissues including the retinal pigment epithelium which causes impairment in the night vision (Avigan et al, 1966; Eldjarn et al, 1966). Visual field impairment generally begins until 20s before the onset of neurologic involvement. The fundus can be granular with areas of depigmentation around the periphery with a subnormal ERG in the early stages. In the more advanced stages, ERG may even be nondetectable (Berson, 1976, 1981).

The treatment is based on restricting dietary phytanic acid in order to reduce serum phytanic acid levels. Refsum has reported the beneficial effect of lowering serum phytanic acid levels in two patients who showed improvement in motor-nerve conduction velocity, some relief of ataxia, at least stabilizing the progression of retinitis pigmentosa. Similarly, Berson et al. reported the stabilizing effect of low phytanic acid diet in ERG (Berson, 1987).

2.1.7 Enhanced S-cone syndrome

In 1990, Marmor et al. reported eight patients who had night blindness, maculopathy, degenerative changes in the region of the vascular arcades, relatively mild visual field loss, and an unusual but characteristic electroretinogram (Marmor et al, 1990). Conventional dark adaptation curves showed a normal initial cone limb, but little or no rod adaptation beyond the cone threshold. The dark-adapted ERG shows no response to low-stimuli that normally activate rods. With high-intensity stimuli that normally activate both rods and cones, the dark-adapted ERG demonstrates large, slow responses. The light-adapted ERG flash cone response also shows similar large, slow waveforms that are nearly identical to those elicited by scotopic high-intensity stimuli (Miyake, 2005) (Figure 7). The ERG responses to stimuli of increasing intensity show several unique characteristics with a large broad a-wave that remains almost constant with respect to b-wave timing under both photopic and, scotopic conditions. Normal scotopic responses show a decrease in b-wave implicit time with increasing stimulus intensity (Marmor et al, 1990). These characteristic ERG responses were found to be related to a larger than usual number of S-cones that apparently replace other cones (Jacobson et al, 1991). For this reason, this condition was termed as "enhanced S-cone syndrome". Abnormalities in the gene NR2E3 are associated with this syndrome in mouse and in man (Haider et al, 2000). The cones develop abnormally at the stage of cellular differentiation when the visual pigment is specified (Weleber, 2002).

The ERG pattern of increased S-cone sensitivity is not unique to enhanced S-cone syndrome but is also found in Goldman-Favre syndrome.

2.1.8 Goldman-Favre syndrome

The Goldman-Favre syndrome is an autosomal recessive disorder characterized by early onset night blindness, atypical peripheral pigmentary degeneration, degenerative changes of the vitreous humor, peripheral and less often central retinoschisis, macular cystic degeneration and, posterior subcapsular lens opacities (Fishman, 2001). Jacobson et al showed that the predominant ERG response was originated mainly from the short-wavelength sensitive cones (Jacobson et al, 1991). This feature of Goldman-Favre syndrome is similar to enhanced S-cone syndrome.

2.2 Cone dystrophies and cone-rod dystrophies

Cone dystrophies and cone-rod dystrophies constitute a major subgroup of hereditary retinal disorders. Cone dystrophies are characterized by impaired central vision and abnormal cone responses in ERG. However, rod-cone dystrophies refer to retinitis pigmentosa, that is, the rod function impairs before the cone function. In contrast, in con-rod dystrophies, cone functions are impaired in advance to rod functions and rod functions is less severely affected than cone functions (Berson et al, 1968; Moore, 1992). The diagnosis of cone dystrophies and cone-rod dystrophies is mainly based on ERG which shows abnormal cone responses.

The most common symptoms of cone dystrophies include photophobia, loss of visual acuity, color vision and central visual fields. Most patients have dark-to-light adaptation problems (Goodmen et al, 1963). "Urban night blindness" is a frequent finding in patients with cone dystrophies. Patients with cone dystrophy who settle in cities cannot see well in the semilighted urban areas, because cone functions are impaired and the semilighted conditions are not dark enough to adapt the rods. Sometimes, patients may have nystagmus. The most frequent fundoscopic finding is the atrophic appearing lesion in the macula. A bull's eye maculopathy may be present. However, in some patients, macula may show only minimal changes or nonspecific mottling of the RPE (Heckenlively, 2006).

In cone-rod dystrophies, diminished visual acuity and loss of color discrimination precedes nyctalopia and progressive visual field loss (Gregory-Evans et al 2000). Autosomal dominant, autosomal recessive and X-linked recessive patterns of inheritance have been described for both cone dystrophy and cone-rod dystrophy (Simunovic, 1998).

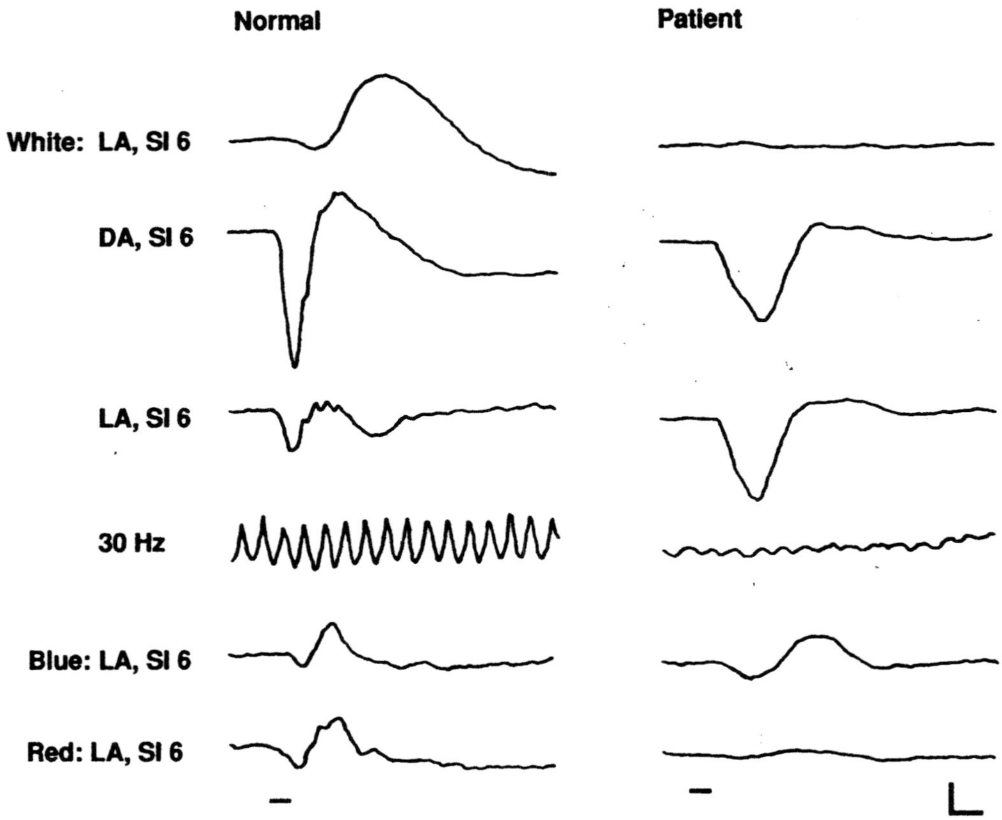

Fig. 7. Full-field electroretinogram in response to white and color stimuli of a normal person and patient with enhanced S-cone syndrome. In the patient, responses at dark and light adaptation are similar, the 30-Hz flicker response is reduced, and responses to blue stimuli are larger than to red. B-wave implicit times are markedly delayed at all stimulus conditions in the patient (DA: dark adaptation, LA: light adaptation, SI: stimulus intensity) (Used with permission of Pergamon Press Ltd. From. Enhanced S cone sensitivity syndrome: long-term follow-up, electrophysiological and psychophysical findings. Clinical Vision Sciences, Vol 8, Number 5, Kellner et al, 1993, permission conveyed through Copyright Clearance Center, Inc).

2.2.1 Cone dystrophy with negative photopic electroretinogram

Kellner and Foerster reported three patients with cone dystrophy who had negative photopic electroretinogram (Kellner & Foerster, 1993). This finding showed that at least in a subset of patients with cone dystrophy, additional inner retinal transmission defect may be present. The differential diagnosis of this condition from incomplete CSNB and X-linked retinoschisis may be performed with dark adaptation testing and fundoscopic examinations.

2.2.2 Cone dystrophy with Mizuo-Nakamura phenomenon

Heckenlively and Weleber described a new X-linked recessive cone dystrophy in which patients have a greenish-golden tapetal-like sheen of the retina (Heckenlively & Weleber, 1986). The authors reported that tapetal-like sheen disappeared after three hours of dark adaptation from greenish-golden shades to orange-red hues. This phenomenon (Mizuo-Nakamura phenomenon) was first described in patients with Oguchi disease. However, distinct electroretinographic and clinical features of Oguchi disease easily differentiates both diseases.

2.2.3 Rod monochromatism

Congenital achromatopsia often called achromatopsia is a rare *non-progressive* cone dysfunction with an autosomal recessive or X-linked recessive inheritance pattern. It can be divided into complete (no functioning cones) and, incomplete (some functioning cones) forms. Complete rod monochromatism has a severe course and, adults have 20/200 visual acuity and no color vision, while the incomplete rod monochromatism is less severe, and adults have 20/50 to 20/200 acuity with abnormal color vision (Moskowitz et al, 2009; Godel et al, 1976; Auerbach et al, 1970). Patients generally complain of photophobia and frequently have nystagmus that usually improves with age. The patients may have blond fundi and, this finding may cause misdiagnosis as ocular albinism. ERG helps distinguish ocular albinism from rod monochromatism which causes a typically diminished ERG response (Heckenlively, 2006).

2.2.4 Blue-cone monochromatism

Normal trichromatic color vision is possible only in the presence of normal functioning blue, green and red cones in the retina. Blue visual pigment is coded by a gene on chromosome 7 (Nathans et al, 1986a), while the green and red visual pigments are coded by highly homologous red and green pigment genes located on the X chromosome (Nathans et al, 1986b).

Blue cone monochromatism is an X-chromosome linked incomplete achromatopsia characterized by the absence of red and green cone function. For this reason, all the color vision is processed by only the blue cones (Ladekjaer-Mikkelsen, 1996). Patients may not discriminate different wavelengths and, but only light intensity. Unlike rod monochromats, blue cone function is selectively preserved. However, ERG responses of blue cone monochromats are similar to those of complete achromats, because blue cones contribute only negligibly to ERG.

2.2.5 Congenital red-green color deficiency

Congenital red-green color deficiency has been routinely diagnosed by psychophsical examinations. The standard ERG responses were reported to be normal under both scotopic and photopic conditions (Fishman, 2001). Figure 8 shows typical examples of the averaged waveform of 40 responses to monochromatic stimuli. The ERG amplitude in a normal subject is maximal around 550 nm, while the maximal amplitude is obtained at 520 to 530 nm in a protane and at around 550 nm in a deutan. The amplitudes are smaller than normal at long wavelengths in the protan subject and larger than normal at long wavelengths in the deutan subject (Nakazato et al, 1986) (Figure 8).

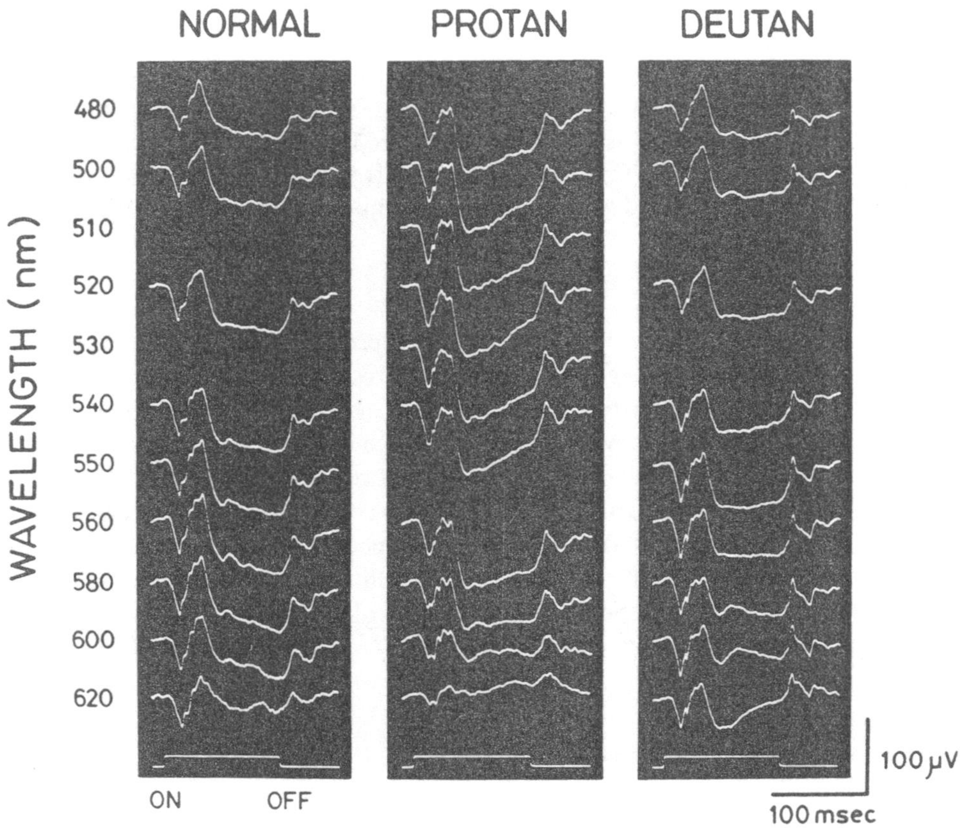

Fig. 8. Typical waveforms in normal subjects, protanopes and deuteranopes (Used with permission of Springer: Documenta Ophthalmologica, Vol 63, Number 2, Nakazato et al, Electroretinographic off-response in congenital red-green color deficiency and its genetic carrier, 1986, permission conveyed through Copyright Clearance Center, Inc).

2.2.6 Cone dystrophy with supernormal rod ERG

Cone dystrophy with supernormal rod electroretinogram was first described in 1983 (Gouras et al, 1983). This autosomal recessively inherited retinal dystrophy is characterized by reduced visual acuity, abnormal color vision, discrete macular changes, and specific alterations of ERG responses. ERG recordings typically show reduced and delayed cone responses, a reduction and marked delay of rod b-waves at low light intensities but elevated rod b-wave amplitudes at higher light intensities (Wissinger et al, 2008). The fundus appearance may be normal at the early stages, however in late stages there may be pigmentary disturbance at the macula and macular atrophy (Robson et al, 2010). This dystrophy was shown to be caused by mutations in KCNV2 gene (Wu et al, 2006; Thiagalingam et al, 2007; Ben Salah et al, 2008), which encodes a subunit of a voltage-gated potassium channel expressed in both rod and cone photoreceptors (Wu et al, 2006). It was speculated that the rapid increase in b-wave amplitude over a short range of stimulus intensity may result from a ''gated'' mechanism, occurring only after an abnormally high threshold has been exceeded, enabling channel activation and ERG b-wave generation.

Robson et al. reported that the ERG to the bright-flash showed a broadened and delayed a-wave through with a rhomboid-like shape (Robson et al, 2010). Figure 9 shows a cone dystrophy patient with supernormal rod electroretinogram (Gundogan et al, 2011).

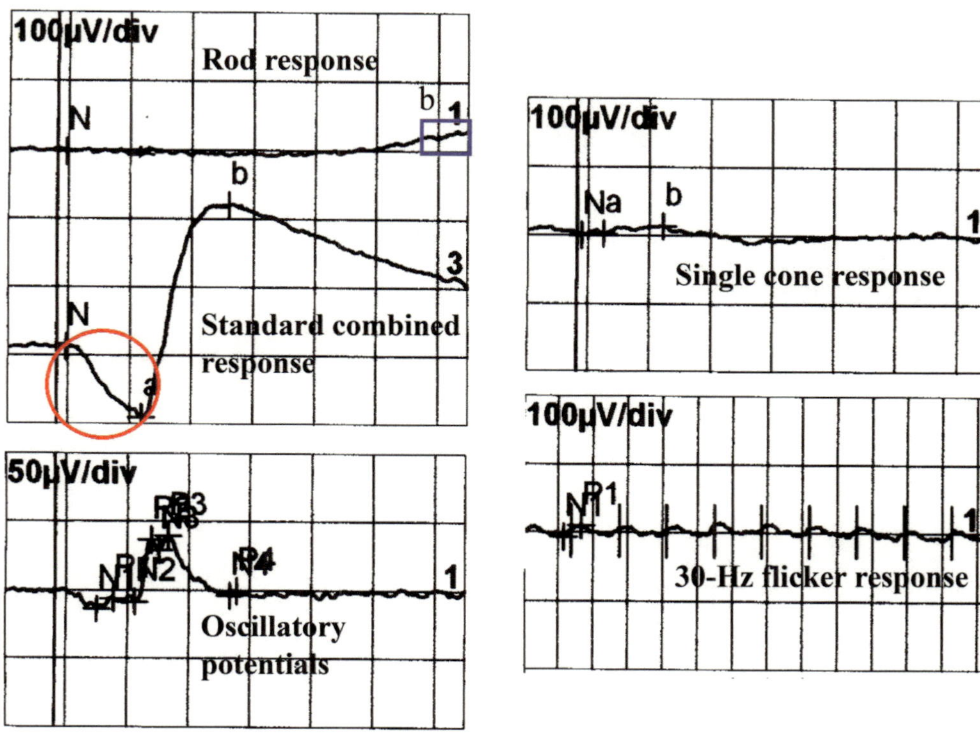

Fig. 9. Full-field electroretinogram with very delayed rod response, a rhomboid a-wave and supernormal b-wave in bright-flash rod-cone response and very reduced cone responses in a patient with KCNV2 mutation (Used with permission of Journal of Retina-Vitreus, 2011).

2.3 Juvenile X-linked retinoschisis

Juvenile X-linked retinoschisis is a hereditary vitreoretinal dystrophy that is the most common cause of macular degeneration in young males (The retinoschisis consortium, 1998). The disease affects 1/5000 to 1/25000 males worldwide and is one of the most common causes of juvenile macular degeneration in boys (George et al, 1995). The disease is thought to be a disorder of the retinal development in the intrauterine life. However visual loss is not recognized until preschool years (Eksandh et al, 2005). The disease is caused by mutations in the RS1 gene (Sauer et al, 1997; The retinoschisis consortium, 1998). Retinoschisin, encoded by RS1 gene, is a protein implicated in cell adhesion and signaling which maintains structural and functional integrity of the retina (Wu et al, 2005).
The disease manifests with cystic changes in the macula causing visual acuity loss. Most of the children are referred to the ophthalmologist because of a failure in school vision tests (Kjellström et al, 2010). The visual acuity loss progresses during the first two decades of life. There is slow progression of severity into the fifth and sixth decades. After the age of 50,

patients generally have a fundoscopic appearance of macular pigmentary changes and/or retinal pigment epithelium atrophy.
The defect in the production of retinoschisin causes lamellar splitting of the retina both in the nerve fiber layer and deeper in the retina. The retinal schisis most commonly occurs in the infero-temporal retina (Eksandh et al, 2000). Recent development of optical coherence tomography increased the clinical sensitivity for detection of retinal splitting (Gerth et al, 2008).

2.3.1 ERG in juvenile X-linked retinoschisis

The characteristic ERG in X-linked retinitis pigmentosa is a reduction in the scotopic b-wave amplitude. The b/a amplitude ratio is typically decreased, when it is below 1.0, a negative ERG pattern is found. However, normal b/a amplitude ratios were reported in the very early stages of the disease (Eksandh et al, 2005) (Figure 10). Therefore, a normal ERG does not absolutely exclude the diagnosis of X-linked retinoschisis.

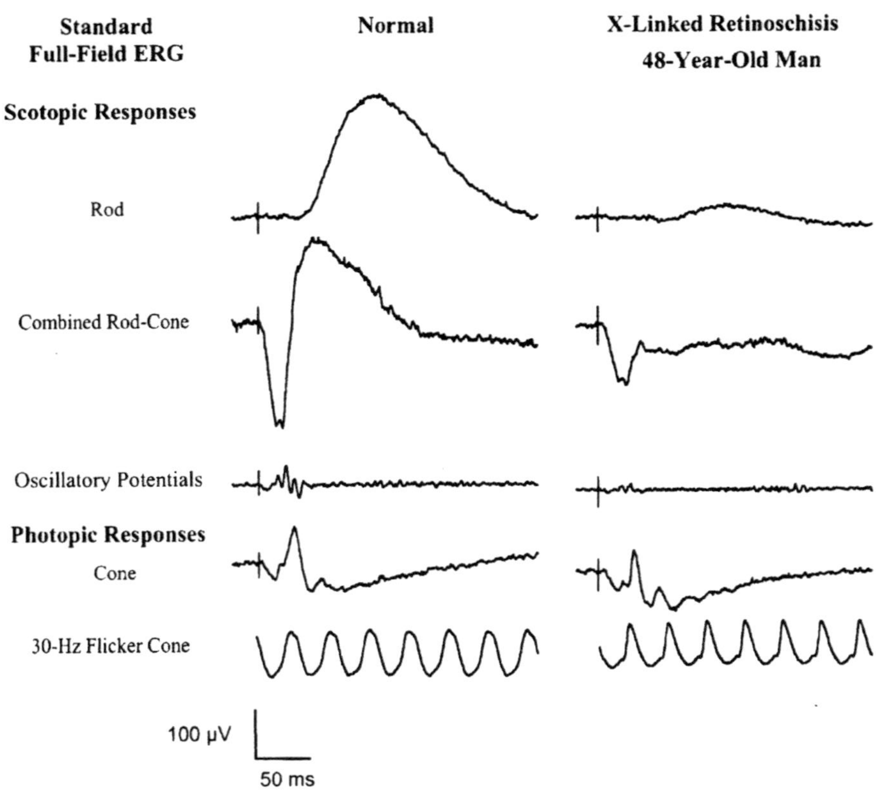

Fig. 10. Reduced and prolonged rod response and negative b-wave in X-linked retinoschisis (Used with permission of Taylor & Francis. From: Electrophysiology of Vision, ISBN: 0-8247-4068-8, Bryan Lam, 2005, permission conveyed through Copyright Clearance Center, Inc).

2.3.2 MfERG in X-linked juvenile retinoschisis

mfERG responses are more impaired in the central than peripheral retina in X-linked retinoschisis. In one study, mfERG measured at the follow-up demonstrated locally subnormal cone function in the macular region in all patients, and significantly delayed implicit time in all ring areas compared with normal controls (Kjelllström et al, 2010). Carriers of X-linked retinoschisis were also reported to have retinal dysfunction by mfERG in the presence of normal-appearing fundus (Kim et al, 2007).

2.4 Congenital stationary night blindness

Hereditary retinal disorders may be stationary or relatively mildly progressive rather than dystrophies with progressive degeneration. Among the stationary disorders, the ERG is an important diagnostic test particularly for congenital stationary night blindness and rod monochromatism. Stationary night blindness disorders may be classified as congenital stationary night blindness (CSNB), fundus albipunctatus, Oguchi disease and fleck retina of Kandori. Stationary cone dysfunction disorders may be classified as hereditary congenital color vision deficiencies, rod monochromatism and blue cone monochromatism (Lam, 2005). Stationary cone dysfunction disorders were mentioned under the title of cone dystrophies in this chapter.

Congenital stationary night blindness is the symptom of a group of hereditary retinal disorders characterized by *non-progressive* night-vision loss present since birth. Other ocular symptoms, such as nystagmus, decreased visual acuity, myopia and hyperopia are generally present (Weleber, 2002; Wutz et al, 2002; Zeitz et al, 2005). The prevalence of CSNB is approximately 1 in 10000 (Rosner et al, 1993). The classification of CSNB is based on both fundus appearance and, hereditary pattern. Some patients have *normal-appearing fundus,* others have some *distinctive fundus abnormalities* (Carr, 1974). Patients with a normal-appearing fundus and CSNB may have an autosomal dominant, autosomal recessive or X-linked recesive inheritance pattern. ERG is the key diagnostic test with distint findings in CSNB.

2.4.1 Schubert-Bornschein type of CSNB

Schubert-Bornschein type of CSNB is characterized by a negative ERG response, that is, the amplitude of the b-wave is smaller than the amplitude of a-wave, causing a b-wave to a-wave amplitude ratio smaller than one (Figure 11). In general, this type of the disease has an autosomal recessive or, X-linked recessive pattern. However, autosomal dominant pedigrees were also reported (Hayakawa et al, 1992; Noble et al, 1990).

In 1986, Miyake studied on patients with X-linked Schubert-Bornscein type CSNB (Miyake, 1986). The author realized that the patients may be classified into two groups as complete and incomplete CSNB with respect to rod function in ERG and subjective dark adaptation testing. The patients with complete type CSNB (or CSNB1) lackes rod function, while the patients with incomplete type CSNB (or CSNB2) have residual rod function. Studies after the discovery of both types of CSNB have documented that both forms are originated from different mutations. Further studies on complete and incomplete type CSNB showed that the two types also differ with respect to cone ERG, long-flash photopic ERG (Miyake et al, 1987; Quigley et al, 1996) and scotopic threshold response (Miyake et al, 1994).

2.4.2 Riggs type CSNB

Riggs type CSNB was first described by Riggs in 1956. The author reported three CSNB patients with detectable, but markedly impaired dark-adaptation (Riggs, 1954). ERG responses of the patients showed reduced b-wave amplitude which was still greater than a-wave amplitude. The b-wave to a-wave amplitude ratios were greater than 1, but still under normal data. Auerbach et al. reported the ERG results of 95 CSNB patients. Fifty-nine of the patients had Schubert-Bornschein type CSNB and 36 patients had Riggs type CSNB (Auerbach et al, 1969). The authors also reported that myopia and nystagmus were less common in Riggs type CSNB patients than Schubert-Bornschein type patients. Riggs type CSNB is inherited as X-linked or autosomal recessively.

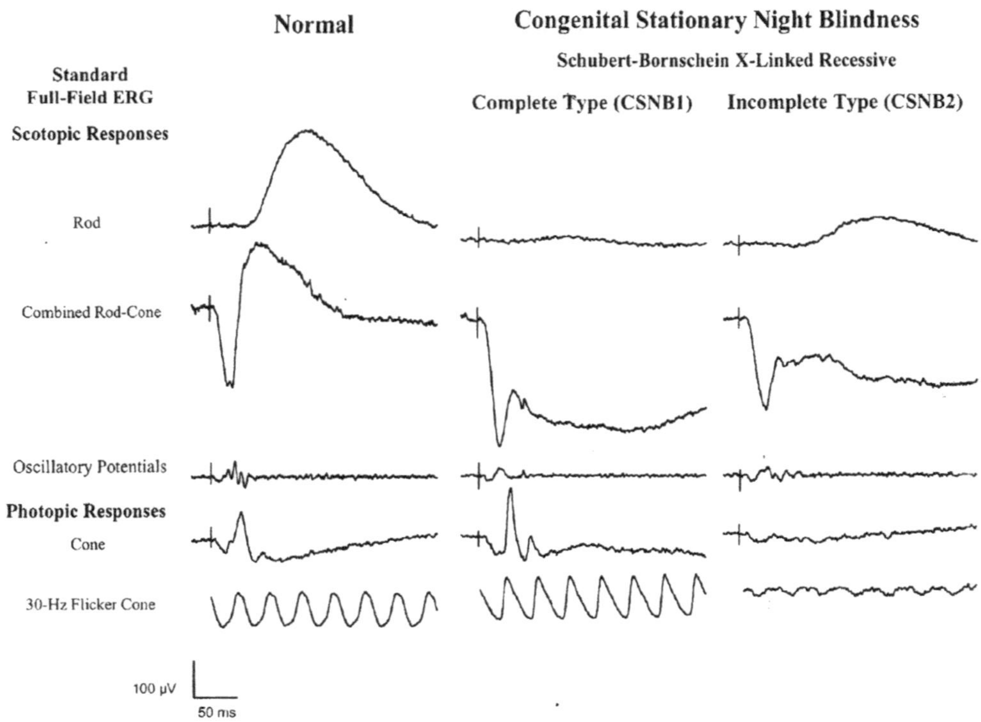

Fig. 11. Complete and incomplete types of X-linked recessively inherited Schubert-Bornschein congenital stationary night blindness. In both types, b/a ratio is below 1.0, however, incomplete type has residual rod function in contrast to complete type (Used with permission of Taylor & Francis. From: Electrophysiology of Vision, ISBN: 0-8247-4068-8, Bryan Lam, 2005, permission conveyed through Copyright Clearance Center, Inc).

2.4.3 Nougaret type CSNB

The first autosomal dominant type of CSNB, Nougaret type, derives its name from the first described patient, Jean Nougaret. Sandberg et al. reported non-detectable scotopic ERG response in a father and son with Nougaret CSNB (Sandberg et al, 1998). The scotopic white bright-flash combined rod-cone responses demonstrated decreased biphasic a-wave with a b-wave amplitude that was positive and at least 50% of normal indicating that the loss of rod function was not complete. The cone responses were only slightly impaired (Lam, 2005). One another autosomal dominant CSNB pedigree was reported by Rambusch in 1909 in a Danish family (Rosenberg et al, 1991). ERG responses in the Rambusch pedigree are similar to those of Nougaret CSNB and resemble the ERG responses of the Riggs CSNB type (Lam, 2005).

2.4.4 Fundus albipunctatus

Fundus albipunctatus is a type of congenital stationary night blindness with an autosomal recessive inheritance pattern. The typical clinical findings include multiple whitish yellow spots at the level of RPE with the exception of the macula, which tend to be scattered as an annulus around the macula. The fundoscopic appearance of the optic disc and retinal vessels are normal and there is no evidence of peripheral clumping of retinal pigment. Fundus albipunctatus is caused by mutations in the RDH5 gene, which encodes for the 11-cis retinal dehydrogenase of the retinal pigment epithelium (Nakamura & Miyake 2002; Nakamura et al, 2003).

The typical pathology is the delayed regeneration of the rod visual pigment. This results in reduced rod responses in ERG, which begin to recover around 30 minutes of dark adaptation and normalizes after 2-3 hours (Carr et al, 1974). Similar to rod responses, delays in the cone visual pigment regeneration was also demonstrated (Petzold & Gordon, 2006).

2.4.5 Oguchi disease

Oguchi disease is a distinct entity under CSNB with characteristic electroretinographic and clinical properties. The disease was first described by Oguchi in 1912. The night vision impairment is typically non-progressive. Typically, dark adaptation is 8-10 times slower than normal (Carr & Ripps, 1967; Cideciyan et al, 1998). Characteristically, fundus has a metallic, phosphorescent-like sheen which disappears after prolonged dark adaptation. This is called Mizuo phenomenon with respect to the author by which this condition was first described in 1913. Scotopic ERG responses were reported to be diminished in amplitude. Photopic ERG responses are normal which gives clue to differentiate Oguchi disease from complete CSNB (Miyake et al, 1996).

2.4.6 Fleck retina of Kandori

Fleck retina of Kandori is an autosomal recessively inherited retinal dystrophy characterized by relatively large yellow irregular shaped flecks in the peripheral retina, minimal dark adaptation abnormality, and normal visual field (Fishman, 2001). ERG responses show a negative pattern suggesting functional impairment within the proximal retina (Kandori et al, 1966).

2.5 Hereditary macular disorders

2.5.1 Stargardt macular dystrophy and fundus flavimaculatus

Stargardt disease which is the first described juvenile-onset hereditary macular degeneration was first defined by the German ophthalmologist Karl Stargardt in 1909, is a familial, progressive, bilateral, and symmetric macular disease leading to partial or complete loss of central vision (Itabashi et al, 1993). All seven patients reported by Stargardt were restricted to one generation suggesting an autosomal recessive inheritance pattern (Aaberg, 1986). The frequently cited incidence of stardardt disease is 1 in 10.000. The typical clinical features of the disease is characterized by the onset of decreased visual acuity, most frequently noted within the first two decades of life, often accompanied by an atrophic-appearing lesion of the macula and a varying degree of yellow-white linear, round, stellate, or pisciform (fishtail) shaped "flecks" at the level of the retinal pigment epithelium (Fishman, 1991). In the 1970s, and 1980s, diffuse blockage of choroidal filling on fluorescein angiography, the so-called 'choroidal silence' or 'dark choroids,' due in part to the accumulation of lipofuscin-like material in the retinal pigment epithelium were recognized

as a feature of Stargardt macular dystrophy. The retinal fleck-like lesions was noted to correspond to hypertrophic retinal pigment epithelial cells with extensive accumulation of lipofuscin-like material (Eagle et al, 1980; Fish et al, 1981).
Later, in 1962, Franceshetti described an autosomal recessively inherited retinal dystrophy characterized with subretinal yellow flecks, which were associated, in 50% of the cases, with macular changes to those seen in Stargardt disease. The author named this condition "fundus flavimaculatus" (Franceschetti, 1965; Franceschetti et al, 1965). However, as Francheschetti recognized, if the flecks are localized at the posterior pole with macular involvement it becomes almost impossible to clinically distinguish fundus flavimaculatus from Stargardt disease. These similar findings caused the investigators to suggest that stargardt macular disease and fundus flavimaculatus reflects the same disease process. For this reason, Deutman suggested the eponym "Stargardt flavimaculatus" as a more accurate identification (Lachapelle et al 1990). The attempts to classify patients into two distinct genetic disorders based on retinal appearance alone was not successful because of overlapping clinical and genetic findings between Stargardt macular dystrophy and fundus flavimaculatus.
In general, ERG rod and cone responses in patients with stargardt macular dystrophy are in the normal range, however, are variable among patients and may demonstrate impaired cone responses as well as impaired rod and cone responses especially in those with more widespread retinal atrophy and fleck-like lesions. In addition, some investigators found prolonged dark adaptation in patients with Stargardt macular dystrophy (Figure 12). For this reason, at least 45-min dark adaptation is suggested before ERG recordings (Fishman et al, 1991).

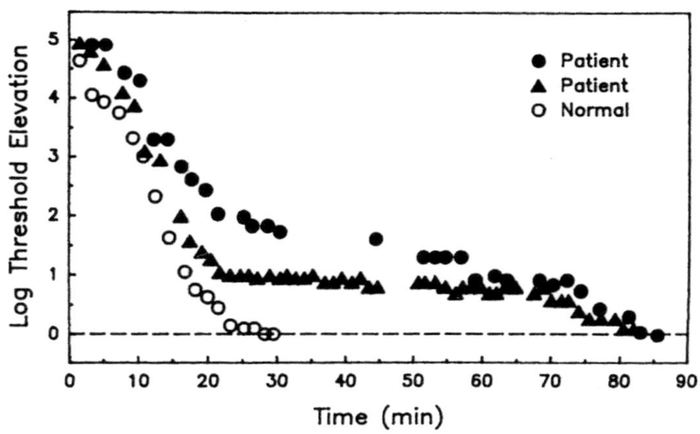

Fig. 12. Dark adaptation curves from a normal subject and two patients with Stargardt macular dystrophy. The initial portions of the slopes are similar, while the latter portion of the dark adaptation curve is prolonged in the patients (Used with permission of Elsevier Inc. From ,'Delayed rod dark adaptation in patients with Stargardt's disease", Fishman et al, Ophthalmology, Volume 98, Number 6, 1991; permission conveyed through Copyright Clearance Center, Inc)

PERG responses are typically diminished regardless of visual acuity (Lois et al, 2001). This striking PERG finding is rather unusual in other macular dystrophies. Multifocal ERGs show markedly diminished or non-detectable foveal response in almost all patients even in those with good visual acuity (Kretschmann et al, 1998) (Figure 13).

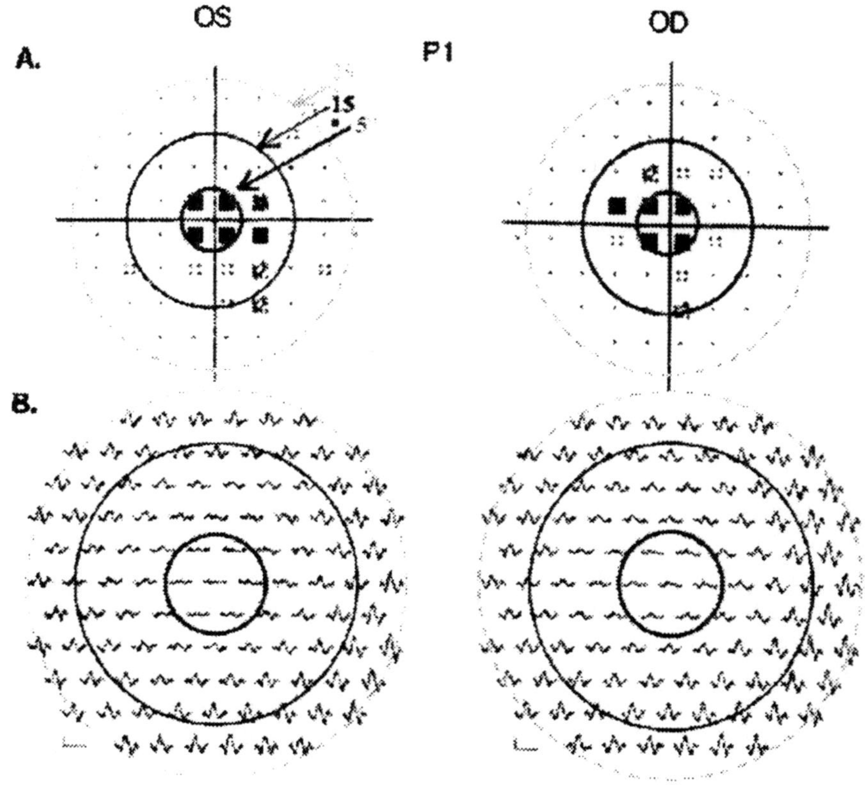

Fig. 13. Humphrey visual fields in Stargardt disease (A). Multifocal electroretinogram responses show reduced central amplitudes, but relatively unchanged implicit times, typical of early Stargardt disease (Used with permission of Wolters Kluwer Health. From ,'The multifocal electroretinogram'', Hood et al, Journal of Neuro-ophthalmology, Volume 23, Number 3, 2003; permission conveyed through Copyright Clearance Center, Inc)

2.5.2 Best vitelliform macular dystrophy

Best vitelliform macular dystrophy is an autosomal dominant, juvenile-onset disorder characterized by ann egg-yellow, slightly elevated macular lesion surrounded by a darker border (Deutman, 1971, 1989). Best disease is associated with a mutation in the VMD2 gene (Palmowski et al, 2003). The macular changes have been staged according to the severity of the macular lesion: previtelliform stage, vitelliform stage, pseudo-hypopyon stage, vitelliruptive stage and atrophic stage. The lesions reflect abnormalities in the retinal pigment epithelium (Weingeist et al, 1982). Histopathologic examinations revealed excessive amounts of lipofuscin accumulation in the retinal pigment epithelium throughout the fundus. Visual acuity is only mildly affected in the early stages of the disease, and is typically better than expected with respect to the appearance of the foveal lesion. However, as the disease progresses, visual acuity decreases parallel to the appearance of macular atrophy.

The functional impairment of retinal pigment epithelium leads to abnormal electro-oculogram which is the key diagnostic test of the disease. The ERG is typically normal in Best vitelliform macular dystrophy. Palmowski et al. studied mfERG responses in three

patients and reported normal implicit times and reduced amplitudes in the central 6 degrees (Palmowski et al, 2003). In contrast, Scholl et al. found decreased amplitudes and delayed implicit times in mfERG in 18 patients with Best vitelliform macular dystrophy (Scholl et al, 2002) (Figure 14, Figure 15). The authors also reported that central mfERG amplitudes were significantly correlated with visual acuity loss and fundoscopic staging.
These findings document the impaired central retinal function which may not be revealed with ERG in these patients.
In one study, the authors divided the patients into two groups according to visual acuities (Jarc-Vidmar et al, 2001). The authors reported normal PERG responses in patients with 0.5 or higher visual acuities and abnormal PERG responses in approximately half of the patients with lower visual acuities. In that study, progression of the disease as assessed by visual acuity decreases and visual field defects were well correlated with the reduction of both PERG P50 and N95 amplitudes. However, there was no correlation with the visual acuity and electro-oculogram which is the key diagnostic test of Best vitelliform macular dystrophy.

2.5.3 Pattern dystrophies

Pattern dystrophies are a group of dominantly inherited retinal disorders which primarily affects the retinal pigment epithelium in the macula. The fundoscopic appearance of the macular lesion is variable and includes butterfly patterns as well as knotted fishnet patterns. The visual prognosis is generally good with a mild disturbance of central vision typically ranging from 20/20 to 20/70 and, metamorphopsia. Pattern dystrophies are divided into morphological subtypes including butterfly dystrophy, fundus pulverulentus, multifocal pattern dystrophy resembling Stargardt disease, and adult-onset vitelliform macular dystrophy (Deutman & Rümke, 1969; Deutman et al, 1970; Hsieh et al, 1972; Slezak & Hommer, 1969). However, some individual patients may not be precisely categorized into one of these groups with respect to fundus abnormalities.
PERG is abnormal due to macular involvement. ERG is generally undisturbed. EOG light-rise to dark-through amplitude ratio is usually reduced but not always abnormal (Hsieh et al, 1972; Daniele et al, 1996; Kingham et al, 1978; Shiono et al, 1990; Watzke et al, 1982). Central retinal dysfunction can be detected by focal ERG or multifocal ERG.

2.5.4 North Carolina macular dystrophy

North Carolina macular dystrophy is an autosomal dominant inherited disease which causes congenital bilateral macular degenerations (Rabb et al, 1998). The disease was first described by Lefler et al in 1972 in the descendants of a large family who lived in the 1800s (Lefler et al, 1971). Lefler reported that ERGs, electro-oculograms and color vision tests were normal in the patients. Lefler named this disease as "dominant macular degeneration and aminoaciduria", however a few years later, Frank et al. showed that aminoaciduria in the cases of Lefler was in fact unrelated to dominant macular degeneration and named the condition as "dominant progressive foveal dystrophy" without evidence of the progression (Frank et al, 1974). Frank et al. also expanded the family history and found that all of the patients were descendants of three Irish brothers who settled in the North Carolina mountains in 1800s.
The fundoscopic findings range from a few yellow drusen-like lesions in the macula to macular colobomas. The disease is generally stable and the visual acuity ranges from 20/20 to 20/800 (Rabb et al, 1998). As the Lefler reported in the first cases, ERG responses are generally normal (Small et al, 1993; Lefler et al, 1971; Frank et al, 1974).

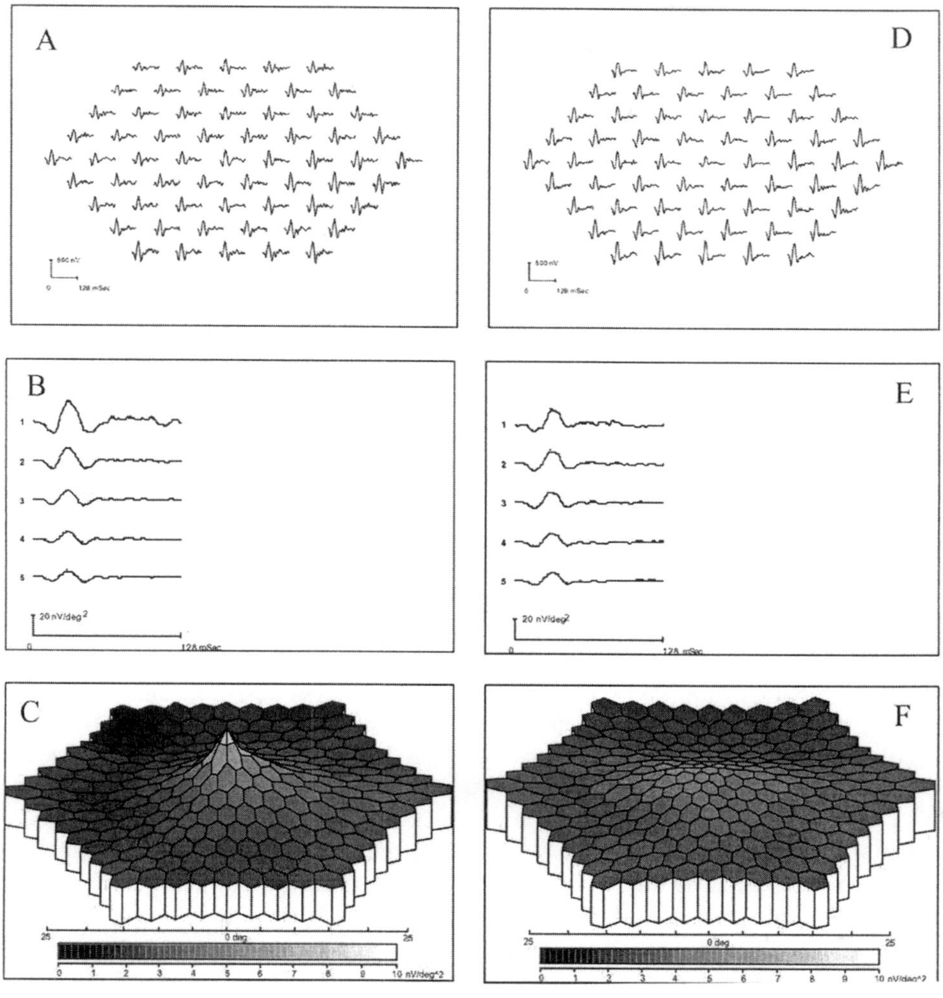

Fig. 14. Multifocal electroretinograms recorded from the left eye of one normal subject (A; representing the median for the central element within the control population of 55 subjects) and from the left eye of Best macular dystrophy patient (D; representing the median for the peak amplitude of the central element within the population of 18 Best macular dystrophy patient). The upper panel (A,D) shows the trace arrays with 61 mfERG waveforms. The patient has a visual acuity of 1.0, however, central peak amplitudes are markedly reduced (D). In the more concentric rings, the amplitudes are normal (E). The three dimensional plots of the response show markedly reduced amplitudes in the fovea (F) (Used with permission of Pergamon. From ,'Mapping of retinal function in Best macular dystrophy using multifocal electroretinography'', Scholl et al, Vision Research, Volume 42, Number 8, 2003; permission conveyed through Copyright Clearance Center, Inc)

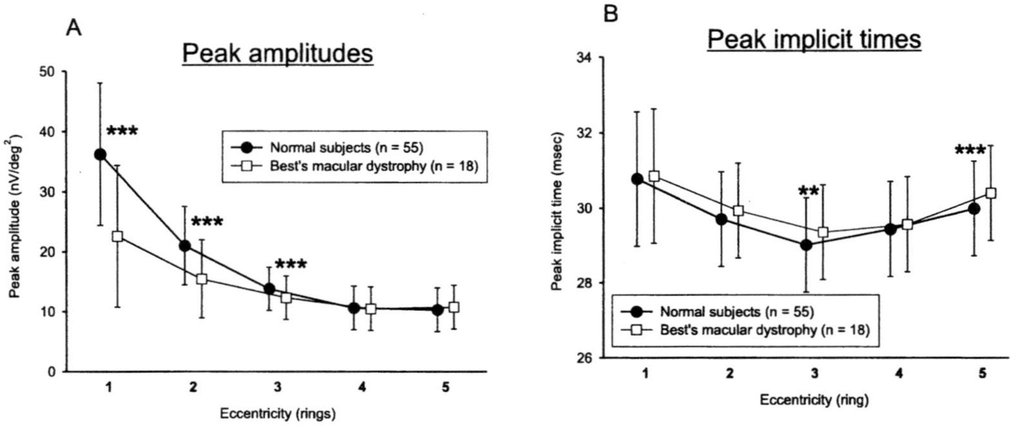

Fig. 15. Multifocal electroretinogram responses are significantly reduced in the central three rings and significantly delayed in the third and fifth rings in patients with Best macular dystrophy (Asterisks indicate significant differences. ***$p<0.001$, **$p<0.01$) (Used with permission of Pergamon. From ,'Mapping of retinal function in Best macular dystrophy using multifocal electroretinography'', Scholl et al, Vision Research, Volume 42, Number 8, 2003; permission conveyed through Copyright Clearance Center, Inc).

2.5.5 Sorsby fundus dystrophy

Sorsby fundus dystrophy, first described by Sorsby and Mason in 1949, is a rare progressive, autosomal dominantly inherited retinal disease (Sivaprasad et al, 2008). Bilateral visual loss occurs generally in the adulthood (from the third to the seventh decade) due to subretinal neovascular membranes causing disciform scarring or chorioretinal atrophy at the macula (Sorsby & Mason, 1949). Night vision impairment may develop in some patients and may precede the development of visible fundus signs.

Both normal and reduced ERG responses were reported in Sorsby fundus dystrophy (Capon et al, 1988; Felbor U et al, 1996). However, Clarke et al. reported markedly abnormal PERG responses even in the presence of a small central island of vision (Clarke et al, 1997).

2.5.6 Central areolar choroidal dystrophy

Central areolar choroidal dystrophy, first described by Nettleship in 1884, is a macular dystrophy characterized by the development of fine, mottled, depigmented retinal pigment epithelium in the macula. After several decades the pathognomonic zone of circumscript atrophy, affecting retina, retinal pigment epithelium and choriocapillaris, develops in the macular region of the eye (Carr, 1965; Hoyng & Deutman, 1996). Although, most cases are sporadic, autosomal dominant and recessive inheritance patterns have been reported (Nagasaka et al, 2003).

ERG responses are generally normal or subnormal in CACD. However, in some cases of central areolar choroidal dystrophy, generalized decrease in both scotopic and photopic ERG is found (Adachi-Usami et al, 1990; Carr, 1965; Noble, 1977). In a recent study, we have showed that mfERG responses were reduced corresponding to the areas of ophthalmoscopically visible lesion and there were significant correlations between foveal retinal sensitivity in the Humprey visual field and mfERG P1/N1 amplitudes (Figure 16) (Gundogan et al, 2010).

2.5.7 Bietti's crystalline dystrophy

Bietti's crystalline dystrophy is characterized by tapetoretinal degeneration with small glistening crystals in the posterior pole. The first cases reported by Bietti in 1937 and 1942 also had corneal crystals (Richards et al, 1991). Later it was understood that paralimbal corneal crystals are found in only one third of the patients. For this reason, the disease are also named as "Bietti's corneal-retinal dystrophy". A study showed circulating crystals in the lymphocytes resembling cholesterol and cholesterol-ester crystals (Wilson et al, 1989). This finding suggested that Bietti's crystalline dystrophy may be due to a systemic abnormality of the lipid metabolism.

The ERG responses may be diminished or minimally abnormal due to the phenotypic heterogeneity of the disease (Fishman, 2001).

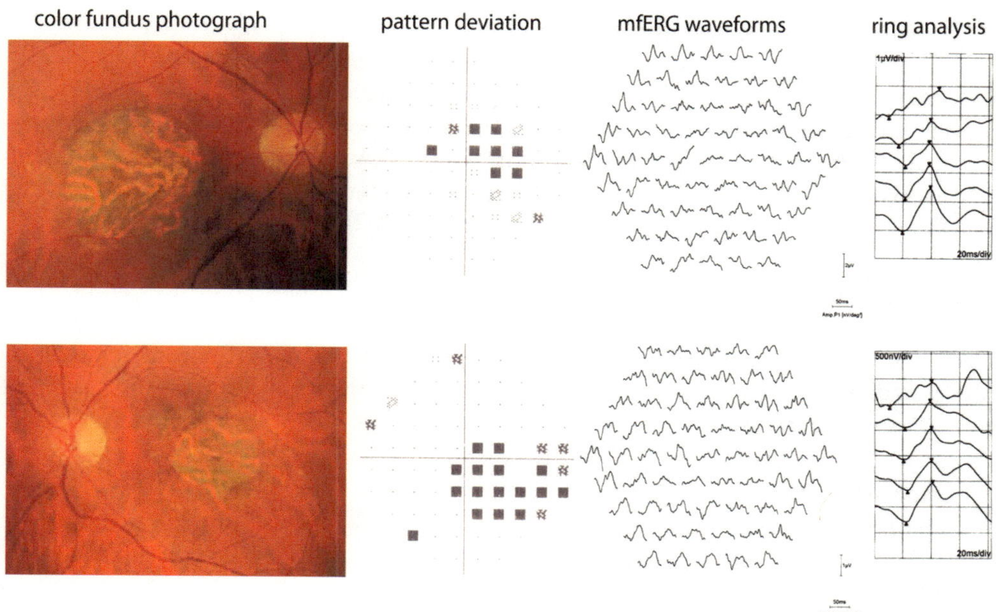

Fig. 16. Color fundus photographs, pattern deviation of Humphrey visual fields and multifocal electroretinogram results of a patient with central areolar choroidal dystrophy. Central responses are markedly reduced and delayed in multifocal electroretinogram (Used with permission of Wichtig Editore. From. 'Multifocal electroretinogram and central visual field testing in central areolar choroidal dystrophy", Gundogan et al, European Journal of Ophthalmology, Volume 20, Number 5, 2010).

2.6 Hereditary vitreoretinal disorders

Hereditary vitreoretinal disorders are a group of diseases with both retinal and vitreal involvement. Electrophysiologic responses typically reflect the degree of retinal involvement in this group of rare conditions.

2.6.1 Stickler syndrome

Stickler syndrome was first described in 1965 (Stickler et al, 1965). The syndrome is characterized by high myopia, premature vitreous syneresis, frequent retinal detachment and premature degenerative changes of articular cartilage. This association of ocular and articular involvement caused to be termed as *hereditary progressive arthro-ophthalmopathy.* ERG responses are generally normal in Stickler syndrome, however, high myopia and retinal detachment may produce reduced amplitudes (Aylward et al, 2008).

2.6.2 Wagner syndrome

Wagner syndrome is a progressive autosomal dominant disorder characterized by vitreous changes including avascular strands and condensed bands, situs inversus of the retinal vessels and atrophic changes of the retinal pigment epithelium and choriocapillaris (Brown et al, 1995). ERG responses may be normal, however, may be reduced if the retinal and choroidal atrophy occurs (Hirose et al, 1973).

2.6.3 Familial exudative vitreoretinopathy

Familial exudative vitreoretinopathy is a rare autosomal dominant or X-linked hereditary pattern characterized by premature termination of retinal vessels in the peripheral temporal retina which causes the development of tractional fibrovascular masses. The clinical findings of familial exudative vitreoretinopahy are quite similar to premature retinopathy. ERG findings are correlated to the extent and severity of the retinal involvement (Ohkubo & Tamino, 1987; Van Noubuys, 1982).

2.7 Hereditary chorioretinal dystrophies

Progressive chorioretinal dystrophies are a group of inherited diseases characterized by the progressive degenerations of the both retinal and choroidal layers. Choroideremia, gyrate atrophy and pigmented paravenous retinochoroidal atrophy are the three most common chorioretinal dystrophies.

2.7.1 Choroideremia

Choroideremia is a X-linked recessive dystrophy characterized by progressive atrophy of the photoreceptors, retinal pigment epithelium, and the choriocapillaris, leading to progressive visual loss (MacDonald et al, 2009). The disease is caused by mutations in the CHM gene, which encodes for the Rab escort protein 1 (REP-1) (Cremers et al, 1990). Night vision impairment and peripheral visual field loss is generally occurs during the first or second decade of life, however, central vision is affected in the late stages of the disease (Mukkamala et al, 2010). Night vision impairment usually progresses to tunnel vision or complete blindness by middle age. The retinas of female carriers are mosaics, containing patches of both mutant and normal cells. As a result of mosaicism, female carriers usually show patchy depigmentation of the retinal pigment epithelium, but can retain good visual function throughout life (Syed et al, 2001).

In the early stages of the disease, both a- and b-wave amplitudes are reduced and the implicit times delayed (Fishman, 2001). In the later stages of the disease, if the ERG responses are recordable, residual retinal function is mostly due to cone functions (Sieving et al, 1986). Female carriers generally have normal ERG responses (Mura et al, 2007).

2.7.2 Gyrate atrophy

Gyrate atrophy is an autosomal recessive dystrophy caused by mutations of the gene encoding ornithine aminotransferase, a vitamin B6 dependent mitochondrial enzyme which catalyzes the conversion of ornithine to glutamate and proline (Mashima et al, 1992). The resultant biochemical abnormality is hypolysinemia, hyperornithinemia, and a marked reduction in ornithine aminotransferase activity in cultured skin fibroblasts and in lymphocytes (Simell & Takki, 1973).

The patients generally begin to experience night blindness between the age of 20 and 40 years. The peripheral fundus has multiple, discrete patches of chorioretinal atrophy areas. With time, these lesions progress toward both centrally and peripherally causing peripheral visual field and visual acuity loss. Myopia and posterior subcapsular cataract are common among patients (Kaiser-Kupfer et al, 1991).

ERG responses are indicative of the extent of the disease and diminishes as the chorioretinal atrophy progresses. In the advanced stages of the disease, the ERG may even be nondetectable.

2.7.3 Pigmented paravenous retinochoroidal atrophy

Pigmented paravenous retinochoroidal atrophy (PPRCA) is a rare bilateral stationary condition of the ocular fundus in which bone corpuscle pigmentation is seen in a paravenous distribution. The first cases were reported by Francessetti under various names, however, the author concluded that the term "pigmented paravenous retinochoroidal atrophy" best describes the condition (Franceschetti, 1962). Although it is not a generalized retinal disorder, the extent and degree of retinal involvement varies significantly between affected patients (Noble & Carr, 1983; Traboulsi & Maumenee, 1986). The disease is usually asymptomatic and diagnosed incidentally during routine fundoscopic examinations. Most reported cases are sporadic, however, familial occurrences were also reported (Traboulsi & Maumenee, 1986; Skalka, 1979). ERG responses are generally variable depending on the extent of the disease (Lam, 2005). Miyake reported that the ERG amplitudes are smaller than normal, however, the implicit times are normal suggesting that the retina is not diffusely involved as it would be in retinitis pigmentosa. MfERG amplitudes are reduced in the affected retinal areas (Miyake, 2006).

3. Conclusion

Electroretinographic testing methods are indispensable parts of the evaluation of patients with hereditary retinal diseases. Full-field ERG has an important role in the diagnosis and follow-up of patients with retinal functional abnormalities and a normal-appearing fundus. In some clinical situations, full-field ERG may also help in the differential diagnosis. This chapter aimed to show some examples of ERGs in hereditary retinal disorders and to show the consistency between function and symptom and signs when appropriate method of ERG technique was chosen.

4. References

Aaberg, TM. (1986). Stargardt's disease and fundus flavimaculatus: evaluation of morphologic progression and intrafamilial co-existence. *Transactions of the American Ophthalmological Society*. Vol.84, pp. 453-87. ISSN 0065-9533

Abraham, FA. (1975). Sector retinitis pigmentosa. Electrophysiological and psychophysical study of the visual system. *Documenta Ophthalmologica*. Vol. 39, No.1, pp.13-28. ISSN 0012-4486

Adachi-Usami, E., Murayama, K. & Yamamoto, Y. (1990). Electroretinograms and pattern visually evoked cortical potentials in central areolar choroidal dystrophy. *Documenta Ophthalmologica*. Vol.75, No.1, pp.33-40. ISSN 0012-4486

Andréasson, SO., Sandberg, MA. & Berson, EL. (1988). Narrow-band filtering for monitoring low-amplitude cone electroretinograms in retinitis pigmentosa. *American Journal of Ophthalmology.* Vol.105, No.5, pp.500-3. ISSN: 0002-9394

Auerbach, E., Godel, V. & Rowe, H. (1969). An electrophysiological and psychophysical study of two forms of congenital night blindness. *Investigative Ophthalmology & Visual Science* . Vol.8, No.3, pp.332-45. ISSN 1552-5783

Auerbach, E. & Kripke, B. (1970). Some studies of rod monochromatism: a dominant pediree. *Electroencephalography and Clinical Neurophysiology.* Vol.28, No.6, pp.643. ISSN:0013-4694

Avigan, J., Steinberg, D., Gutman, A., Mize, CE. & Milne, GW. (1966). Alpha-decarboxylation, an important pathway for degradation of phytanic acid in animals. *Biochemical and Biophysical Research Communications.* Vol.24, No.6, pp.838-44. ISSN 0006-291X

Aylward, B., daCruz, L., Ezra, E., Sullivan, P., MacLaren, RE., Charteris, D., Gregor, Z., Bainbridge, J. & Minihan, M. (2008). Stickler syndrome. *Ophthalmology.* Vol.115, No.9, pp.1636-7. ISSN 0161-6420

Berson, EL. (1981). Retinitis pigmentosa and allied diseases: applications of electroretinographic testing. *International Ophthalmology.* Vol.4, No.1-2, pp.7-22. ISSN 0165-5701

Berson, EL., Gouras, P. & Gunkel, RD. (1968). Progressive cone degeneration, dominantly inherited. *Archives of Ophthalmology.* Vol.80, No.1, pp.77-83. ISSN 0093-0326

Berson, EL. & Howard, J. (1971). Temporal aspects of the electroretinogram in sector retinitis pigmentosa. *Archives of Ophthalmology.* Vol.86, No.6, pp.653-65. ISSN 0093-0326

Berson, EL. (1987). Electroretinographic findings in retinitis pigmentosa. *Japanese Journal of Ophthalmology.* Vol.31, No.3, pp.327-48. ISSN 0021-5155

Berson, EL. (1976). Retinitis pigmentosa and allied retinal diseases: electrophysiologic findings. *Transaction. Section on Ophthalmology. American Academy of Ophthalmology and Otolaryngology.* Vol.81, No.4 Pt 1, pp.659-666. ISSN 0002-7154

Birch, DG. & Sandberg, MA. (1987). Dependence of cone b-wave implicit time on rod amplitude in retinitis pigmentosa. *Vision Research.* Vol.27, No.7, pp.1105-12. ISSN 0042-6989

Birch, DG. (2006). Retinitis pigmentosa. In. *Principles and practice of clinical electrophysiology of vision,* Heckenlively, JR., Arden, GB., pp. (781-794), The MIT pres, 0-262-08346-9, Cambridge.

Bishara, S., Merin, S., Cooper, M., Azizi, E., Delpre, G. & Deckelbaum, RJ. (1982). Combined vitamin A and E therapy prevents retinal electrophysiological deterioration in abetalipoproteinaemia. *British Journal of Ophthalmology.* Vol.66, No.12, pp.767-70. ISSN 0007-1161

Boughman, JA., Conneally, PM. & Nance, WE. (1980). Population genetic studies of retinitis pigmentosa. *American Journal of Human Genetics.* Vol.32, No.2, pp.223-35. ISSN 0002-9297

Brown, DM., Graemiger, RA., Hergersberg, M., Schinzel, A., Messmer, EP., Niemeyer, G., Schneeberger, SA., Streb, LM., Taylor, CM., Kimura, AE., et al. (1995). Genetic linkage of Wagner disease and erosive vitreoretinopathy to chromosome 5q13-14. *Archives of Ophthalmology.* Vol.113, No.5, pp.671-5. ISSN 0093-0326

Bunker, CH., Berson, EL., Bromley, WC., Hayes, RP. & Roderick, TH. (1984). Prevalence of retinitis pigmentosa in Maine. *American Journal of Ophthalmology.* Vol.97, No.3, pp.357-65. ISSN 0002-9394

Capon, MR., Polkinghorne, PJ., Fitzke, FW. & Bird, AC. (1988). Sorsby's pseudoinflammatory macula dystrophy--Sorsby's fundus dystrophies. *Eye (London).* Vol.2, No. Pt 1, pp.114-22. ISSN 0950-222X

Carr, RE., Ripps, H., Siegel, IM. & Weale, RA. (1966). Rhodopsin and the electrical activity of the retina in congenital night blindness. *Investigative Ophthalmology & Visual Science* . Vol.5, No.5, pp.497-507. ISSN 1552-5783

Carr, RE. (1965). Central Areolar Choroidal Dystrophy. *Archives of Ophthalmology.* Vol.73, pp.32-5. ISSN 0093-0326

Carr, RE. (1974). Congenital stationary nightblindness. *Transactions of the American Ophthalmological Society.* Vol.72, pp.448-87. ISSN 0065-9533

Chan, HL. & Brown, B. (1998). Investigation of retinitis pigmentosa using the multifocal electroretinogram. *Ophthalmic & Physiological Optics.* Vol.18, No.4, pp.335-50. ISSN 0275-5408

Cideciyan, AV., Zhao, X., Nielsen, L., Khani, SC., Jacobson, SG. & Palczewski, K. (1998). Null mutation in the rhodopsin kinase gene slows recovery kinetics of rod and cone phototransduction in man. *Proceedings of the National Academy of Sciences of the United States of America.* Vol.95, No.1, pp.328-33. ISSN 0027-8424

Clarke, MP., Mitchell, KW. & McDonnell, S. (1996-1997). Electroretinographic findings in macular dystrophy. *Documenta Ophthalmologica.* Vol.92, No.4, pp.325-39. ISSN 0303-6405

Cremers, FP., van de Pol, DJ., van Kerkhoff, LP., Wieringa, B. & Ropers, HH. (1990). Cloning of a gene that is rearranged in patients with choroideraemia. *Nature.* Vol.347, No.6294, pp.674-7. ISSN 0028-0836

Daniele, S., Carbonara, A., Daniele, C., Restagno, G. & Orcidi, F. (1996). Pattern dystrophies of the retinal pigment epithelium. *Acta Ophthalmologica Scandinavica.* Vol.74, No.1, pp.51-5. ISSN:1395-3907

Deutman, AF. & Rümke. AM. (1969). Reticular dystrophy of the retinal pigment epithelium. Dystrophia reticularis laminae pigmentosa retinae of H. Sjogren. *Archives of Ophthalmology.* Vol.82, No.1, pp.4-9. ISSN 0093-0326

Deutman, AF., van Blommestein, JD., Henkes, HE., Waardenburg, PJ. & Solleveld-van Driest, E. (1970). Butterfly-shaped pigment dystrophy of the fovea. *Archives of Ophthalmology.* Vol.83, No.5, pp.558-69. ISSN 0093-0326

Deutman, AF. (1989) Macular dystrophies. In *Retina.* Vol.2(Ed.Ryan, SJ.) pp.264-268. CV Mosby, St. Louis, MO USA.

Deutman, AF. (1971) *The hereditary Dystrophies of the posterior pole of the eye.* pp.198-299. Thomas CC, Springfield.

Eagle, RC Jr., Lucier, AC., Bernardino, VB Jr. & Yanoff, M. (1980). Retinal pigment epithelial abnormalities in fundus flavimaculatus: a light and electron microscopic study. *Ophthalmology.* Vol.87, No.12, pp.1189-200. ISSN 0161-6420

Eksandh, L., Andréasson, S. & Abrahamson, M. (2005). Juvenile X-linked retinoschisis with normal scotopic b-wave in the electroretinogram at an early stage of the disease. *Ophthalmic genetics.* Vol.26, No.3, pp.111-7. ISSN 1381-6810

Eksandh, LC., Ponjavic, V., Ayyagari, R., Bingham, EL., Hiriyanna, KT., Andréasson, S., Ehinger, B. & Sieving, PA. (2000). Phenotypic expression of juvenile X-linked retinoschisis in Swedish families with different mutations in the XLRS1 gene. *Archives of Ophthalmology.* Vol.118, No.8, pp.1098-104. ISSN 0093-0326

Eldjarn, L., Stokke, O. & Try, K. (1966). Alpha-oxidation of branched chain fatty acids in man and its failure in patients with Refsum's disease showing phytanic acid accumulation. Scandinavian Journal of Clinical and Laboratory Investigation. Vol.18, No.6, pp.694-5. ISSN:0036-5513

Felbor, U., Stöhr, H., Aman, T., Schönherr, U., Apfelstedt-Sylla, E. & Weber, BH. (1996). A second independent Tyr168Cys mutation in the tissue inhibitor of metalloproteinases-3 (TIMP3) in Sorsby's fundus dystrophy. *Journal of Medical Genetics.* Vol.33, No.3, pp.233-6. ISSN 0022-2593

Felius, J. & Swanson, WH. (1999). Photopic temporal processing in retinitis pigmentosa. *Investigative Ophthalmology & Visual Sciences.* Vol.40, No.12, pp.2932-44. ISSN 0146-0404

Fish, G., Grey, R., Sehmi, KS. & Bird, AC. (1981). The dark choroid in posterior retinal dystrophies. *British Journal of Ophthalmology.* Vol.65, No.5, pp.359-63. ISSN 0007-1161

Fishman, GA., Alexander, KR. & Anderson, RJ. (1985). Autosomal dominant retinitis pigmentosa. A method of classification. *Archives of Ophthalmology.* Vol.103, No.3, pp.366-74. ISSN 0093-0326

Fishman, GA., Farbman, JS. & Alexander, KR. (1991). Delayed rod dark adaptation in patients with Stargardt's disease. *Ophthalmology.* Vol.98, No.6, pp.957-62. ISSN 0161-6420

Fishman, GA., Kumar, A., Joseph, ME., Torok, N. & Anderson, RJ. (1983). Usher's syndrome. Ophthalmic and neuro-otologic findings suggesting genetic heterogeneity. *Archives of Ophthalmology.* Vol.101, No.9, pp.1367-74. ISSN 0093-0326

Fishman, GA. (2001). The electroretinogram, In: *Electrophysiologic testing in disorders of the retina, optic nerve, and visual pathways*, Fishman GA, Birch DG, Holder GE, Brigell MG, pp. (1-155), American Academy of Ophthalmology, 1-56055-198-4, Singapore.

Franceschetti, A. & François, J. (1965). Fundus flavimaculatus. *Archives d'ophtalmologie et revue gènèrale d'ophtalmologie.* Vol.25, No.6, pp.505-30. ISSN 0003-973X

Franceschetti, A. (1962). A curious affection of the fundus oculi: helicoid peripapillar chorioretinal degeneration. Its relation to pigmentary paravenous chorioretinal degeneration. *Documenta Ophthalmologica.* Vol.16, pp.81-110. ISSN 0012-4486

Franceschetti, A. (1965). A special form of tapetoretinal degeneration: fundus flavimaculatus. *Transaction. Section on Ophthalmology. American Academy of Ophthalmology and Otolaryngology.* Vol.69, No.6, pp.1048-53. ISSN 0002-7154

Frank, HR., Landers, MB 3rd., Williams, RJ. & Sidbury, JB. (1974). A new dominant progressive foveal dystrophy. *American Journal of Ophthalmology.* Vol.78, No.6, pp.903-16. ISSN: 0002-9394

George, ND., Yates, JR. & Moore, AT. (1995). X linked retinoschisis. *British Journal of Ophthalmology.* Vol.79, No.7, pp.697-702. ISSN 0007-1161

Gerth, C., Zawadzki, RJ., Werner, JS. & Héon, E. (2008). Retinal morphological changes of patients with X-linked retinoschisis evaluated by Fourier-domain optical coherence tomography. *Archives of Ophthalmology*. Vol.126, No.6, pp.807-11. ISSN 0093-0326

Godel, V., Regenbogen, L., Adam, A. & Stein, R. (1976). Rod monochromatism -- an incomplete form. *Journal of Pediatric Ophthalmology*. Vol.13, No.4, pp.221-5. ISSN 0022-345X

Goodman, G., Ripps, H. & Siegel, IM. (1963). Cone Dysfunction Syndromes. *Archives of Ophthalmology*. Vol.70, pp.214-31. ISSN 0093-0326

Gouras, P., Carr, RE & Gunkel, RD. (1971). Retinitis pigmentosa in abetalipoproteinemia: Effects of vitamin A. *Investigative Ophthalmology & Visual Sciences*. Vol. 10, Number.10, pp. 784-793. ISSN 0146-0404.

Gouras, P., Eggers, HM. & MacKay, CJ. (1983). Cone dystrophy, nyctalopia, and supernormal rod responses. A new retinal degeneration. *Archives of Ophthalmology*. Vol.101, No.5, pp.718-24. ISSN 0093-0326

Gregory-Evans, K., Kelsel, RE., Gregory-Evans, CY., Downes, SM., Fitzke, FW., Holder, GE., Simunovic, M., Mollon, JD., Taylor, R., Hunt, DM., Bird, AC. & Moore, AT. (2000). Autosomal dominant cone-rod retinal dystrophy (CORD6) from heterozygous mutation of GUCY2D, which encodes retinal guanylate cyclase. *Ophthalmology*. Vol.107, No.1, pp.55-61. ISSN 0161-6420

Gundogan, FC., Dinç, UA., Erdem, U., Ozge, G. & Sobaci, G. (2010). Multifocal electroretinogram and central visual field testing in central areolar choroidal dystrophy. *European Journal of Ophthalmology. Vol.* 20, Number. 5, pp.919-24. ISSN 1120-6721.

Gundogan, FC., Tas, A & Sobaci G (2011). Cone dystrophy with supernormal rod electroretinogram. In print *Journal of Retina Vitreous*. ISSN 1300-1256

Haider, NB., Jacobson, SG., Cideciyan, AV., Swiderski, R., Streb, LM., Searby, C., Beck, G., Hockey, R., Hana, DB., Gorman, S., Duhl, D., Carmi, R., Bennett, J., Weleber, RG., Fishman, GA., Wright, AF., Stone, EM. & Sheffield, VC. (2000). Mutation of a nuclear receptor gene, NR2E3, causes enhanced S cone syndrome, a disorder of retinal cell fate. *Nature Genetics*. Vol.24, No.2, pp.127-31. ISSN 1061-4036.

Hamel, C. (2006). Retinitis pigmentosa. *Orphanet Journal of Rare Disease*. Vol.11, pp.1:40. ISSN 1750-1172.

Hayakawa, M.,Imai, Y., Wakita, M., Kato, K., Yanashima, K., Miyake, Y. & Kanai, A. (1992). A Japanese pedigree of autosomal dominant congenital stationary night blindness with variable expressivity. *Ophthalmic Paediatrics and Genetics*. Vol.13, No.4, pp.211-7. ISSN 0167-6784.

Heckenlively, JR. & Weleber, RG. (1986). X-linked recessive cone dystrophy with tapetal-like sheen. A newly recognized entity with Mizuo-Nakamura phenomenon. *Archives of Ophthalmology*. Vol.104, No.9, pp.1322-8. ISSN 0093-0326.

Heckenlively, JR. (2006). Cone dystrophies and degenerations, In: *Principles and practice of clinical electrophysiology of vision*, Heckenlively, JR., Arden, GB., pp. (795-802), The MIT pres, 0-262-08346-9, Cambridge.

Hirose, T., Lee, KY. & Schepens, CL. (1973). Wagner's hereditary vitreoretinal degeneration and retinal detachment. *Archives of Ophthalmology*. Vol.89, No.3, pp.176-85. ISSN 0093-0326

Holder, GE. (2001). Pattern electroretinography (PERG) and an integrated approach to visual pathway diagnosis. *Progress in Retinal and Eye Research*. Vol.20, No.4, pp.531-61. ISSN 1350-9462

Holder, GE. (2001). The pattern electroretinogram, In: *Electrophysiologic testing in disorders of the retina, optic nerve, and visual pathways*, Fishman GA, Birch DG, Holder GE, Brigell MG, pp. (197-235), American Academy of Ophthalmology, 1-56055-198-4, Singapore.

Holopigian, K., Seiple, W., Greenstein, VC., Hood, DC. & Carr, RE. (2001). Local cone and rod system function in patients with retinitis pigmentosa. *Investigative Ophthalmology & Visual Sciences*. Vol.42, No.3, pp.779-88. ISSN 0146-0404

Hood, DC., Holopigian, K., Greenstein, V., Seiple, W., Li, J., Sutter, EE. & Carr, RE. (1998). Assessment of local retinal function in patients with retinitis pigmentosa using the multi-focal ERG technique. *Vision Research*. Vol.38, No.1, pp.163-79. ISSN 0042-6989

Hoyng, CB. & Deutman, AF. (1996). The development of central areolar choroidal dystrophy. *Graefe's Archive for Clinical and Experimental Ophthalmology*. Vol.234, No.2, pp.87-93. ISSN 0721-832X

Hsieh, RC., Fine, BS. & Lyons, JS. (1977). Patterned dystrophies of the retinal pigment epithelium. *Archives of Ophthalmology*. Vol.95, No.3, pp.429-35. ISSN 0093-0326

Humphries, P., Kenna, P. & Farrar, GJ. (1992). On the molecular genetics of retinitis pigmentosa. *Science*. Vol.256, No.5058, pp.804-8. ISSN 0036-8075

Iijima, H., Yamaguchi, S. & Hosaka, O. (1993). Photopic electroretinogram implicit time in retinitis pigmentosa. *Japanese Journal of Ophthalmology*. Vol.37, No.2, pp.130-5. ISSN 0021-5155

Itabashi, R., Katsumi, O., Mehta, MC., Wajima, R., Tamai, M. & Hirose, T. (1993). Stargardt's disease/fundus flavimaculatus: psychophysical and electrophysiologic results. *Graefe's Archive for Clinical and Experimental Ophthalmology*. Vol.231, No.10, pp.555-62. ISSN 0721-832X

Jacobson, SG., Román, AJ., Román, MI., Gass, JD. & Parker, JA. (1991). Relatively enhanced S cone function in the Goldmann-Favre syndrome. *American Journal of Ophthalmology*. Vol.111, No.4, pp.446-53. ISSN: 0002-9394

Jarc-Vidmar, M.,Popović, P.,Hawlina, M., Brecelj, J (2001). Pattern ERG and psychophysical functions in Best's disease. Documenta Ophthalmologica. Vol. 103, No: 1, pp: 47-61. ISSN 0012-4486

Kaiser-Kupfer, MI., Caruso, RC. & Vale, D. (1991). Gyrate atrophy of the choroid and retina. Long-term reduction of ornithine slows retinal degeneration. *Archives of Ophthalmology*. Vol.109, No.11, pp.1539-48. ISSN 0093-0326

Kandori, F., Setogawa, T. & Tamai, A. (1966). Electroretinographical studies on "fleck retina with congenital nonprogressive nightblindness". *Yonago Acta Medica*. Vol.10, No.2, pp.98-108. ISSN 0513-5710

Kandori, F., Tamai, A., Watanabe, T. & Kurimoto, S. (1968). Unilateral pigmentary degeneration of the retina. Report of two cases. *American Journal of Ophthalmology*. Vol.66, No.6, pp.1091-101. ISSN: 0002-9394

Keating, D., Parks, S. (2006). Multifocal Techniques, In: *Principles and practice of clinical electrophysiology of vision*, Heckenlively, JR., Arden, GB., pp. (319-351), The MIT pres, 0-262-08346-9, Cambridge.

Kellner, U. & Foerster, MH. (1993). Cone dystrophies with negative photopic electroretinogram. *British Journal of Ophthalmology.* Vol.77, No.7, pp.404-9. ISSN 0007-1161

Kim, LS., Seiple, W., Fishman, GA & Szlyk, JP (2007). Multifocal ERG findings in carriers of X- linked retinoschisis. *Documenta Ophthalmologica.* Vol. 114, Number. 1, pp.:21-26.ISSN 0012-4486

Kimberling, WJ., Möller, CG., Davenport, SL., Lund, G., Grissom, TJ., Priluck, I., White, V., Weston, MD., Biscone-Halterman, K. & Brookhouser, PE. (1989). Usher syndrome: clinical findings and gene localization studies. The *Laryngoscope.* Vol.99, No.1, pp.66-72. ISSN 0023-852X

Kingham, JD., Fenzl, RE., Willerson, D. & Aaberg, TM. (1978). Reticular dystrophy of the retinal pigment epithelium. A clinical and electrophysiologic study of three generations. *Archives of Ophthalmology.* Vol.96, No.7, pp.1177-84. ISSN 0093-0326

Kjellström, S., Vijayasarathy, C., Ponjavic, V., Sieving, PA. & Andréasson, S (2010). Long-term 12 year follow-up of X-linked congenital retinoschisis. *Ophthalmic genetics.* Vol.31, No.3, pp.114-25. ISSN 1381-6810

Kolb, H. & Galloway, NR. (1964). Three Cases Of Unilateral Pigmentary Degeneration. *British Journal of Ophthalmology.* Vol.48, pp.471-9. ISSN 0007-1161

Kondo, M., Miyake, Y., Horiguchi, M., Suzuki, S. & Tanikawa, A. (1995). Clinical evaluation of multifocal electroretinogram. *Investigative Ophthalmology & Visual Sciences.* Vol.36, No.10, pp.2146-50. ISSN 0146-0404

Kretschmann, U., Seeliger, MW., Ruether, K., Usui, T., Apfelstedt-Sylla, E. & Zrenner, E. (1998). Multifocal electroretinography in patients with Stargardt's macular dystrophy. *British Journal of Ophthalmology.* Vol.82, No.3, pp.267-75. ISSN 0007-1161

Lachapelle, P., Little, JM. & Roy, MS. (1989). The electroretinogram in Stargardt's disease and fundus flavimaculatus. *Documenta Ophthalmologica.* Vol.73, No.4, pp.395-404. ISSN 0012-4486

Ladekjaer-Mikkelsen AS, Rosenberg T, Jørgensen AL. A new mechanism in blue cone monochromatism. *Hum Genet.* 1996 Oct;98(4):403-8.

Lam BL. (2005). *Electrophysiology of Vision: Clinical testing and applications,* Taylor & Francis, 0-8247-4068-8, New York.

Lefler, WH., Wadsworth, JA. & Sidbury, JB Jr. (1971). Hereditary macular degeneration and amino-aciduria. *American Journal of Ophthalmology.* Vol.71(1 Pt 2), pp.224-30. ISSN: 0002-9394

Lois, N., Holder, GE., Bunce, C., Fitzke, FW. & Bird, AC. (2001). Phenotypic subtypes of Stargardt macular dystrophy-fundus flavimaculatus. *Archives of Ophthalmology.* Vol.119, No.3, pp.359-69. ISSN 0093-0326

MacDonald, IM., Russell, L. & Chan, CC. (2009). Choroideremia: new findings from ocular pathology and review of recent literature. *Survey of Ophthalmology.* Vol.54, No.3, pp.401-7. ISSN 0039-6257

Marmor, MF., Jacobson, SG., Foerster, MH., Kellner, U. & Weleber, RG. (1990). Diagnostic clinical findings of a new syndrome with night blindness, maculopathy, and enhanced S cone sensitivity. *American Journal of Ophthalmology.* Vol.110, No.2, pp.124-34. ISSN: 0002-9394

Marmor, MF. (1989). Large rod-like photopic signals in a possible new form of congenital night blindness. *Documenta Ophthalmologica.* Vol.71, No.3, pp.265-9. ISSN 0012-4486

Marmor, MF. (1979). The electroretinogram in retinitis pigmentosa. *Archives of Ophthalmology*. Vol.97, No.7, pp.1300-4. ISSN 0093-0326

Marmor, MF., Fulton, AB., Holder, GE., Miyake, Y. & Brigell, M. (2009). ISCEV Standard for full-field clinical electroretinography (2008 update). *Documenta Ophthalmologica,* Vol. 118, No. 1, pp. 69-77. ISSN 0012-4486

Mashima, Y., Murakami, A., Weleber, RG., Kennaway, NG., Clarke, L., Shiono, T. & Inana, G. (1992). Nonsense-codon mutations of the ornithine aminotransferase gene with decreased levels of mutant mRNA in gyrate atrophy. *American Journal of Human Genetics*. Vol.51, No.1, pp.81-91. ISSN 0002-9297

Miyake, Y., Horiguchi, M., Suzuki, S., Kondo, M. & Tanikawa, A. (1996). Electrophysiological findings in patients with Oguchi's disease. *Japanese Journal of Ophthalmology*. Vol.40, No.4, pp.511-9. ISSN 0021-5155

Miyake, Y., Horiguchi, M., Terasaki, H. & Kondo, M. (1994). Scotopic threshold response in complete and incomplete types of congenital stationary night blindness. *Investigative Ophthalmology & Visual Sciences*. Vol.35, No.10, pp.3770-5. ISSN 0146-0404

Miyake, Y., Yagasaki, K., Horiguchi, M., Kawase, Y. & Kanda, T. (1986). Congenital stationary night blindness with negative electroretinogram. A new classification. *Archives of Ophthalmology*. Vol.104, No.7, pp.1013-20. ISSN 0093-0326

Miyake, Y., Yagasaki, K., Horiguchi, M. & Kawase, Y. (1987). On- and off-responses in photopic electroretinogram in complete and incomplete types of congenital stationary night blindness. *Japanese Journal of Ophthalmology*. Vol.31, No.1, pp.81-7. ISSN 0021-5155

Miyake, Y. (2006). Chorioretinal disorders, In: *Electrodiagnosis of retinal diseases,* Miyake, Y, pp. (331-342), Springer, 4-431-25466-8, Japan.

Miyake, Y. (2006). Retinitis pigmentosa and pigmentary retinopathies In: *Electrodiagnosis of retinal diseases,* Miyake, Y, pp. (191-242), Springer, 4-431-25466-8, Japan.

Moore, AT. (1992). Cone and cone-rod dystrophies. *Journal of Medical Genetics*. Vol.29, No.5, pp.289-90. ISSN 0022-2593

Moskowitz, A., Hansen, RM., Akula, JD., Eklund, SE. & Fulton, AB. (2009). Rod and rod-driven function in achromatopsia and blue cone monochromatism. *Investigative Ophthalmology & Visual Sciences*. Vol.50, No.2, pp.950-8. ISSN 0146-0404

Mukkamala, K., Gentile, RC., Willner, J. & Tsang, S. (2010). Choroideremia in a woman with ectodermal dysplasia and complex translocations involving chromosomes X, 1, and 3. *Ophthalmic genetics*. Vol.31, No.4, pp.178-82. ISSN 1381-6810

Mura, M., Sereda, C., Jablonski, MM., MacDonald, IM. & Iannaccone, A. (2007). Clinical and functional findings in choroideremia due to complete deletion of the CHM gene. *Archives of Ophthalmology*. Vol.125, No.8, pp.1107-13. ISSN 0093-0326

Nagasaka, K., Horiguchi, M., Shimada, Y. & Yuzawa, M. (2003). Multifocal electroretinograms in cases of central areolar choroidal dystrophy. *Investigative Ophthalmology & Visual Sciences*. Vol.44, No.4, pp.1673-9. ISSN 0146-0404

Nakamura, M. & Miyake, Y. (2002). Macular dystrophy in a 9-year-old boy with fundus albipunctatus. *American Journal of Ophthalmology*. Vol.133, No.2, pp.278-80. ISSN: 0002-9394

Nakamura, M., Skalet, J. & Miyake, Y. (2003). RDH5 gene mutations and electroretinogram in fundus albipunctatus with or without macular dystrophy: RDH5 mutations and

ERG in fundus albipunctatus. *Documenta Ophthalmologica.* Vol.107, No.1, pp.3-11. ISSN 0012-4486

Nakazato, H., Hanazaki, H., Kawasaki, K., Tanabe, J & Yonemura D (1986). Electroretinographic off-response in congenital red-green color deficiency and its genetic carrier. *Documenta Ophthalmologica* Vol. 63, No.2 , pp. 179-186 ISSN 0012-4486

Nathans, J., Piantanida, TP., Eddy, RL., Shows, TB. & Hogness, DS. (1986). Molecular genetics of inherited variation in human color vision. *Science.* Vol.232, No.4747, pp.203-10. ISSN 0036-8075

Nathans, J., Thomas, D. & Hogness, DS. (1986). Molecular genetics of human color vision: the genes encoding blue, green, and red pigments. *Science.* Vol.232, No.4747, pp.193-202. ISSN 0036-8075

Noble, KG., Carr, RE. & Siegel, IM. (1990). Autosomal dominant congenital stationary night blindness and normal fundus with an electronegative electroretinogram. *American Journal of Ophthalmology.* Vol.109, No.1, pp.44-8. ISSN: 0002-9394

Noble, KG. & Carr, RE. (1983). Pigmented paravenous chorioretinal atrophy. *American Journal of Ophthalmology.* Vol.96, No.3, pp.338-44. ISSN: 0002-9394

Noble, KG. (1977). Central areolar choroidal dystrophy. *American Journal of Ophthalmology.* Vol.84, No.3, pp.310-8. ISSN: 0002-9394

Nussbaum, JJ., Ferencz, JR., Maeda, K. & Weiss, L. (1991). Autosomal dominant crystalline dystrophy. Richards BW, Brodstein DE. *Ophthalmology.* Vol.98, No.5, pp.658-65. ISSN 0161-6420

Ohkubo, H. & Tanino, T. (1987). Electrophysiological findings in familial exudative vitreoretinopathy. *Documenta Ophthalmologica.* Vol.65, No.4, pp.461-9. ISSN 0012-4486

Palmowski, AM., Allgayer, R., Heinemann-Vernaleken, B., Scherer, V. & Ruprecht, KW. (2003). Detection of retinal dysfunction in vitelliform macular dystrophy using the multifocal ERG (MF-ERG). *Documenta Ophthalmologica.* Vol.106, No.2, pp.145-52. ISSN 0012-4486

Petzold, A. & Plant, GT. (2006). Clinical disorders affecting mesopic vision. *Ophthalmic & Physiological Optics.* May;26(3):326-41. ISSN 0275-5408

Ponjavic, V., Andréasson, S. & Ehinger, B. (1994). Full-field electroretinograms in patients with central areolar choroidal dystrophy. *Acta Ophthalmologica (Copenh).* Vol.72, No.5, pp.537-44. ISSN 0001-639X

Quigley, M., Roy, MS., Barsoum-Homsy, M., Chevrette, L., Jacob, JL. & Milot, J. (1996-1997). On- and off-responses in the photopic electroretinogram in complete-type congenital stationary night blindness. *Documenta Ophthalmologica.* Vol.92, No.3, pp.159-65. ISSN 0012-4486

Rabb, MF., Mullen, L., Yelchits, S., Udar, N. & Small, KW. (1998). A North Carolina macular dystrophy phenotype in a Belizean family maps to the MCDR1 locus. *American Journal of Ophthalmology.* Vol.125, No.4, pp.502-8. ISSN 0002-9394

Refsum, S. (1981). Heredopathia atactica polyneuritiformis phytanic-acid storage disease, Refsum's disease:" a biochemically well-defined disease with a specific dietary treatment. *Archives of Neurology.* Vol.38, No.10, pp.605-6. ISSN 0003-9942

Riggs, LA. (1954). Electroretinography in cases of night blindness. *American Journal of Ophthalmology.* Vol.38, No.1:2, pp.70-8. ISSN: 0002-9394

Robson, AG., Webster, AR., Michaelides, M., Downes, SM., Cowing, JA., Hunt, DM., Moore, AT. & Holder, GE. (2010). "Cone dystrophy with supernormal rod electroretinogram": a comprehensive genotype/phenotype study including fundus autofluorescence and extensive electrophysiology. *Retina.* Vol.30, No.1, pp.51-62. ISSN 0275-004X

Rosenberg, T., Haim, M., Piczenik, Y. & Simonsen, SE. (1991). Autosomal dominant stationary night-blindness. A large family rediscovered. *Acta Ophthalmologica (Copenh).* Vol.69, No.6, pp.694-702. ISSN 0001-639X

Rosner, M., Hefetz, L. & Abraham, FA. (1993). The prevalence of retinitis pigmentosa and congenital stationary night blindness in Israel. *American Journal of Ophthalmology.* Vol.116, No.3, pp.373-4. ISSN: 0002-9394

Runge, P., Muller, DP., McAllister, J., Calver, D., Lloyd, JK. & Taylor, D. (1986). Oral vitamin E supplements can prevent the retinopathy of abetalipoproteinaemia. *British Journal of Ophthalmology.* Vol.70, No.3, pp.166-73. ISSN 0007-1161

Sandberg, MA., Pawlyk, BS., Dan, J., Arnaud, B., Dryja, TP. & Berson, EL. (1998). Rod and cone function in the Nougaret form of stationary night blindness. *Archives of Ophthalmology.* Vol.116, No.7, pp.867-72. ISSN 0093-0326

Sankila, EM., Pakarinen, L., Kääriäinen, H., Aittomäki, K., Karjalainen, S., Sistonen, P. & de la Chapelle, A. (1995). Assignment of an Usher syndrome type III (USH3) gene to chromosome 3q. *Human Molecular Genetics.* Vol.4, No.1, pp.93-8. ISSN 0964-6906

Scholl, HP., Schuster, AM., Vonthein, R. & Zrenner, E. (2002). Mapping of retinal function in Best macular dystrophy using multifocal electroretinography. *Vision Research.* Vol.42, No.8, pp.1053-61. ISSN 0042-6989

Seeliger, MW., Zrenner, E., Apfelstedt-Sylla, E. & Jaissle, GB. (2001). Identification of Usher syndrome subtypes by ERG implicit time. *Investigative Ophthalmology & Visual Sciences.* Vol.42, No.12, pp.3066-71. ISSN 0146-0404

Shiono, T., Ishikawa, A., Hara, S. & Tamai, M. (1990). Pattern dystrophy of the retinal pigment epithelium. *Retina.* Vol.10, No.4, pp.251-4. ISSN 0275-004X

Sieving, PA., Niffenegger, JH. & Berson, EL. (1986). Electroretinographic findings in selected pedigrees with choroideremia. *American Journal of Ophthalmology.* Vol.101, No.3, pp.361-7. ISSN 0002-9394

Simell, O. & Takki, K. (1973). Raised plasma-ornithine and gyrate atrophy of the choroid and retina. *Lancet.* Vol.1, No.7811, pp.1031-3. ISSN 0140-6736

Simunovic, MP. & Moore, AT. (1998). The cone dystrophies. *Eye (London, England).* Vol.12, No. (Pt 3b), pp.553-65. ISSN 0950-222X

Sivaprasad, S., Webster, AR., Egan, CA., Bird, AC. & Tufail, A. (2008). Clinical course and treatment outcomes of Sorsby fundus dystrophy. *American Journal of Ophthalmology.* Vol.146, No.2, pp.228-234. Epub 2008 May 23. ISSN: 0002-9394

Skalka, HW. (1979). Hereditary pigmented paravenous retinochoroidal atrophy. *American Journal of Ophthalmology.* Vol.87, No.3, pp.286-91. ISSN 0002-9394

Slezak, H. & Homer, K. (1969). [Fundus pulverulentus]. *Albrecht Von Graefe's Archive for Clinical and Experimental Ophthalmology.* Vol.178, No.2, pp.176-82. ISSN 0065-6100

Small, KW., Weber, J., Roses, A. & Pericak-Vance, P. (1993). North Carolina macular dystrophy (MCDR1). A review and refined mapping to 6q14-q16.2. *Ophthalmic Paediatrics and Genetics.* Vol.14, No.4, pp.143-50. ISSN 0167-6784

Sorsby, A. & Mason, ME. (1949). A fundus dystrophy with unusual features. *British Journal of Ophthalmology*. Vol.33, No.2, pp.67-97. ISSN 0007-1161

Stickler, GB., Belau, PG., Farrell, FJ., Jones, JD., Pugh, DG., Steinberg, AG. & Ward, LE. (1965). Hereditary Progressive Arthro-Ophthalmopathy. *Mayo Clinic Proceedings*. Vol.40, pp.433-55. ISSN 0025-6196

Sutter, EE. & Tran, D. (1992). The field topography of ERG components in man--I. The photopic luminance response. *Vision Research*. Vol.32, No.3, pp.433-46. ISSN 0042-6989

Swain, PK., Chen, S., Wang, QL., Affatigato, LM., Coats, CL., Brady, KD., Fishman, GA., Jacobson, SG., Swaroop, A., Stone, E., Sieving, PA. & Zack, DJ. (1997). Mutations in the cone-rod homeobox gene are associated with the cone-rod dystrophy photoreceptor degeneration. *Neuron*. Vol.19, No.6, pp.1329-36. ISSN 0896-6273

Syed, N., Smith, JE., John, SK., Seabra, MC., Aguirre, GD. & Milam, AH. (2001). Evaluation of retinal photoreceptors and pigment epithelium in a female carrier of choroideremia. *Ophthalmology*. Vol.108, No.4, pp.711-20. ISSN 0161-6420

The Retinoschisis Consortium. (1998). Functional implications of the spectrum of mutations found in 234 cases with X-linked juvenile retinoschisis. *Human Molecular Genetics*. Vol.7, No.7, pp.1185-92. ISSN 0964-6906

Van Aarem, A., Wagenaar, M., Pinckers, AJ., Huygen, PL., Bleeker-Wagemakers, EM., Kimberling, BJ. & Cremers, CW. (1995). Ophthalmologic findings in Usher syndrome type 2A. *Ophthalmic genetics*. Vol.16, No.4, pp.151-8. ISSN 1381-6810

van Nouhuys, CE. (1982). Dominant exudative vitreoretinopathy and other vascular developmental disorders of the peripheral retina. *Documenta Ophthalmologica*. Vol.54, No.(1-4), pp.1-414. ISSN 0012-4486

Watzke, RC., Folk, JC. & Lang, RM. (1982). Pattern dystrophy of the retinal pigment epithelium. *Ophthalmology*. Vol.89, No.12, pp.1400-6. ISSN 0161-6420

Weingeist, TA., Kobrin, JL. & Watzke, RC. (1982). Histopathology of Best's macular dystrophy. *Archives of Ophthalmology*. Vol.100, No.7, pp.1108-14. ISSN 0093-0326

Weleber, RG. (2002). Infantile and childhood retinal blindness: a molecular perspective (The Franceschetti Lecture). *Ophthalmic genetics*. Vol.23, No.2, pp.71-97. ISSN 1381-6810

Weleber, RG., Francis, P. (2006). Differential diagnosis of the electronegative electroretinogram, In: *Principles and practice of clinical electrophysiology of vision*, Heckenlively, JR., Arden, GB., pp. (809-822), The MIT pres, 0-262-08346-9, Cambridge.

Wilson, DJ., Weleber, RG., Klein, ML., Welch, RB. & Gren, WR. (1989). Bietti's crystalline dystrophy. A clinicopathologic correlative study. *Archives of Ophthalmology*. Vol.107, No.2, pp.213-21. ISSN 0093-0326

Wissinger, B., Dangel, S., Jägle, H., Hansen, L., Baumann, B., Rudolph, G., Wolf, C., Bonin, M., Koeppen, K., Ladewig, T., Kohl, S., Zrenner, E. & Rosenberg, T. (2008). Cone dystrophy with supernormal rod response is strictly associated with mutations in KCNV2. *Investigative Ophthalmology & Visual Sciences*. Vol.49, No.2, pp.751-7. ISSN 0146-0404

Wu, WW., Wong, JP., Kast, J., Molday, RS. (2005). RS1, a discoidin domain-containing retinal cell adhesion protein associated with X-linked retinoschisis, exists as a novel disulfide-linked octamer. The *Journal of Biological Chemistry*. Vol.280, No.11, pp.10721-30. ISSN 0021-9258

Wutz, K., Sauer, C., Zrenner, E., Lorenz, B., Alitalo, T., Broghammer, M., Hergersberg, M., de la Chapelle, A., Weber, BH., Wissinger, B., Meindl, A. & Pusch, CM. (2002). Thirty distinct CACNA1F mutations in 33 families with incomplete type of XLCSNB and Cacna1f expression profiling in mouse retina. *European Journal of Human Genetics.* Vol.10, No.8, pp.449-56. ISSN 1018-4813

Zeitz, C., van Genderen, M., Neidhardt, J., Luhmann, UF., Hoeben, F., Forster, U., Wycisk, K., Mátyás, G., Hoyng, CB., Riemslag, F., Meire, F., Cremers, FP. & Berger, W. (2005). Mutations in GRM6 cause autosomal recessive congenital stationary night blindness with a distinctive scotopic 15-Hz flicker electroretinogram. *Investigative Ophthalmology & Visual Sciences.* Vol.46, No.11, pp.4328-35. ISSN 0146-0404

7

Molecular Modeling of Protein Structure, Biology of Disease and Clinical Electroretinography in Human X-Linked Retinoschisis (XLRS)

Yuri V. Sergeev[1], Kristen E. Bowles[1],
Lucia Ziccardi[2] and Paul A. Sieving[1,2]
[1]*Ophthalmic Genetics and Visual Function Branch, National Eye Institute*
[2]*Section of Translational Research in Retina & Macular Degeneration*
National Institute on Deafness and Other Communication Disorders
National Institutes of Health, Bethesda, Maryland
USA

1. Introduction

We describe a promising approach using *in silico* structure-function studies of protein atomic structure and computational medicine to understand disease. *In silico* studies use an atomic structure of proteins and molecular modeling for structure-function analysis. This approach is critical for large-scale genetic studies in order to understand a possible functional role of genetic mutations. Indeed, structural changes associated with missense mutations might impact protein folding, protein-protein interaction sites, or solubility or stability of protein molecules. The structural effect of mutational changes can be analyzed *in silico* on the basis of 3-dimensional structure, multiple alignments of homologous sequences, molecular modeling, and molecular dynamics simulations. The parameters derived from 3-dimensional protein structure could be used in clinical studies to predict a severity of protein structure-function changes caused by genetic mutations and evaluate genotype-to-phenotype relationships. In this chapter, we use X-linked retinoschisis (XLRS) as our disease model. XLRS is a form of juvenile macular and retinal degeneration in which schisis or splitting within the retinal layers leads to early and progressive vision loss. XLRS is a rare disease estimated to affect 1:5000 males (George et al., 1995; Wang et al., 2002) and is a disease with considerable clinical and electrophysiological variation. Precise analysis of XLRS is pertinent to identify disease severity and genotype-phenotype correlation. Due to the lack of a protein assay, a correlation between phenotype and genotype is difficult. Advances in molecular modeling give new insight to mutation severity at atomic level and provide a possible connection between genotype-phenotype correlations. This creates the hope that disease risk assessment at the atomic level will be a reality in the future. For our study, we use the electroretinogram (ERG) for our phenotypical data set, which we correlated with expected mutation severity.

2. Biological factors and electroretinography of XLRS

2.1 Biology of retinoschisin protein: secretion and expression, hypothesized function, underlying mechanisms of functional loss of RS1 protein

Retinoschisin (RS1) is a retinal secreted photoreceptor disulphide-linked oligomeric protein. A number of mutations in RS1 co-segregate with XLRS providing strong evidence that the disease is caused by mutations in the *RS1* gene (Sauer et al., 1997). Although inherited mutations in the *RS1* gene have been shown to cause an XLRS phenotype, the functional impact of most missense variants that result in a single amino acid change is less well defined. RS1 is a 24-kDa secreted protein which is expressed exclusively in the retina (Reid et al., 1999), pineal gland (Takada et al., 2006), and uterus (Huopaniemi et al., 1999). In retinal layers it is found in photoreceptor cells and in neurons of the inner retina (Figure 1). It encodes a conserved discoidin domain homologous to proteins involved in cell adhesion and cell–cell interactions. Based on its structural features, RS1 is believed to hold retinal cells together, to preserve the retinal architecture, and to function as an adhesive protein for the structural and functional integrity of the retina (Molday et al., 2007; Vijayasarathy et al., 2007). It may mediate the association of the extracellular matrix with the surface of photoreceptors and other retinal cells to promote cell adhesion and thereby stabilize the cellular architecture of the highly structured retinal tissues. There exist three primary mechanisms that may be responsible for the loss of function of the RS1 protein: the misfolding of the discoidin domain, which negatively influences the putative adhesive properties of the protein; the defective disulfide-linked subunit assembly of RS1 into dimers and octamers; or the inability of RS1 to insert into endoplasmic reticulum membrane as part of the protein secretion process.

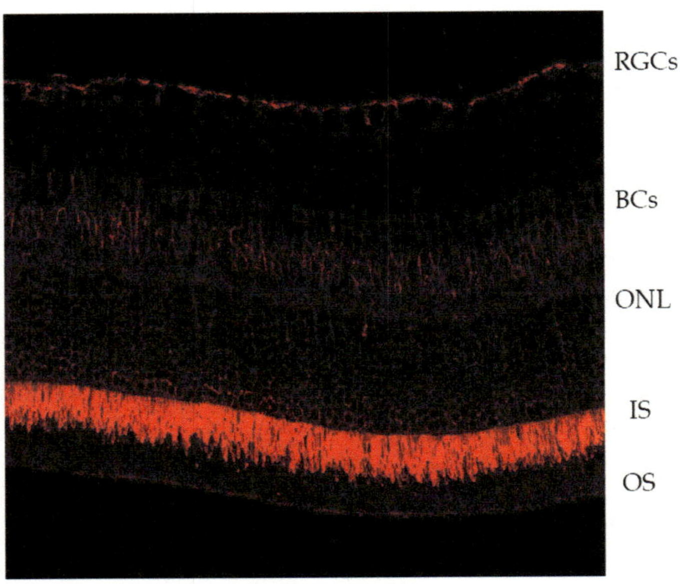

Fig. 1. RS1 labeling in a wild-type mouse. Immunohistochemistry with antibody raised against RS1 protein. RS1 labeling in a normal adult C57BL/6J mouse retina, displayed by confocal microscopy, is observed in all retinal layers. On the right are shown RGCs: retinal ganglion cells, BCs: bipolar cells, ONL: outer nuclear layer, IS: inner segments, OS: outer segments.

2.2 Retinal morphology in retinoschisis: photoreceptors disruption and altered photoreceptor/bipolar cells synapse in the RS1-KO mouse

Currently, there are three mouse models of human XLRS. One has been generated by homologus DNA insertion across the endogenous *RS1* gene (Weber et al., 2002), presenting a phenotype consisting of abnormal retinal architecture with schisis in the inner nuclear layer, reduced outer segment layer thickness, loss of photoreceptors, and a selective ERG b-wave reduction with relative sparing of the a-wave similar to XLRS male subjects. A second *RS1* knock-out mouse model (Zeng et al., 2004) was created by substituting a neomycin resistance cassette for exon 1 and 1.6 kb in intron 1 of RS1h, the murine orthologue of the human *RS1* gene. This model also displayed structural and functional features similar to those of human XLRS, including the electronegative ERG waveform and splitting in the inner nuclear layer similar to retinoschisis cavities by 6 months of age. They also demonstrated displacement of cells from the photoreceptor outer nuclear layer (ONL) and reduced thickness of the outer segment layer (Zeng et al., 2004). More recently, a third mouse model was generated using an ENU mutagenesis approach (Jablonski et al., 2005) derived from an induced mutation in intron 2 of RS1h, which leads to two novel splice variants. It is remarkable that, similar to the human condition, male homozygous mutant mice have retinal abnormalities as early as two weeks of age which do not appear to progress up to 38 weeks.

2.3 Clinical features of XLRS disease: visual acuity, visual field, OCT, fundus appearance, ERG

XLRS classical phenotype is present in two-thirds or more of affected males (George et al., 1996) and consists in an early-onset central vision loss from bilateral foveo-macular cystic cavities involving the inner retina and additional retinal layers (Gregori et al., 2009) that extend from the fovea in a spoke-wheel pattern for approximately 1-1.5 disc diameter (Figure 2).

XLRS patients often have hyperopic refractive error with astigmatism (Roesch et al., 1998; Kato et al., 2001; Vijayasarathy et al., 2009). Visual acuity ranging between 20/20 to 20/200 in young patients, who come to ophthalmological attention because of reading difficulty, due to the macular involvement of the disease. Patients typically exhibit modest severity at a young age (cystic form), with a slow progression until the second decade, when most retain around 20/70 vision. It worsens through the teenage years and stabilizes in adulthood when the atrophic stage can lead to legal blindness (Lesch et al., 2008). However, some XLRS males exhibit unpredictable, severe disease even at very early age, and surprisingly, the ERG can show an unexpected preservation of the scotopic b-wave (Eksandh et al., 2005; Sieving et al., 1999a).

XLRS is a highly penetrant disease condition (Forsius et al., 1973). In some cases subtle retinal changes are difficult to identify by ophthalmoscopy and can be detected only by optical coherence tomography (OCT) scans (Eriksson et al., 2004) (Figure 2). In the late stages of the disease when macular atrophy starts, a hyperfluorescent window defect of the retinal pigment epithelium (RPE) on fluoresceine angiography (FA) can be observed. This feature, however, can mimic retinal abnormalities seen in age-related macular degeneration or Stargardt maculopathy. In such cases, the combination of ERG, FA, and OCT is needed to determine the correct diagnosis. The electronegative scotopic ERG is pathognomonic of XLRS; the FA will not exhibit the dark choroid sign that is typically present in Stargardt's maculopathy; and the OCT can detect cysts otherwise undetectable by standard ophthalmoscopy. Peripheral retinoschisis can be found in half of affected males. Retinal splitting can involve all the retinal layers through the nerve fiber layer. The consequent abnormal visual signaling causes an dense scotoma in the involved areas (Li et al., 2007). Sometimes peripheral retinal scars, possibly to be considered pre-existing areas of self-limited schisis, can be observed.

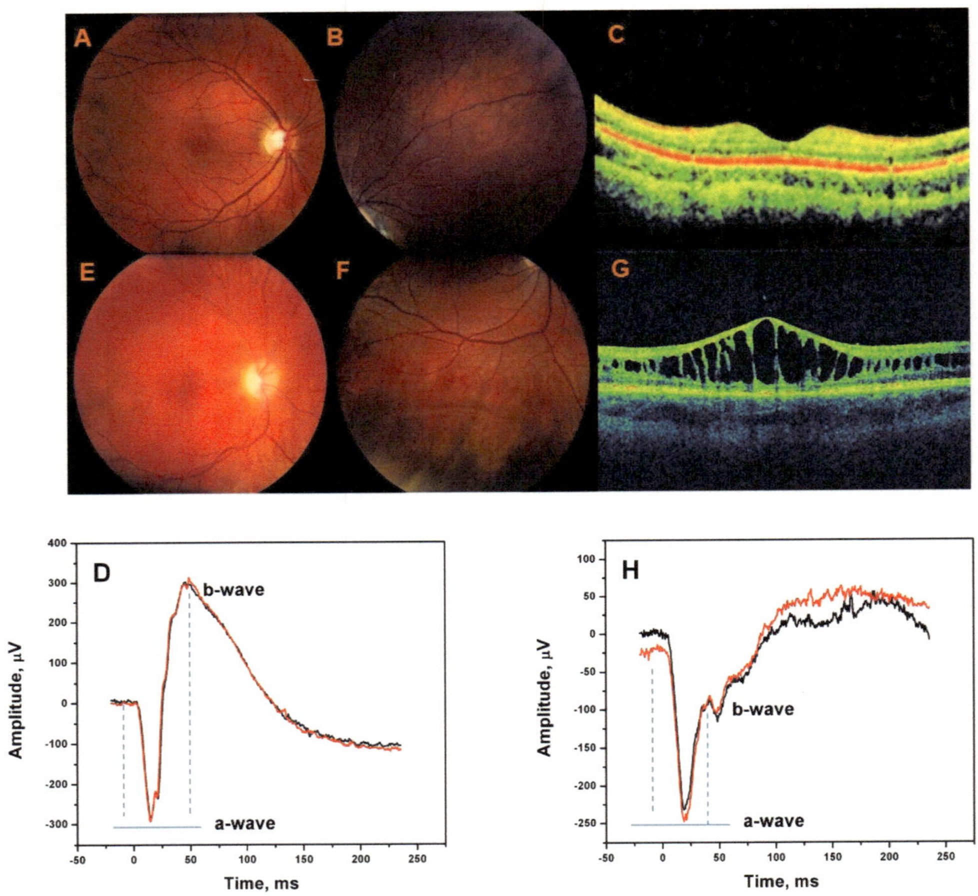

Fig. 2. Collage of Prototypical Fundus (A, B, E, F), OCT (C, G) and ERG (D, H) in normal and in affected by XLRS individuals. Panels A-D and E-H correspond to the normal and the XLRS affected individuals, respectively.

2.4 Photoreceptor and bipolar cell function as seen in the full field ERG

The ERG is a useful tool for evaluate outer retinal function and may assist in identifying the primary sight of XLRS pathology. Through the interpretation of the ERG, one can pinpoint disease at the cellular level in outer retinal visual loss and monitor disease progression. The ERG is a good phenotypical measurement in wide spread disease due to its objective nature and ability to measure function of the entire retina. To better understand the pathology behind the characteristic electronegative ERG in XLRS, one must first understand normal retinal physiology. In a dark-adapted retina, free flowing ions move to and from the rod photoreceptor. When rhodopsin in the rod photoreceptor captures a photon of light, it undergoes a conformational change causing a cascade of intracellular events within the photoreceptor outer segment resulting in hyperpolarization of the cell. Rod hyperpolarization causes an increased ionic potential towards the distal retina that results in the a-wave (Breton et al., 1994; Hagins et al., 1970). The rod then signals the on-bipolar cell which depolarizes and causes an influx of ions into the proximal retina. This forms the ERG b-wave. In XLRS, the b-wave amplitude is smaller than the a-wave amplitude (i.e. does not return to pre-flash baseline) and is deemed 'electronegative' (Figure 2H). An electronegative ERG suggests dysfunction proximal to the rod outer segment.

2.5 Bipolar cell dysfunction and "electronegative" b-wave in both human and murine model of XLRS

In the retina of the RS1-deficient mouse and the XLRS human the reduced scotopic ERG b-wave amplitude (Figure 2H) suggests an effect on bipolar-cell function, perhaps initiated from an altered photoreceptor/bipolar-cell synapse activity. This implies primary involvement of the inner retina where schisis cavities occur in XLRS. The identification of L-type voltage-gated calcium channels (Shi et al., 2009), Na/K ATPase (alpha3, beta2 isoforms) (Friedrich et al.), the sterile alpha and TIR motif-containing protein SARM1 (Molday, 2007), and phospholipids/Ca^{2+} (Vijayasarathy et al., 2007) as potential RS1 interacting ligands corroborate a role for RS1 in cell signaling events as well. However, ERG show considerable variation in this disease and ophthalmologists have to be aware about the possibility of relative ERG b-wave preservation especially in presence of atypical or mild manifestation of the disease (Eksandh et al., 2005; Sieving et al., 1999a; Vijayasarathy et al., 2009). These observations may imply that the degree of ERG dysfunctions may not correlate with the extent of fundus involvement and that synaptic integrity might be impaired secondarily over a greater extent of the fundus. In addition, because disruption of the inner segment architecture due to the loss of RS1 might be the basic mechanism that underlies the displacement and disorganization of photoreceptors in RS1-deficient mouse retina, reduced ERG a-wave responses can be found (Kjellstrom et al., 2007b). Clinically, abnormal photoreceptor function has been described in some XLRS subjects (Bradshaw et al., 1999; Kellner et al., 1990) mostly related to the advanced stages of the disease (Peachey et al., 1987) when the outer retinal atrophy may occur.

2.6 The significance of phenotypic b/a-wave ratio

In retina electrophysiology signal transmission between rod photoreceptors and the post-synaptic bipolar cell neurons is measured by the amplitudes of the a-wave and b–wave, respectively (Newman and Odette, 1984; Robson and Frishman, 1995; Stockton and Slaughter, 1989). To account for any compromise of the photoreceptor layer in XLRS, a ratio of photoreceptor to bipolar-cell synaptic transmission compared to photo-transduction quality can be used: the b-wave amplitude to a-wave amplitude ratio (b/a-wave ratio). One can use the b/a-wave ratio to adjust for any photoreceptor dysfunction affect on the b-wave amplitude, and can imply the quantity of dysfunction in bipolar cells. Normally the b-wave amplitude is greater than the a-wave in the dark-adapted ERG for bright stimuli, but in XLRS the b-wave naturally is reduced (Peachey et al., 1987). Thus, a reduced b/a-wave ratio is characteristic of inner retinal disease such as XLRS.

2.7 Natural history and disease progression: role of age

Several reports based on visual acuity loss (Apushkin et al., 2005), fundus changes with schisis cavities modification (Lesch et al., 2008), and retinal function deterioration (Vijayasarathy et al., 2010; Vijayasarathy et al., 2009) have focused on the "progressive" nature of XLRS disease. In detail, visual acuity is mostly impaired starting in grade school (Apushkin et al., 2005) due to macular schisis. However, even if 20% of XLRS children (Roesch et al., 1998) present significant vision loss in early childhood, half of these patients may have poor vision due to complications of the disorder, such as retinal detachment or vitreous hemorrhage. A bimodal age is a characteristic of presentation of XLRS in childhood (George et al., 1996). One group presented strabismus and nystagmus at an age less than 2 years, and the other group presented only poor vision at approximately 7 years of age. Exotropia and esotropia were in the same proportion, and in the group with exotropia the occurrence of poor vision from severe schisis was highest. Rhegmatogenous (tractional retinal detachment) may also be the initial presentation of XLRS. Other XLRS males may present during infancy peripheral bullous elevation of the inner retinal layer accompanied with vitreous hemorrhage (George et al., 1996). In such cases it is difficult to assess a "progressive" trait of the disease.

Retinal appearance at funduscopy, OCT scans and ERG b-wave amplitude reduction (Figure 2, E-H) provide an estimate of the retinal changes in XLRS patients. A substantial change from the "cystic" (< 25 years old) to the "atrophic" (> 25 years old) pattern of the retina with age was recently described (Lesch et al., 2008). We also showed (Vijayasarathy et al., 2009) worsening of retinal function by age in a family harboring a null mutation in exon 5 of the *RS1* gene indicating disease progression with age. In this study, the two younger males, ages 1.5 and 5 years, had well preserved b-waves extending above the pre-flash baseline and nearly normal ERG a-wave and b-wave configuration with a classical XLRS fundus appearance. However, four older affected male relatives, ages 32, 43, 43, and 48 years, showed the classic "electronegative" ERG with advanced XLRS retinal changes with reduced electronegative, b-waves. This suggests that older subjects had markedly decreased b-wave amplitudes compared to the younger subjects.

In addition, disease progression has also been observed in natural history studies of the *RS1* knockout-mouse model (Kjellstrom et al., 2007b): progressive loss of photoreceptor nuclei and shortening of the outer segments with age has been found with a considerably reduction of the ERG a-wave amplitude by 16 months. An exact understanding of how XLRS disease progresses with age is not clear. In a recent study (Kjellstrom et al., 2010), 10 XLRS subjects underwent baseline ERG testing between the ages of 6 and 15 years. Follow up ERG testing was preformed 8 to 14 years later. For the cohort, no difference was found either between the b-wave amplitude or b/a-wave ratio from the first to second visit.

2.8 Clinical severity (metanalysis of severity grade systems) and genotype-phenotype correlation in human XLRS

Wide phenotypic heterogeneity is one of the remarkable characteristic of this disease, and it is possibly related to the increasing number of mutations identified in the *RS1* gene (1998). Currently, there is no standard method to grade the severity of XLRS disease. The clinical presentation of XLRS patients can vary based on the age of patients. Strabismus, nystagmus, hyperopia associated with severe cystic macular lesion with or without peripheral schisis, and subnormal ERG b-waves are findings more frequently reported at a very young age, while retinal detachment or progressive macular atrophy with or without peripheral retinal scar, low visual acuity, and non-detectable ERG b-wave with reduced a-wave are instead mostly found in older ages. The OCT has been used to classify XLRS clinical severity. For example, clinical severity was determined by retinal examination and OCT scans in a cohort of 19 males, disregarding the genotype of the examined group (Prenner et al., 2006). Retinal tomography was more recently used (Lesch et al., 2008) to assess the prevalence of "cystic" and "atrophic" forms of the disease, variable with age. Visual acuity changes have been also considered valuable for predicting the extent of XLRS disease. However, Apushkin (Apushkin et al., 2005) analyzed the natural course of visual acuity changes in 38 XLRS patients, aged 9 to 65 years, finding only limited progression of vision loss over a mean follow-up period of 10 years.

Investigators have explored whether the type of mutations on the *RS1* gene predict the severity of the disease. More than 160 mutations have been identified in the *RS1* gene so far (1998). Mutations cause loss of protein function either due to the absolute loss of protein expression or to the presence of conformationally defective misfolded protein. The majority is missense mutations in exons 4–6; deletions, insertions, nonsense, and splice-site mutations have also been reported (Table 1). Several other studies have been conducted to ascertain correlations between genotype and phenotype in XLRS (Bradshaw et al., 1999; Eksandh et al., 2000a; Hiriyanna et al., 1999; Hotta et al., 2001; Lesch et al., 2008; Roesch et al., 1998; Shinoda et al., 2000; Sieving et al., 1999b); however, no clear link between genetic mutations and clinical phenotype have been firmly established. Furthermore, 145 unrelated XLRS families were examined in search of a correlation in severity of clinical phenotypes with the associated gene mutations (Hiriyanna et al., 1999). They found that mutations able to produce truncated RS1 protein (from deletions, splice-site and frame-shift mutations) are clearly related with severe phenotype.

Moreover three Japanese XLRS patients were described with retinal detachment or severe macular lesion and low visual acuity at a very young age; two of them harbored deletions of exon 1 or of the boundary region between exon 3 and intron 3 (Shinoda et al., 2000). The authors also reported (Shinoda et al., 2004) a progressive XLRS phenotype in two siblings harboring a deletion of RS1 exon 4 and summarized that severe cases of XLRS are usually associated with upstream deletions (exons 1–3) in the *RS1* gene which prevent the formation of functional mRNA (Hiriyanna et al., 1999; Shinoda et al., 2000), whereas the mild cases have relatively well preserved visual function and are usually associated with downstream deletions (exon 4). Two XLRS patients harboring "donor splice" mutation in exon 4, known to produce a null biochemical phenotype, with peripheral and central schisis, subnormal or non-detectable b-wave, and reduced a-wave, whereas another four patients, carrying missense mutations (R200C and R102W) resulted in more preserved ERG b-wave and almost normal retinal periphery with slight macular changes were reported (Bradshaw et al., 1999). We recently described (Vijayasarathy et al., 2010) a considerable difference between the severe clinical phenotype in subjects harboring RS1 null-protein signal-sequence mutations and the less compromised retinal function in XLRS patients carrying missense mutation. These findings suggest that mutations, like deletions and frame shifts that putatively cause protein truncation, result in greater clinical severity of the disease, even if there is no univocal classification system for XLRS. All these mutations related to a partial or full loss of protein suggests a severe XLRS phenotype, and therefore, might be unified in a one group of non-missense severe variants (Table 1).

Mutations	No[a]	DNA structure	Protein structure	Protein function
Missense	>110	Change a single nucleotide	Code for a different amino acid	Affects protein folding, sorting, loss of protein
Nonsense	9	Codes for a stop codon	Could truncate the protein	Full or partial loss-of-function
Splice site	16	A genetic mutation that inserts or deletes a number of nucleotides in the specific site at which splicing of an intron takes place during the processing of precursor messenger RNA into mature messenger RNA	The abolishment of the splicing site results in one or more introns remaining in mature mRNA	Production of aberrant proteins
Deletions	26	Delete one or more nucleotides in DNA	In-frame deletions or frameshifts	Full or partial loss-of-function
Insertions	4	Insert one or more nucleotides into DNA	In-frame deletions or frameshifts	Full or partial loss-of-function
Silent	6	Change a single nucleotide	Code for the same amino acid	Native-like protein

Table 1. Genetic mutations in X-linked retinoschisis and their role in protein structure/function. [a]http://www.retina-international.org/sci-news/xlrsmut.htm.

3. Molecular modeling, functional role and severity of pathogenic mutations in human XLRS

Genetic mutations often cause a change in protein expression. As described above several primary mechanisms might be responsible for the loss of RS1 function due to genetic mutations. The first mechanism is the misfolding of the discoidin domain, which changes the putative adhesive properties of the protein. Caused by missense mutations, RS1 misfolding might initiate formation of aberrant proteins in non-native conformation. The second mechanism is the defective disulfide-linked subunit assembly of RS1 into dimers and octamers which results in abnormal protein secretion caused by missense changes affecting reactive thiol groups. The third mechanism is the inability of RS1 to insert into endoplasmic reticulum (ER) membrane as part of the protein secretion process. This is caused by severe changes associated with the insertion or the removal of large fragments in protein molecule, protein truncations, and null mutations.

According to analysis in Paragraph 2.6 and Table 2 the majority of XLRS mutations could be divided in two large groups of (a) missense mutations and (b) non-missense changes with a severe XLRS phenotype. Although a severe role of non-missense changes is confirmed in numerous cases, the severity of XLRS phenotype for missense changes is less obvious. Here we imply molecular modeling of protein structure as described by ERGs clinical severities of XLRS via the computational evaluation of impact of pathogenic missense mutations.

3.1 Protein folding/misfolding in ER and protein folding landscapes

The effect of missense mutations on a protein fold is difficult to understand without some basics of the native protein folding. Over one-third of newly synthesized proteins are translocated into the ER, which ensures their delivery into the secretory pathway. The ER lumen contains molecular chaperones that maintain polypeptide solubility, enzymes that are necessary for post-translational modification of proteins, and factors that directly assist in the folding of newly synthesized polypeptides such as foldases and isomerases. Proteins that not attain their native conformations, because of genetic mutations, cellular stress or other random events, may harm the cell. Therefore, protein systems within the ER lumen mediate quality control, that resulting in the resolution of terminally misfolded proteins from correctly folded proteins and folding intermediates. To compensate for the potentially disastrous consequences of misfolded protein accumulation, ER-retained species are most commonly destroyed.

There are numerous observations of retinoschisins modified by missense mutations and expressed in cell culture which demonstrate the absence of modified RS1 bands from SDS-PAGE or native gels and associated with a loss of protein due to misfolding and rapid degradation (Wang et al., 2002; Wang et al., 2006; Wu and Molday, 2003; Wu et al., 2005). Several major mechanisms lead to degradation of misfolded protein. About 30% of cytosolic proteins carry specific KFERQ-targeting motifs in their sequences allowing for selective targeting of cytosolic proteins to the lysosome for degradation by chaperone-mediated autophagy (Kaushik and Cuervo, 2006, 2008). However, the absence of the specific targeting motif in the RS1 sequence suggests another option. As a result, misfolded or unassembled proteins are retained in the ER bound to chaperones or lectins until they are delivered to the cytosol for degradation in the ubiquitin-proteasome pathway (Goldberg, 2003). Mutant variants with significant changes in protein fold caused by missense mutations or deletions could generate misfolded proteins susceptible to hydrolysis similar to that of human haemoglobin in which about one-fifth of missense proteins undergo rapid degradation (Goldberg, 2003). Therefore, the severe mutant variants are expected to have a markedly perturbed non-native protein fold causing misfolding in the ER and later digestion in the proteasome (Vijayasarathy et al., 2010).

The mechanism by which a polypeptide chain folds to a specific three-dimensional protein structure was recently discussed (Dobson, 2004). In the ER, proteins fold into their native conformations and undergo different post-translational modifications and the formation of disulphide bonds. Native states of proteins almost always correspond to the structures that are most thermodynamically stable under physiological conditions. The primary sequence of protein is the major determinant for proper folding of protein (Anfinsen et al., 1961). The protein folds along several competing pathways into intermediate, non-native structures with decreasing free energies until it achieves a conformation with the lowest energy to form a protein with native interactions (Dobson, 2004). The total number of possible conformations of any polypeptide chain is so large that a systematic search for this particular structure would be impractical. The folding process involves a random search of many protein folds accessible to a polypeptide chain.

The natural fluctuations in the conformation of an unfolded or incompletely folded polypeptide chain cause highly separated residues in the amino-acid sequence to come into contact with one other. In addition, if the energy surface of protein or 'landscape' has the correct shape, only a small number of all possible conformers needs to be tested by any given protein molecule during its transition from a random coil to a native structure. The landscape is encoded by the amino-acid sequence of protein. Therefore, natural selection has enabled proteins to change so that polypeptides are able to fold rapidly and efficiently. Such a description is often referred to as the 'new view' of protein folding (Dobson, 1999, 2003, 2004). On average, native-like interactions between residues are more determined and the polypeptide chain is finding lowest-energy structure by a process of trial and error. Misfolded or intermediate non-native proteins never achieve this lowest energy minimum. Pathogenic mutations produce a severe or mild effect in a protein structure and cause the protein to stay in an intermediate or even misfolded conformation with a relatively higher free energy.

3.2 Role of cysteine residues and disulphide bonds in protein stability

Cysteine residues normally form disulphide bonds which significantly constrain the number of possible conformers from finding a lowest-energy structure. The disulphide bond or disulphide bridge is formed by the pairing of two thiol groups of cysteines as a result of protein oxidation. A disulfide bond is a strong covalent bond of about 2.05 Å in length connecting two sulfur $S\gamma$ atoms which dissociate with energy of 60 kcal/mole. The structure of a disulfide bond can be described by its χ_{ss} dihedral angle between the $C\beta - S\gamma - S\gamma - C\beta$ atoms, which is in majority close to ±90°. When the dihedral angle approaches 0° or 180°, then the disulfide is a better oxidant. Rotation about the $S\gamma - S\gamma$ axis has a low energy barrier.

The disulfide bond holds two fragments of the protein chain together. This stabilizes the native fold of a protein by lowering entropy of the polypeptide chain and by condensing hydrophobic residues around the bond into local hydrophobic core using hydrophobic interactions. The disulfide bond increases the effective local concentration of hydrophobic residues causing a decrease of the local concentration of water molecules in the hydrophobic core. Since water molecules break up hydrogen bonds, their low concentration stabilizes a protein secondary structure.

The native disulphide bonds are critical for proper protein folding. The native structure of a protein typically has a single disulfide bind. In proteins with more than two cysteines, non-native disulfide species may be created. Non-disulphide species are almost always unfolded. As the number of cysteines increases, the number of non-native species increases significantly. Indeed, RS1 monomer has 10 cysteines which can form up to five disulphide bonds. In general, 10 cysteine residues can form ${}_{10}C_2$=45 distinct disulphide bonds. A protein with ten-cysteines, such as RS1, could form 945 [$=10!/(10/2)!2^{10/2}$] different five-disulfide species, only one of which is the protein with native disulfide bonds. All other 944 proteins are the non-native disulphide species!

In the cell in order to avoid non-native disulphides formation, protein disulphide isomerases (PDI) are necessary to catalyze the inter-conversion of disulfide species and accelerate the formation of the native disulfide species. In the ER, PDI has a function of a cellular chaperone with the essential foldase activity to maintain a native protein fold (Noiva, 1999; Tsai et al., 2001). PDI catalyzes oxidation and reshuffling (isomerization) of disulphides in substrate proteins by using the catalytic CxxC motif (Gruber et al., 2006). Current data suggest that PDI docks close to two $S\gamma$ cysteines in the substrate protein, forms a native disulphide bridge between those cysteines, and possibly stabilizes native contacts in that area by utilizing a chaperone function. Thus, we might conclude that PDI's are an essential interaction partners of RS1 in ER in order to form a structure with native disulphide bonds.

Hence, we suggest that genetic mutations which are associated with the cysteine insertion/removal might interfere with suitable PDI binding in the vicinity of missense change. This might cause the appearance of new non-native disulphide bonds previously corrected by the foldase action. The insertion or deletion of cysteine residues should be taken into account when the severity of damage to protein molecule caused by the pathogenic missense change is evaluated.

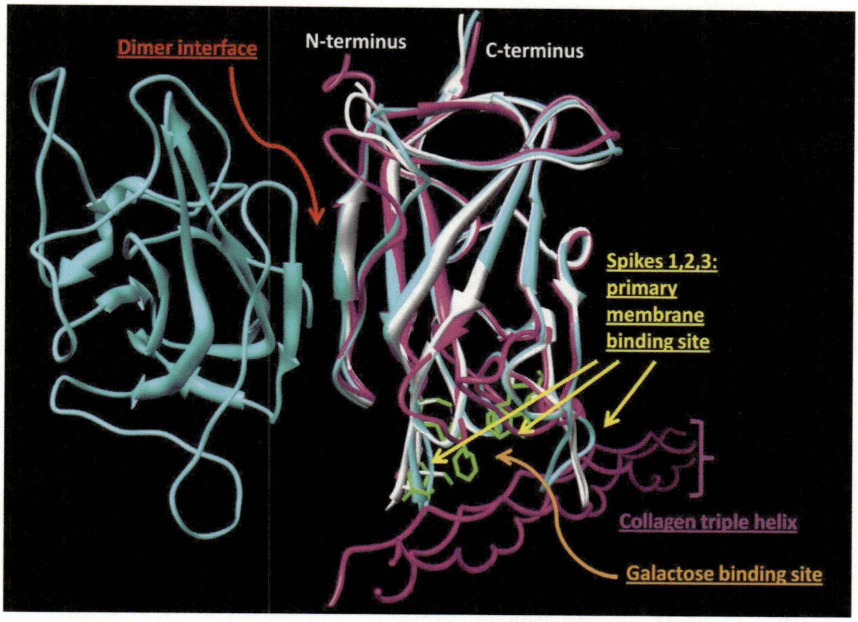

Fig. 3. A superposition of 3 discoidin ribbon structures to demonstrate the areas involved in interactions of discoidin domains with other molecules. Structures of the DDR2 discoinin domain bound to a triple-helical collagen peptide (magenta), the dimeric (cyan) and monomeric (white) forms of the membrane-binding C2 domain of human coagulation factor V (cyan) are shown.

3.3 Discoidin domains and molecular modeling of RS1 protein structure

Currently more than 72,000 protein structures have been determined by protein crystallography and deposited in the RCSB protein data bank. This list could be significantly expanded if structural genomic approaches such as a sequence homology and molecular modeling are used to generate protein structures. These computational methods were used successfully to predict the effect of thermodynamics experiments, to simulate the dynamics of protein folding and unfolding, and to explain a functional and structural role of elements of protein structure and other areas.

Similar methods could be used to evaluate an impact of missense mutations on protein structure stability and function. We used molecular modeling to predict a structure of mature retinoschisin which is formed by Rs1 and discoidin domains (Sergeev et al., 2010). Discoidin domains have a similar fold with elements of spatial structure in a shape of a β-sandwich, shown schematically in Figure 3 (Baumgartner et al., 1998) as the superposition of three structures demonstrating a binding to different molecules. The galactose, phospholipids, and collagen binding sites are located in shown in the lower part of this figure (area of spikes) suggesting a high conformational flexibility in this area (Carafoli et al., 2009; Macedo-Ribeiro et al., 1999). Moreover, the discoidin domains are able to form a dimeric structure shown by the cyan ribbon (Macedo-Ribeiro et al., 1999). Therefore binding to galactose, membrane, collagen, and a dimer formation could be potentially expected for the discoidin domain of retinoschisin. In general, the discoidin fold is conserved in more than 9 different proteins. The discoidin domain is present in single or multiple copies in extracellular or trans-membrane proteins implicated in cell-cell adhesion, and cell-cell interaction such as the coagulation factors V (FaV) and VIII (FaVIII), milk fat globule, neuropilin and neurexins, and implicated in phospholipid binding (Adams et al., 2004). In different species they have 47 highly conserved residues (~30% sequence identity) including 2 cysteines forming a disulphide bridge and several tryptophans maintaining a stable hydrophobic core of a discoidin domain β-sandwich (Kiedzierska et al., 2007). The structure of mature retinoschisin is shown in Figure 4A. In this structure the Rs1 domain is located in residues 25-64 and the folded, β-sandwich discoidin domain occupies residues 65-224 (Wu and Molday, 2003). The structure of the mature retinoschisin was equilibrated using molecular dynamics (MD). Usually MD is used to obtain an 'idealized' or equilibrated protein structure with stereochemistry close to perfect. The main justification of the MD method is that statistical ensemble averages are equal to time averages of the system, so-called the ergodic hypothesis. MD by computer simulation of physical movements by atoms and molecules take into account physical interactions between atoms of the protein structure and molecules of surrounding waters. Whereas it is possible to take "still snapshots" of crystal structures using X-Ray crystallography and NMR, no current experimental technique allows access to all the time scales of motion at atomic resolution.

MD can be used to refine the location of cysteine residues in the RS1 structure which is necessary to understand retinoschisin function (Wang et al., 2002; Wang et al., 2006; Wu and Molday, 2003; Wu et al., 2005). The structure of mature RS1 contains 10 cysteines in positions 38, 40, 42, 59, 63, 83, 110, 142, 219, and 223, which are shared in an even proportion between Rs1 and discoidin domains (Figure 4A). The structure of the discoidin domain and the positions of 5 cysteines were reported in several cases (Fraternali et al., 2003; Wang et al., 2006; Wu and Molday, 2003). The other 5 cysteines are located in the Rs1 domain of mature retinoschisin. In a protein structure, 7 cysteines are predicted to be concentrated in an area close to amino- and carboxy-termini, and 3 cysteines are located close to a spike area shown at the top (terminal extensions) and the bottom (discoidin domain) parts of Figure 4A, respectively. Nearly 70% of the RS1 surface is formed by non-polar groups (see Figures 4B and C, rotation of ~180°) suggesting that non-polar groups (green) could be important for the RS1 normal function.

Although numerous experiments have demonstrated that retinoschisin is secreted as a monomer, dimer, or octamer in model cell systems (Wang et al., 2006; Wu et al., 2005) this protein is secreted *in vivo* as a homo-oligomeric complex. A structural model of secreted RS1 homo-oligomeric protein complex currently is not available. Oligomerization is critical for the functioning of retinoschisin as an extracellular adhesion protein (Wu et al., 2005) where non-polar surface of RS1 could play a role. In contrast, protein misfolding caused by pathogenic mutation could interrupt proper secretion of a functional protein (Wang et al., 2002; Wang et al., 2006; Wu and Molday, 2003).

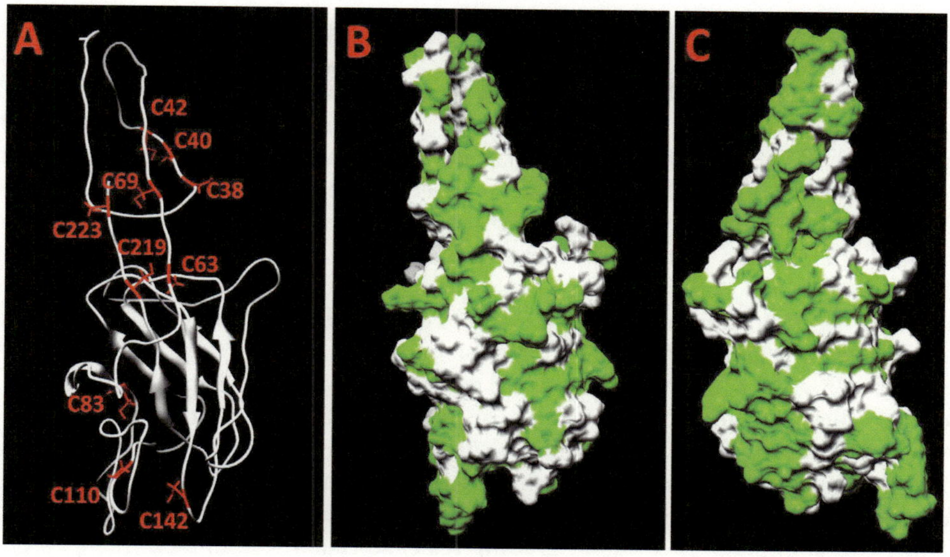

Fig. 4. RS1 structure is a monomer with a significant fraction of non-polar surface. RS1 structure is shown by a ribbon (Panel A). Positions of cysteines are shown in red. Accessible surface area of RS1 demonstrates a significant proportion of exposed non-polar areas shown by green (Panels B and C).

3.4 Computational assessment of severity of protein damage caused by the pathogenic missense change

in the last decade, new approaches using semi-empirical force-fields were developed in molecular modeling. Stability of native protein structure and protein complexes is defined by non-polar interactions, disulphide covalent bonds, salt bridges, and hydrogen bonds. Semi-empirical methods imply simplified forces and potentials are taken into account for these interactions within protein structure. Semi-empirical methods generate values of protein stabilization energies that correlate well with an experimental data for a majority of tested proteins. This approach might help to grade severities of molecular perturbations due to missense changes and explain how a genetic mutation could impact protein structure in quantitative manner.

The free energy of protein stabilization (in kcal mol^{-1}) is a function of several parameters. The first term includes a solvation energy contribution from hydrophobic and polar groups of protein (Eisenberg and McLachlan, 1986) based on a concept of accessible surface area (Lee and Richards, 1971) which could be evaluated using a fast geometry algorithm (Tsodikov et al., 2002). The second term is the energy of hydrogen bonds with regard to simple geometric considerations (Petukhov et al., 1999). Additional terms include Van der Waals energy which takes into account the experimental transfer energies from water to vapor; the electrostatic coulomb free energy term, which describes electrostatic interactions in protein; the crude entropy of protein chain to obtain a measure of free energy and free energy of the steric overlaps between atoms in protein structure (Abagyan and Totrov, 1994; Munoz and Serrano, 1994).

Currently, all these terms are combined in the FoldX force field (Schymkowitz et al., 2005; Schymkowitz et al., 2002). The rapid evaluation of protein stabilization free energy change due to missense mutations could be accessed with this field based on an empirical energy function derived from experimental work on proteins. The predictive power of this approach has been successfully tested with experimental thermodynamics data of 1000 mutant proteins (Guerois et al., 2002) from the ProTherm database (Gromiha et al., 2000; Gromiha et al., 1999; Gromiha et al., 2002). Recently a combination of molecular dynamics folding simulations and FoldX potential has been suggested as an approach of *in silico* analysis of missense substitutions (Tavtigian et al., 2008). In our work, the changes in energy of protein stabilization due to missense change were evaluated using semi-empirical methods using the FoldX force field.

In addition, we used information about differences between amino acids replacing each other in order to achieve a correct estimate for mutations involving cysteine residues. The amino acids differ by combination of several chemical factors like composition, polarity and molecular volume which correlate best with protein residue substitution frequencies as observed (Grantham, 1974). The Grantham difference for each amino acid pair could be used to characterize a physiochemical differences between wild-type and missense variant amino acid residues (Karchin et al., 2007; Tavtigian et al., 2008).

Therefore, we suggested a molecular grading scale, so-called a computed impact score, *CI* (Sergeev et al., 2010), which considers changes in protein conformation and the Grantham differences between amino acids. Graphically, with these two categories as axes, the computed impact shows the characteristic distance between two amino acids involved in the mutation change. The axes are made orthogonal to facilitate the calculation of the difference in distance between amino acids. The overall difference, which is described by the *CI*, demonstrates the overall difference between two amino acids for the same position in wild-type protein and mutant variant. The changes in energy of protein stabilization, *ΔΔGstab*, the *CI*, and accessible surface areas, ASA, were determined in our XLRS cohort, as shown in Table 2 for several mutations. Finally, the computed impact score used to grade an impact of each pathogenic mutation at the protein level was compared with severity of XLRS estimated from ERG data.

Missense mutation	*ΔΔGstab*, kcal/mol	CI	ASA, Å^2	Missense mutation	*ΔΔGstab*, kcal/mol	CI	ASA, Å^2
E72K	12.7	0.24	102	R141C	19.8	0.54	48
W92C	20.7	0.61	209	N179D	21.6	0.36	8
R102W	12.8	0.32	41	R200C	16.1	0.50	53
L127P	27.7	0.50	6	R213W	12.6	0.32	0
I136T	22.2	0.42	0	R213Q	10.6	0.20	0
G140E	12.1	0.30	0	C219W	3.9	0.52	4

Table 2. Computed impact, surface accessibility and protein stabilization energy change caused by the pathogenic missense mutations selected from our XLRS cohort. ASA is characterizing the residue exposure (>40 Å^2) or location in the protein hydrophobic core (≤40 Å^2).

3.5 Molecular grading scale: protein structure-based classification of the pathogenic missense mutations impact in human XLRS

We applied molecular modeling of the RS protein and consider perturbations caused by mutations found in human XLRS affected subjects. Computational analysis has predicted that pathogenic missense mutations could be separated in two groups by using the molecular grading scale.

The ERG b/a-wave ratios were sorted by patient age and by the impact of mutation on protein atomic structure. This analysis was applied independently to ERG b/a-wave ratios as a function of average patient age versus severity of XLRS phenotype (Figure 5A). To minimize the effect of statistical errors and to improve a signal-to-noise ratio in experimental ERG data, we used the method described previously (Sergeev et al., 2010) to a new XLRS cohort of patients. All b/a-wave ratios were divided into groups by age (younger, older) and by mutation severity (low-impact, high-impact) (Figure 5A). The b/a-wave ratio in older (37-43 y/o) XLRS patients was greater than younger (13-17 y/o) for severe missense variants with the b-wave unchanged as the a-wave declined similarly to that observed in the *Rs1b-KO* mouse (Kjellstrom et al., 2007b) and in the NEI dataset (Sergeev et al., 2010). In the mouse model, the decline of a-wave amplitude with age coincided with the loss of outer nuclear layer cells, whereas the decline in the b-wave and the b/a-wave ratio was associated with increasing severity of schisis cavities in younger ages (Kjellstrom et al., 2007a). As result, phenotypic b/a-wave ratios declined for younger individuals accompanied by a corresponding rise of computed impact score, a measure of the structural severity of the mutation (Figure 5A). Although this change is statistically less significant for older patients, a common trend showing a slight decrease with computed impact seems to be similar to that of described for younger individuals.

Differences in phenotypes were verified for low- and high-impact missense changes and severe non-missense mutations (Figure 5B). Low-impact missense changes show average b/a-wave ratio close to 1.0 for a maximum with 15 XLRS patients of different ages (labeled by star in bottom panel). This ratio corresponds to a maximum of 10 patients with an average value of approximately 0.6, which is consistent with more severe XLRS phenotype as expected for high-impact missense variants. In addition, the severity of high impact missense changes is confirmed by identical correspondence to 15 patients with the severe non-missense variants (top panel). Thus, low- and high-impact missense changes in protein structure might be associated with mild and severe changes in the XLRS phenotype.

Earlier we demonstrated that maximum structure perturbations associated with severe XLRS phenotype arise from either the removal or insertion of cysteine residues or from changes in the hydrophobic core (Sergeev et al., 2010). Less severe or mild changes were associated with missense mutations targeting a significant part of protein surface. Our present study, which was uses different datasets, has demonstrated that mild phenotypic changes could be associated with mutations in the water inaccessible residues when polar-to-polar or the hydrophobic-to-hydrophobic changes has appeared.

Our computational analysis has predicted that pathogenic missense mutations could be separated in mild and severe groups of XLRS phenotype by using the molecular grading scale. The results for the expected phenotypes of 109 missense changes which are currently available for XLRS are shown in the Table 3. In order to understand how the phenotype of XLRS disease described by b/a-wave ratios is related to missense changes, we analyzed mutant residue accessibilities (ASA) in the RS1 structure similar to that of shown in the Table 2. All mutations were ranked according to their computed impact. These mutations were separated into two groups, low-impact and high-impact, by their computed severity threshold (~0.4) as previously demonstrated (Sergeev et al., 2010). From this analysis, half of the mild mutations could be considered as mutations which were partially or fully exposed at the protein surface; another half are the mutations predicted to be buried in the hydrophobic core. Mutations from this latter group were variants related to insertion, exchange, or removal of charged residues or replacement with a homologous hydrophobic or polar residue. In only two cases, C223S and C83S, cysteines were affected by a mild missense change. In contrast, the majority of missense variants were predicted to cause severe changes, related to insertion or removal of cysteine residues (23 mutations) and/or buried in the hydrophobic core.

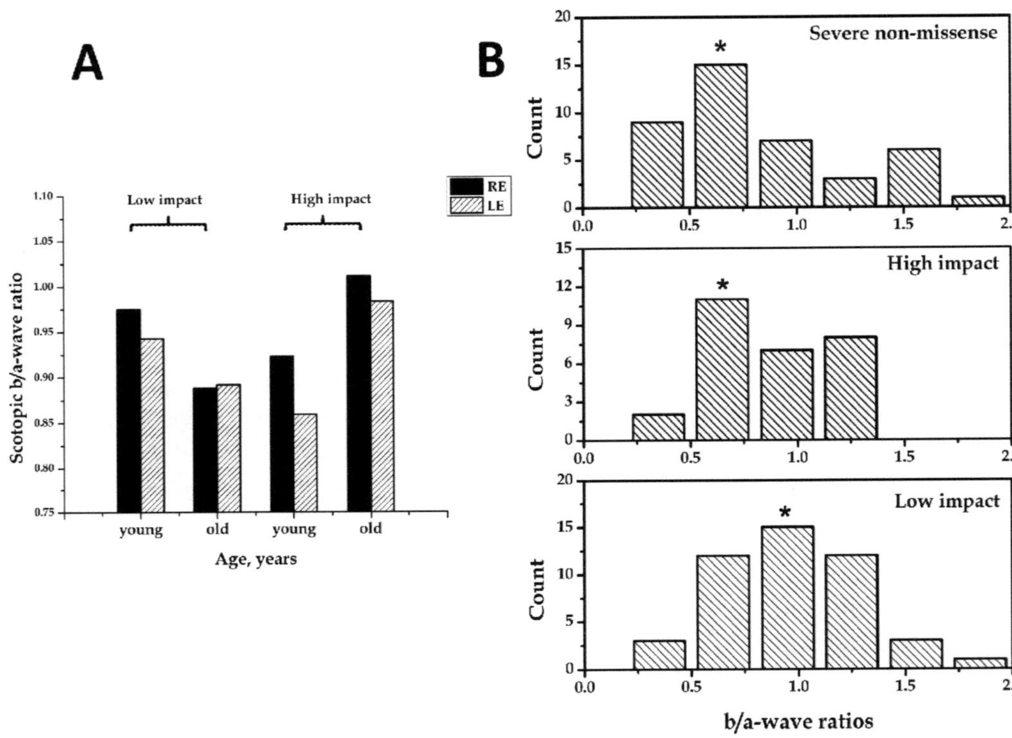

Fig. 5. Severity of the XLRS phenotype is associated with the expected impact of missense changes on the RS1 protein structure. **Panel A:** ERG average b/a-wave ratios as a function of average patient age and severity of XLRS phenotype. Average b/a-wave ratios obtained for patients divided into 4 groups by missense mutations classes (low-impact, high-impact) and by patient age (young, old). Scotopic b/a-wave ratios for 4 groups of patients are shown. ERG b/a-wave ratios for right (RE) and left (LE) eyes in each group are black and shaded, respectively. **Panel B:** Histogram of the XLRS patient b/a-wave ratios divided in groups of a low- and a high-impact missense, and severe non-missense genetic mutations as predicted using by a molecular grading scale. No differences in age were considered in this case. Histograms bars with maximum counts are labeled by asterisks (*). The ratios were obtained for the same XLRS cohort of patients (< 55 years old).

XLRS phenotype	Missense variants*)
Mild	R209H, D158N, R213Q, S73P, E146D, G70S, T185K, H207Q, I133F, A101P, R141H, E72K, G178D, E72D, Q154R, D168H, L113F, H207D, E72Q, E146K, G70A, A211T, G109A, R200H, R209L, E215Q, G109E, G140E, K167N, H222N, N104K, R141G, R102Q, R213W, R102W, P203L, T138A, P192A, A98E, G109R, C223S, W96R, P192T, I199T, P193L, R191P, C83S, A211F, P192S, R102E, E215K, D145H, P192R
Severe	C59S, R197P, G70R, I195V, P192L, N179D, L69P, R197H, V76G, G74V, G135V, G140R, L137P, R209P, L216P, R209G, E72A, P193S, R156G, E215V, C219S, I136T, D143V, P68R, C142R, G109W, C110R, L103R, Y89C, F176S, C223R, C110Y, C219G, R209C, N99C, R200C, L127P, R197C, G70D, C219W, R182C, C219R, R141C, W163C, W122C, Y65C, W112C, Y155C, I81N, I81D, W92C, W96C, F108C, C142W, C223Y

Table 3. Classes of XLRS phenotypes as predicted using the molecular grading scale for 110 pathogenic missense variants. *) Human Gene Mutation, Retina News International, and X-linked Retinoschisis Sequence Variation databases were used.

Finally, this study confirms results of our previous work that severe phenotype maximum structure perturbations are related to dramatic changes in a protein hydrophobic core or to the deletion or insertion of cysteine residues affecting in general the stability of protein fold. The kinetics of the disease progression might depend on the degree of the mutation impact on protein stability caused by the pathogenic missense change. Thus, we have to incorporate age, genotype, and molecular modeling into ERG analysis to understand a functional role of pathogenic mutations.

4. Incorporating age and genotype into ERG analysis

In our study, the effect of high-impact missense mutations could be recognized as severe at an earlier age when compared to low-impact missense mutations. In order to recognize the predicted affect of mutations we look to kinetics of the disease progression and incorporate patient age into the analysis of the relationship between genotype and phenotype. An exact understanding of how XLRS disease progresses with age is not clear. A 15-year, longitudinal XLRS study suggests that XLRS is a more stationary disease up to age 35 years, as seen in baseline and follow up ERG testing of 10 subjects. The first examination was performed on subjects between 6 to 15 years of age. A follow up examination was preformed 8 to 14 years later. In both exams, all 10 subjects showed reduced b-wave amplitudes, and no difference was found between the b-wave amplitude of the first or second visit (Kjellstrom et al., 2010). With these studies in mind, we raised the question of what role XLRS mutation severity plays in the dark-adapted ERG response. We preformed a retrospective cross-sectional study on 73 XLRS subjects who were seen at the National Eye Institute between 2004 and 2010. All subjects underwent ocular examination including a full-field ERG with ISCEV standard, dark-adapted response. All subjects were genotyped for *RS1* mutations. By separating subjects into two mutation severity groups (low-impact, high-impact), our data suggest that null protein or severity dysfunctional protein is associated with more retinal dysfunction than mildly dysfunctional protein. Greater dysfunction of subjects with severe mutations was seen in the b-wave amplitude and b/a-wave ratio (70.2 μV, $p = 0.02$, less severe = 54 eyes, more severe = 79 eyes; excluding those >55 y/o). In our XLRS cohort, subjects maintained a-wave amplitudes within normal limits, or slightly below normal limits, suggesting little to no change in photoreceptor number or function in older subjects compared to younger subjects. Also, mutation severity did not play a role in a-wave amplitude (more severe n = 44 subjects, less severe n = 30, difference =-2.29 μV, p=0.89, excluding those >55 y/o). This data suggest that the outer segment of the photoreceptor was only minimally affected at most, and that mutation burden lies at the level of the photoreceptor-to-bipolar cell synapse.

Our cohort also displayed an earlier aging effect due to mutation than what would be expected from aging alone. The rise and fall of the b-wave amplitude with age in normal populations has been thoroughly studied (Birch and Anderson, 1992). At birth, the maximum response is minimal, but increases approximately 5 fold by age 4 months. By 5 years of age, children have normal adult b-wave amplitudes. The b-wave was not statistically affected from 5 years to 55 years of age, showing less than 25 μV decline per decade. Between ages 45-55 and 55-65, a significant decline of approximately 100 μV b-wave amplitude was seen. Birch's study showed that subjects ages 68 years have b-wave amplitudes approximately half those of subjects between the ages of 15 to 24 years.

For some time, investigators have questioned the possibility of photoreceptor disease in XLRS. One study found decreased a-wave amplitudes in 1/3 of their XLRS cohort, suggesting that rod photoreceptor dysfunction or loss could be a more primary manifestation of XLRS that first thought (Bradshaw et al., 1999). However, the majority of studies suggest complete or relative preservation of the a-wave in XLRS (Eksandh et al., 2000b; Kellner et al., 1990; Peachey et al., 1987). To look further into the question, Khan et al. modeled the leading edge of the a-wave to assess for pathology in the photo-transduction pathway (Khan et al., 2001). By modeling the first 15 ms of the waveform Khan found no difference between XLRS and normal subjects in sensitivity (S) and photoreceptor maximum amplitude (K_{max}) in the majority of XLRS waveforms measured.

4.1 The b/a-wave ratio can be a useful tool to quantify rod bipolar cell dysfunction relationship to rod function

To account for any compromise of the photoreceptor layer in XLRS, a ratio of photoreceptor-to-bipolar cell synaptic transmission compared to photo-transduction quality can be used (b/a-wave ratio). One can use the b/a-wave ratio to adjust for any photoreceptor dysfunction affect on the b-wave amplitude and can amplify the quantity of dysfunction in bipolar cells.

A reduced b/a-ratio is a characteristic of XLRS. The clinical lower limit of normal for the b/a ratio is 1.2 (Sergeev et al., 2010). Given normal b-wave amplitudes previous discussed, one would expect preservation of b/a-ratios in normal subjects until approximately 55 years of age (Birch and Anderson, 1992). In our study, no change in b/a ratio was due to aging alone (n=143 eyes, difference = 0.0039/year, p=0.17; excluding those >55 y/o); however, subjects with low-impact mutations maintained an overall higher b/a-ratio up to 55 years of age than did subjects with high-impact mutations (difference 0.3, p = 0.005, less severe = 54 eyes, more severe = 79 eyes; excluding those >55 y/o; Figure 6).

At first glance, it might appear that our study contradicts the XLRS longitudinal study by Kjellstrom (2010). However, had the longitudinal study identified the genetic mutations of all subjects (only three subjects were genotyped), a decrease in b/a-ratio could have been expected in subjects with severe mutations. Of the three subjects who underwent genotyping, two had severe mutations and had decreased b/a-wave ratio at the follow up visit (ratios decreased from 1.2 to 0.8, and 1.1 to 0.77). According to our data, subjects with low-impact mutations would have only a modest change within the 10 to 15 year followup period.

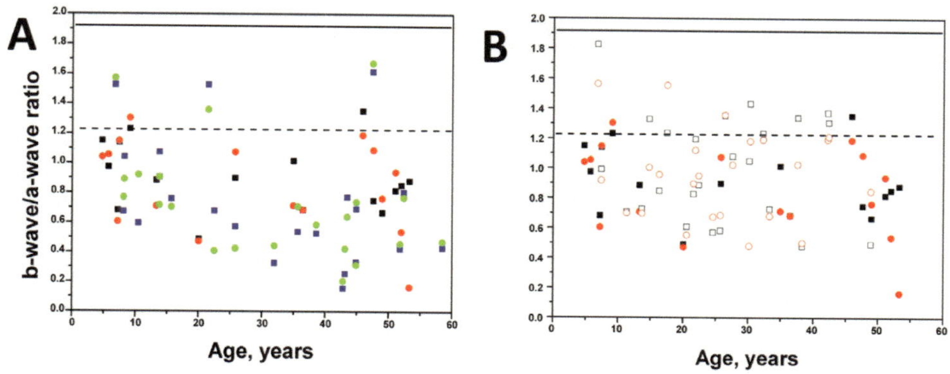

Fig. 6. Phenotypic data on clinical ERG b/a-wave ratios are shown for the cohort of X-linked retinoschisis patients as a function age (0-60 years old). Panel A: a superposition of ERG's b/a-wave ratios for patients with severe non-missense and high-impact missense variants. Panel B: a superposition of ERG's b/a-wave ratios for patients with the high-impact missense and low-impact missense variants. All data colored according to predicted severity: solid blue squares and green circles, solid black squares and red circles, open black squares and red circles are severe non-missense, high-impact missense and low-impact missense mutations. Squares and circles stand for right (OD) and left (OS) eye, respectively. The solid line and short dashes shows mean b/a-wave ratio and the mean minus two standard deviations, respectively, calculated from a group of 96 normal individuals (Sergeev et al., 2010).

5. Conclusion

Our computational analysis has suggested that the disease risk assessment at the atomic level could be implied in clinical studies. The combination of clinical electrophysiology, biology of retinal disease and molecular modeling provide a useful approach for evaluation of possible associations between the predicted structural alteration and/or damage to retinoschisin and the severity of XLRS disease.

6. Acknowledgment

We thank Sean Finnegan from the National Eye Institute for his valuable editorial help.

7. References

The Retinoschisis Consortium. (1998). Functional implications of the spectrum of mutations found in 234 cases with X-linked juvenile retinoschisis. HumMolGenet 7, 1185-1192.

Abagyan, R., and Totrov, M. (1994). Biased probability Monte Carlo conformational searches and electrostatic calculations for peptides and proteins. J Mol Biol *235,* 983-1002.

Adams, T.E., Hockin, M.F., Mann, K.G., and Everse, S.J. (2004). The crystal structure of activated protein C-inactivated bovine factor Va: Implications for cofactor function. ProcNatlAcadSciUSA *101,* 8918-8923.

Anfinsen, C.B., Haber, E., Sela, M., and White, F.H., Jr. (1961). The kinetics of formation of native ribonuclease during oxidation of the reduced polypeptide chain. ProcNatlAcadSciUSA *47,* 1309-1314.

Apushkin, M.A., Fishman, G.A., and Rajagopalan, A.S. (2005). Fundus findings and longitudinal study of visual acuity loss in patients with X-linked retinoschisis. Retina *25,* 612-618.

Baumgartner, S., Hofmann, K., Chiquet-Ehrismann, R., and Bucher, P. (1998). The discoidin domain family revisited: new members from prokaryotes and a homology-based fold prediction. Protein Sci *7,* 1626-1631.

Birch, D.G., and Anderson, J.L. (1992). Standardized full-field electroretinography. Normal values and their variation with age. Arch Ophthalmol *110,* 1571-1576.

Bradshaw, K., George, N., Moore, A., and Trump, D. (1999). Mutations of the XLRS1 gene cause abnormalities of photoreceptor as well as inner retinal responses of the ERG. DocOphthalmol *98,* 153-173.

Breton, M.E., Schueller, A.W., Lamb, T.D., and Pugh, E.N., Jr. (1994). Analysis of ERG a-wave amplification and kinetics in terms of the G-protein cascade of phototransduction. Invest OphthalmolVisSci *35,* 295-309.

Carafoli, F., Bihan, D., Stathopoulos, S., Konitsiotis, A.D., Kvansakul, M., Farndale, R.W., Leitinger, B., and Hohenester, E. (2009). Crystallographic insight into collagen recognition by discoidin domain receptor 2. Structure *17,* 1573-1581.

Dobson, C.M. (1999). Protein misfolding, evolution and disease. Trends BiochemSci *24,* 329-332.

Dobson, C.M. (2003). Protein folding and misfolding. Nature *426,* 884-890.

Dobson, C.M. (2004). Principles of protein folding, misfolding and aggregation. SeminCell DevBiol *15,* 3-16.

Eisenberg, D., and McLachlan, A.D. (1986). Solvation energy in protein folding and binding. Nature *319,* 199-203.

Eksandh, L., Andreasson, S., and Abrahamson, M. (2005). Juvenile X-linked retinoschisis with normal scotopic b-wave in the electroretinogram at an early stage of the disease. Ophthalmic Genet *26,* 111-117.

Eksandh, L.C., Ponjavic, V., Ayyagari, R., Bingham, E.L., Hiriyanna, K.T., Andreasson, S., Ehinger, B., and Sieving, P.A. (2000a). Phenotypic expression of juvenile X-linked retinoschisis in Swedish families with different mutations in the XLRS1 gene. Arch Ophthalmol *118,* 1098-1104.

Eksandh, L.C., Ponjavic, V., Ayyagari, R., Bingham, E.L., Hiriyanna, K.T., Andreasson, S., Ehinger, B., and Sieving, P.A. (2000b). Phenotypic expression of juvenile X-linked retinoschisis in Swedish families with different mutations in the XLRS1 gene. ArchOphthalmol *118,* 1098-1104.

Eriksson, U., Larsson, E., and Holmstrom, G. (2004). Optical coherence tomography in the diagnosis of juvenile X-linked retinoschisis. Acta Ophthalmol Scand *82,* 218-223.

Forsius, H., Krause, U., Helve, J., Vuopala, V., Mustonen, E., Vainio-Mattila, B., Fellman, J., and Eriksson, A.W. (1973). Visual acuity in 183 cases of X-chromosomal retinoschisis. Can J Ophthalmol *8,* 385-393.

Fraternali, F., Cavallo, L., and Musco, G. (2003). Effects of pathological mutations on the stability of a conserved amino acid triad in retinoschisin. FEBS Lett *544*, 21-26.

Friedrich, U., Stohr, H., Hilfinger, D., Loenhardt, T., Schachner, M., Langmann, T., and Weber, B.H. The Na/K-ATPase is obligatory for membrane anchorage of retinoschisin, the protein involved in the pathogenesis of X-linked juvenile retinoschisis. Hum Mol Genet.

George, N.D., Yates, J.R., Bradshaw, K., and Moore, A.T. (1995). Infantile presentation of X linked retinoschisis. BrJOphthalmol *79*, 653-657.

George, N.D., Yates, J.R., and Moore, A.T. (1996). Clinical features in affected males with X-linked retinoschisis. Arch Ophthalmol *114*, 274-280.

Goldberg, A.L. (2003). Protein degradation and protection against misfolded or damaged proteins. Nature *426*, 895-899.

Grantham, R. (1974). Amino acid difference formula to help explain protein evolution. Science *185*, 862-864.

Gregori, N.Z., Berrocal, A.M., Gregori, G., Murray, T.G., Knighton, R.W., Flynn, H.W., Jr., Dubovy, S., Puliafito, C.A., and Rosenfeld, P.J. (2009). Macular spectral-domain optical coherence tomography in patients with X linked retinoschisis. Br J Ophthalmol *93*, 373-378.

Gromiha, M.M., An, J., Kono, H., Oobatake, M., Uedaira, H., Prabakaran, P., and Sarai, A. (2000). ProTherm, version 2.0: thermodynamic database for proteins and mutants. Nucleic Acids Res *28*, 283-285.

Gromiha, M.M., An, J., Kono, H., Oobatake, M., Uedaira, H., and Sarai, A. (1999). ProTherm: Thermodynamic Database for Proteins and Mutants. Nucleic Acids Res *27*, 286-288.

Gromiha, M.M., Uedaira, H., An, J., Selvaraj, S., Prabakaran, P., and Sarai, A. (2002). ProTherm, Thermodynamic Database for Proteins and Mutants: developments in version 3.0. Nucleic Acids Res *30*, 301-302.

Gruber, C.W., Cemazar, M., Heras, B., Martin, J.L., and Craik, D.J. (2006). Protein disulfide isomerase: the structure of oxidative folding. Trends BiochemSci *31*, 455-464.

Guerois, R., Nielsen, J.E., and Serrano, L. (2002). Predicting changes in the stability of proteins and protein complexes: a study of more than 1000 mutations. Journal of Molecular Biology *320*, 369-387.

Hagins, W.A., Penn, R.D., and Yoshikami, S. (1970). Dark current and photocurrent in retinal rods. Biophys J *10*, 380-412.

Hiriyanna, K.T., Bingham, E.L., Yashar, B.M., Ayyagari, R., Fishman, G., Small, K.W., Weinberg, D.V., Weleber, R.G., Lewis, R.A., Andreasson, S., *et al.* (1999). Novel mutations in XLRS1 causing retinoschisis, including first evidence of putative leader sequence change. Hum Mutat *14*, 423-427.

Hotta, Y., Nakamura, M., Okamoto, Y., Nomura, R., Terasaki, H., and Miyake, Y. (2001). Different mutation of the XLRS1 gene causes juvenile retinoschisis with retinal white flecks. Br J Ophthalmol *85*, 238-239.

Huopaniemi, L., Fellman, J., Rantala, A., Eriksson, A., Forsius, H., De La Chapelle, A., and Alitalo, T. (1999). Skewed secondary sex ratio in the offspring of carriers of the 214G > A mutation of the RS1 gene. Ann Hum Genet *63*, 521-533.

Jablonski, M.M., Dalke, C., Wang, X., Lu, L., Manly, K.F., Pretsch, W., Favor, J., Pardue, M.T., Rinchik, E.M., Williams, R.W., *et al.* (2005). An ENU-induced mutation in Rs1h causes disruption of retinal structure and function. Mol Vis *11*, 569-581.

Karchin, R., Monteiro, A.N., Tavtigian, S.V., Carvalho, M.A., and Sali, A. (2007). Functional impact of missense variants in BRCA1 predicted by supervised learning. PLoSComputBiol *3*, e26.

Kato, K., Miyake, Y., Kachi, S., Suzuki, T., Terasaki, H., Kawase, Y., and Kanda, T. (2001). Axial length and refractive error in X-linked retinoschisis. Am J Ophthalmol *131*, 812-814.

Kaushik, S., and Cuervo, A.M. (2006). Autophagy as a cell-repair mechanism: activation of chaperone-mediated autophagy during oxidative stress. MolAspects Med *27*, 444-454.

Kaushik, S., and Cuervo, A.M. (2008). Chaperone-mediated autophagy. Methods MolBiol *445*, 227-244.

Kellner, U., Brummer, S., Foerster, M.H., and Wessing, A. (1990). X-linked congenital retinoschisis. Graefes ArchClinExpOphthalmol *228*, 432-437.

Khan, N.W., Jamison, J.A., Kemp, J.A., and Sieving, P.A. (2001). Analysis of photoreceptor function and inner retinal activity in juvenile X-linked retinoschisis. Vision Res *41*, 3931-3942.

Kiedzierska, A., Smietana, K., Czepczynska, H., and Otlewski, J. (2007). Structural similarities and functional diversity of eukaryotic discoidin-like domains. BiochimBiophysActa *1774*, 1069-1078.

Kjellstrom, S., Bush, R.A., Zeng, Y., Takada, Y., and Sieving, P.A. (2007a). Retinoschisin gene therapy and natural history in the Rs1h-KO mouse: long-term rescue from retinal degeneration. Invest Ophthalmol Vis Sci *48*, 3837-3845.

Kjellstrom, S., Bush, R.A., Zeng, Y., Takada, Y., and Sieving, P.A. (2007b). Retinoschisin gene therapy and natural history in the Rs1h-KO mouse: long-term rescue from retinal degeneration. Invest OphthalmolVisSci *48*, 3837-3845.

Kjellstrom, S., Vijayasarathy, C., Ponjavic, V., Sieving, P.A., and Andreasson, S. (2010). Long-term 12 year follow-up of X-linked congenital retinoschisis. Ophthalmic Genet *31*, 114-125.

Lee, B., and Richards, F.M. (1971). The interpretation of protein structures: estimation of static accessibility. J Mol Biol *55*, 379-400.

Lesch, B., Szabo, V., Kanya, M., Somfai, G.M., Vamos, R., Varsanyi, B., Pamer, Z., Knezy, K., Salacz, G., Janaky, M., *et al.* (2008). Clinical and genetic findings in Hungarian patients with X-linked juvenile retinoschisis. Mol Vis *14*, 2321-2332.

Li, X., Ma, X., and Tao, Y. (2007). Clinical features of X linked juvenile retinoschisis in Chinese families associated with novel mutations in the RS1 gene. Mol Vis *13*, 804-812.

Macedo-Ribeiro, S., Bode, W., Huber, R., Quinn-Allen, M.A., Kim, S.W., Ortel, T.L., Bourenkov, G.P., Bartunik, H.D., Stubbs, M.T., Kane, W.H., *et al.* (1999). Crystal structures of the membrane-binding C2 domain of human coagulation factor V. Nature *402*, 434-439.

Molday, L.L., Wu, W.W., and Molday, R.S. (2007). Retinoschisin (RS1), the protein encoded by the X-linked retinoschisis gene, is anchored to the surface of retinal photoreceptor and bipolar cells through its interactions with a Na/K ATPase-SARM1 complex. JBiolChem *282*, 32792-32801.

Molday, R.S. (2007). Focus on molecules: retinoschisin (RS1). ExpEye Res *84*, 227-228.

Munoz, V., and Serrano, L. (1994). Intrinsic secondary structure propensities of the amino acids, using statistical phi-psi matrices: comparison with experimental scales. Proteins *20*, 301-311.

Newman, E.A., and Odette, L.L. (1984). Model of electroretinogram b-wave generation: a test of the K+ hypothesis. JNeurophysiol *51*, 164-182.

Noiva, R. (1999). Protein disulfide isomerase: the multifunctional redox chaperone of the endoplasmic reticulum. SeminCell DevBiol *10*, 481-493.

Peachey, N.S., Fishman, G.A., Derlacki, D.J., and Brigell, M.G. (1987). Psychophysical and electroretinographic findings in X-linked juvenile retinoschisis. ArchOphthalmol *105*, 513-516.

Petukhov, M., Cregut, D., Soares, C.M., and Serrano, L. (1999). Local water bridges and protein conformational stability. Protein Sci *8*, 1982-1989.

Prenner, J.L., Capone, A., Jr., Ciaccia, S., Takada, Y., Sieving, P.A., and Trese, M.T. (2006). Congenital X-linked retinoschisis classification system. Retina *26*, S61-S64.

Reid, S.N., Akhmedov, N.B., Piriev, N.I., Kozak, C.A., Danciger, M., and Farber, D.B. (1999). The mouse X-linked juvenile retinoschisis cDNA: expression in photoreceptors. Gene *227*, 257-266.

Robson, J.G., and Frishman, L.J. (1995). Response linearity and kinetics of the cat retina: the bipolar cell component of the dark-adapted electroretinogram. VisNeurosci *12*, 837-850.

Roesch, M.T., Ewing, C.C., Gibson, A.E., and Weber, B.H. (1998). The natural history of X-linked retinoschisis. Can J Ophthalmol *33*, 149-158.

Sauer, C.G., Gehrig, A., Warneke-Wittstock, R., Marquardt, A., Ewing, C.C., Gibson, A., Lorenz, B., Jurklies, B., and Weber, B.H. (1997). Positional cloning of the gene associated with X-linked juvenile retinoschisis. NatGenet *17*, 164-170.

Schymkowitz, J., Borg, J., Stricher, F., Nys, R., Rousseau, F., and Serrano, L. (2005). The FoldX web server: an online force field. Nucleic Acids Res *33*, W382-W388.

Schymkowitz, J.W., Rousseau, F., and Serrano, L. (2002). Surfing on protein folding energy landscapes. ProcNatlAcadSciUSA *99*, 15846-15848.

Sergeev, Y.V., Caruso, R.C., Meltzer, M.R., Smaoui, N., MacDonald, I.M., and Sieving, P.A. (2010). Molecular modeling of retinoschisin with functional analysis of pathogenic mutations from human X-linked retinoschisis. HumMolGenet *19*, 1302-1313.

Shi, L., Jian, K., Ko, M.L., Trump, D., and Ko, G.Y. (2009). Retinoschisin, a new binding partner for L-type voltage-gated calcium channels in the retina. J Biol Chem *284*, 3966-3975.

Shinoda, K., Ishida, S., Oguchi, Y., and Mashima, Y. (2000). Clinical characteristics of 14 japanese patients with X-linked juvenile retinoschisis associated with XLRS1 mutation. Ophthalmic Genet *21*, 171-180.

Shinoda, K., Ohde, H., Ishida, S., Inoue, M., Oguchi, Y., and Mashima, Y. (2004). Novel 473-bp deletion in XLRS1 gene in a Japanese family with X-linked juvenile retinoschisis. Graefes Arch Clin Exp Ophthalmol *242*, 561-565.

Sieving, P.A., Bingham, E.L., Kemp, J., Richards, J., and Hiriyanna, K. (1999a). Juvenile X-linked retinoschisis from XLRS1 Arg213Trp mutation with preservation of the electroretinogram scotopic b-wave. AmJOphthalmol *128*, 179-184.

Sieving, P.A., Bingham, E.L., Kemp, J., Richards, J., and Hiriyanna, K. (1999b). Juvenile X-linked retinoschisis from XLRS1 Arg213Trp mutation with preservation of the electroretinogram scotopic b-wave. Am J Ophthalmol *128*, 179-184.

Stockton, R.A., and Slaughter, M.M. (1989). B-wave of the electroretinogram. A reflection of ON bipolar cell activity. JGenPhysiol *93*, 101-122.

Takada, Y., Fariss, R.N., Muller, M., Bush, R.A., Rushing, E.J., and Sieving, P.A. (2006). Retinoschisin expression and localization in rodent and human pineal and consequences of mouse RS1 gene knockout. Mol Vis *12*, 1108-1116.

Tavtigian, S.V., Greenblatt, M.S., Lesueur, F., and Byrnes, G.B. (2008). In silico analysis of missense substitutions using sequence-alignment based methods. HumMutat *29*, 1327-1336.

Tsai, B., Rodighiero, C., Lencer, W.I., and Rapoport, T.A. (2001). Protein disulfide isomerase acts as a redox-dependent chaperone to unfold cholera toxin. Cell *104*, 937-948.

Tsodikov, O.V., Record, M.T., Jr., and Sergeev, Y.V. (2002). Novel computer program for fast exact calculation of accessible and molecular surface areas and average surface curvature. JComputChem *23*, 600-609.

Vijayasarathy, C., Sui, R., Zeng, Y., Yang, G., Xu, F., Caruso, R.C., Lewis, R.A., Ziccardi, L., and Sieving, P.A. (2010). Molecular mechanisms leading to null-protein product from retinoschisin (RS1) signal-sequence mutants in X-linked retinoschisis (XLRS) disease. Hum Mutat *31*, 1251-1260.

Vijayasarathy, C., Takada, Y., Zeng, Y., Bush, R.A., and Sieving, P.A. (2007). Retinoschisin is a peripheral membrane protein with affinity for anionic phospholipids and affected by divalent cations. Invest OphthalmolVisSci *48*, 991-1000.

Vijayasarathy, C., Ziccardi, L., Zeng, Y., Smaoui, N., Caruso, R.C., and Sieving, P.A. (2009). Null retinoschisin-protein expression from an RS1 c354del1-ins18 mutation causing progressive and severe XLRS in a cross-sectional family study. Invest Ophthalmol Vis Sci *50*, 5375-5383.

Wang, T., Waters, C.T., Rothman, A.M., Jakins, T.J., Romisch, K., and Trump, D. (2002). Intracellular retention of mutant retinoschisin is the pathological mechanism underlying X-linked retinoschisis. HumMolGenet *11*, 3097-3105.

Wang, T., Zhou, A., Waters, C.T., O'Connor, E., Read, R.J., and Trump, D. (2006). Molecular pathology of X linked retinoschisis: mutations interfere with retinoschisin secretion and oligomerisation. BrJOphthalmol *90*, 81-86.

Weber, B.H., Schrewe, H., Molday, L.L., Gehrig, A., White, K.L., Seeliger, M.W., Jaissle, G.B., Friedburg, C., Tamm, E., and Molday, R.S. (2002). Inactivation of the murine X-linked juvenile retinoschisis gene, Rs1h, suggests a role of retinoschisin in retinal cell layer organization and synaptic structure. ProcNatlAcadSciUSA *99*, 6222-6227.

Wu, W.W., and Molday, R.S. (2003). Defective discoidin domain structure, subunit assembly, and endoplasmic reticulum processing of retinoschisin are primary mechanisms responsible for X-linked retinoschisis. JBiolChem *278*, 28139-28146.

Wu, W.W., Wong, J.P., Kast, J., and Molday, R.S. (2005). RS1, a discoidin domain-containing retinal cell adhesion protein associated with X-linked retinoschisis, exists as a novel disulfide-linked octamer. JBiolChem *280*, 10721-10730.

Zeng, Y., Takada, Y., Kjellstrom, S., Hiriyanna, K., Tanikawa, A., Wawrousek, E., Smaoui, N., Caruso, R., Bush, R.A., and Sieving, P.A. (2004). RS-1 Gene Delivery to an Adult Rs1h Knockout Mouse Model Restores ERG b-Wave with Reversal of the Electronegative Waveform of X-Linked Retinoschisis. Invest Ophthalmol Vis Sci *45*, 3279-3285.

8

Electroretinogram Alterations in Diabetes?

María Miranda[1], María Victoria Sánchez-Villarejo[1], Raquel Álvarez-Nölting[1], Concha Vilela[2] and Francisco Javier Romero[2,3]

[1]Universidad CEU-Cardenal Herrera, Moncada, Valencia

[2]Fundación Oftalmológica del Mediterráneo

[3]Universidad Católica de Valencia 'San Vicente Mártir'

Spain

1. Introduction

Diabetes mellitus is a heterogeneous metabolic disorder characterized by hyperglycemia resulting from defective insulin secretion (type 1), resistance to insulin action (type 2), or both. It is often associated with complications, such as cardiovascular disease, kidney failure, retinopathy, as well as peripheral and autonomic neuropathies. Retinopathy is the most common microvascular complication of diabetes, and it remains a major cause of visual impairment worldwide. Vascular lesions in the early stages of diabetic retinopathy are characterized by the presence of capillary microaneurysms, pericyte deficient capillaries, and obliterated and degenerated capillaries. Proliferative diabetic retinopathy is the more advanced form of the disease, when circulation problems cause the retina to become oxygen deprived. As a result, new fragile blood vessels can begin to grow in the retina and into the vitreous. Therefore, diabetic retinopathy has long been recognized as a vascular disease. However, it is becoming increasingly clear that neuronal cells of the retina are also affected by diabetes. Electroretinogram (ERG) is the neurophysiological test used in order to measure electric changes that happen in the retina after a light stimulus. Changes in the ERG may be due to an impairment of any of the retinal cell types: photoreceptors (a-wave ERG), and amacrine, bipolar, and, mainly, Müller cells (b-wave ERG). Moreover, oscillatory potentials are likely to be due to inner retinal neurotransmission. Though it may seem that diverse studies have presented contradictory results, it is important to point that most of the studies in diabetic experimental animals point to a very early alteration in the b-wave amplitude and reductions in oscillatory potentials. The nervous potential originated in the retina after a light stimulus is transmitted to the visual cortex via the optic nerve. Retinal ganglion cells (RGCs), which form this optic nerve, are the best studied of the retinal neurons with respect to the effect of diabetes. The aim of this work is to summarize recent clinical and laboratory findings about several experimental therapies that have been used to minimize neural changes in retina of different animal models of diabetes.

2. Diabetic retinopathy: a microvascular or a neuronal disease?

The prevalence of diabetes mellitus (DM) worldwide is increasing rapidly in association with the increase of obesity. Complications are a major fear of patients with diabetes. Retinopathy is the most feared complication of diabetes, compromising quality of life in most sufferers. Almost all patients with type 1 diabetes will develop retinopathy over a 15- to 20-year period, and approximately 20-30% will advance to the blinding stage of the disease. More than 60% of patients with type 2 diabetes will have retinopathy. However, current therapeutic options for the treatment of diabetic retinopathy (DR) such as photocoagulation and vitrectomy are limited by their considerable side effects and far from satisfactory.

Retinal changes in diabetes are thought to be initiated by sustained hyperglycemia leading to biochemical abnormalities, that include alterations of various vasoactive and growth factors (Brownlee, 2001), nonenzymatic glycation (Bierhaus et al., 1998), increase in the polyol pathway and redox imbalance (Engerman et al., 1993; Ido et al., 1997), oxidative stress (Arnal et al., 2009; Johnsen-Soriano et al, 2008; Miranda et al., 2006), and activation of protein kinase C (PKC) (Koya & King, 1998).

In addition, DR has long been recognized as a vascular disease, but it is becoming increasingly clear that neuronal cells of the retina are also affected by diabetes.

Diabetic retinopathy is classified into an early, nonproliferative stage, and a latter, proliferative stage. Histologically, vascular lesions in the early stages of diabetic retinopathy in man and animals are characterized by the presence of capillary microaneurysms, pericyte deficient capillaries, and obliterated and degenerated capillaries.

Non-proliferative diabetic retinopathy (NPDR) is the early stage of the disease in which symptoms will be mild or non-existent. NPDR is characterized by the presence of: (i) microaneurysms, (ii) intraretinal hemorrhages, (iii) exudates, (iv) intraretinal vascular abnormalities (IRMA), (v) vascular changes of veins, (vi) alterations in the foveal avascular zone (FAZ), (vii) macular edema.

Approximately 50% of patients with very severe NPDR progress to PDR within 1 year. Proliferative diabetic retinopathy (PDR) is the more advanced form of the disease. At this stage, circulation problems cause the retina to become oxygen deprived. As a result new fragile blood vessels can begin to grow in the retina and into the vitreous. New vessels may proliferate on the optic nerve head and along the course of the major vascular arcades. The new vessels mostly grow along the posterior hyaloid and sudden vitreous contraction may result in rupture of these fragile vessels. When the vitreous detachment occurs, the new vessels are pulled anteriorly along with the underlying retina, resulting in tractional retinal detachment. On the other hand, vitreous might detach completely without any pull on the retina and the new vessels disappear. Diabetic macular edema is now the principal cause of vision loss in diabetes and involves leakage from a disrupted blood-retinal barrier. The intraretinal fluid comes from leaking microaneurysms or diffuses from capillary incompetent areas. In the clinical course of PDR, rubeosis may appear as a result of the progression of neovascularization in the front of the iris and the angle of the chamera, and finally result in neovascular glaucoma.

The final metabolic pathway causing diabetic retinopathy is not known. Numerous researchers have suggested that pathogenesis of diabetic retinopathy includes microvascular damage induced by glucose. Currently, there has been a great interest in vasoproliferative factors, which induce neovascularization. It has been shown that retinal ischemia stimulates a pathological neovascularization mediated by angiogenic factors, such as vascular endothelial growth factor (VEGF), which results in PDR. VEGFs are released by retinal pigment epithelium, pericytes and endothelial cells of the retina.

Evidence has begun to point to the fact that even before vascular complications begin to manifest, neuronal cell death and dysfunction have already begun.

Retinal ganglion cells (RGCs) are the best studied of the retinal neurons with respect to the effect of diabetes. Loss of ganglion cells has been detected in diabetic rats, mice and humans (Asnaghi et al., 2003; Barber et al., 1998; Martin et al., 2004). Barber et al. (1998) studied retinal sections from streptozotocin diabetic rats after 7.5 months of diabetes and identified 22% and 14% reductions in the thickness of the inner plexiform and inner nuclear layers, respectively, and a 10% reduction in the number of surviving ganglion cells. An increase in the frequency of retinal apoptosis was also obesrved in whole-mounted rat retinas after 1, 3, 6, and 12 months of diabetes and TUNEL-positive cells were not associated with blood vessels. Some researchers suggest that this "retinal neuropathy" require severe hyperglycemia and high activity of aldose reductase (Asnaghi et al., 2003).

Consistent with a possible role of apoptosis in the death of retinal neurons, numerous initiator and effector caspases have been found to become activated in retinas of both patients and diabetic animals. Upregulation of Bax, caspase-9 and -3 expression in the ganglion cell layer has been associated with neuronal degeneration in human diabetic retinopathy (Oshitari et al., 2008), suggesting that RGCs undergo apoptosis in diabetic patients leading to a reduction in the thickness of the nerve fibre layer (Kern et al., 2008). In streptozotocin (STZ) diabetic rats an increase in TUNEL-positive and caspase 3-positive cells have been observed in the ganglion cell layer (Arnal et al., 2009), and this was accompanied by a reduction in the thickness of all the layers of the retina. The mitochondria- and caspase-dependent cell-death pathway may be, in part, associated with neuronal degeneration in diabetic retinas.

Kern (Kern et al., 2010) induced diabetes in three different strains of rats with streptozotocin: Sprague Dawley, Lewis, and Wistar rats. After 8 months a significant loss of cells in the GCL occurred only in diabetic Lewis rats, whereas Wistar and Sprague Dawley rats showed little change, though all type of rats showed alterations in the electroretinogram.

Although RGC are the best studied, other neuronal cells can be damaged by diabetes, like horizontal cells, amacrine cells and photoreceptors (Park et al., 2003; Kusner et al., 2004; Seki, et al., 2004). In this sense, apoptosis has been observed in a few photoreceptor cells 4 weeks after the induction of diabetes in rats, and the number of apoptotic photoreceptors increased thereafter (Park et al., 2003). Others (Zhang et al., 2008) observed an increase in the number of TUNEL-positive cells espetially in the outer nuclear layer (ONL) 1 week after diabetes onset and reached a peak at 4 to 6 weeks, at the same time retinal ONL thickness was reduced significantly. With regard to photoreceptor function in diabetes, decreased amplitudes of the photoreceptor response 12 weeks after diabetes induction in rats and significantly faster dark adaptation than controls have been observed (Lieth et al, 2008); this faster relative recovery found in diabetes after bleach, in the presence of normal pigment dynamics, may reflect a decrease in outer segment lengths. Animal studies also show glial activation (Lieth et al., 2008), impaired glial cell metabolism (Li et al., 2002), and microglial cell activation (Layton et al., 2005).

3. Electroretinogram (ERG) and diabetic retinopathy.

The onset of vision loss is insidious in diabetes. While clinical diagnosis of diabetic retinopathy requires detection of vascular pathology, diabetes also induces changes in retinal function; indeed, functional changes occur in the retina prior to clinical symptoms of the disease.

Electrophysiological studies of humans with diabetes could be used to assess alterations such as dysfunction of ganglion cells and loss of colour and contrast sensitivity (Roy et al., 1986; Ghirlanda et al., 1991), moreover alterations in oscillatory potentials have been shown to predict the onset of proliferative retinopathy better than vascular lesions seen on fundus photographs (Bresnick & Palta, 1987). Recently Luu (Luu et al., 2010) performed full-field electroretinograms in subjects with nonproliferative diabetic retinopathy, diabetic subjects without retinopathy, and normal control subjects and found that all the oscillatory potential (OP) components (OP1-OP4) were significantly reduced in amplitude and increased in implicit time in the no-DR and NPDR groups. OP4 amplitude correlated significantly with the retinal arteriolar caliber suggesting a correlation between retinal neuronal dysfunction and microvasculature changes. Interestingly, one study has assessed the effect of short-term strict glycemic control on OP amplitude (Frost-Larsen et al, 1983) and reported that OP amplitudes, which were initially abnormal in a group of aretinopathic subjects with IDDM, were normalized after 11 days of strict glycemic control.

Other studies have concluded that neuroretinal function is affected before the onset of vascular lesions in humans. The amplitude of the b-wave of the scotopic full-field (flash) ERG, reflecting largely the activity of the bipolar cells are abnormal in diabetes in the absence of visible fundus signs of retinopathy (Coupland, 1987; Hardy et al., 1995). Although functional changes can occur in the absence of retinopathy, this does not mean that function is not related to retinopathy, it is more a sign of the retinopathy severity and the magnitude of the functional loss.

The origin of the electroretinogram anomalies is not known, though it can be related to apoptosis of retinal ganglionar cells (RGCs) and the morphological alterations in the surviving RGCs.

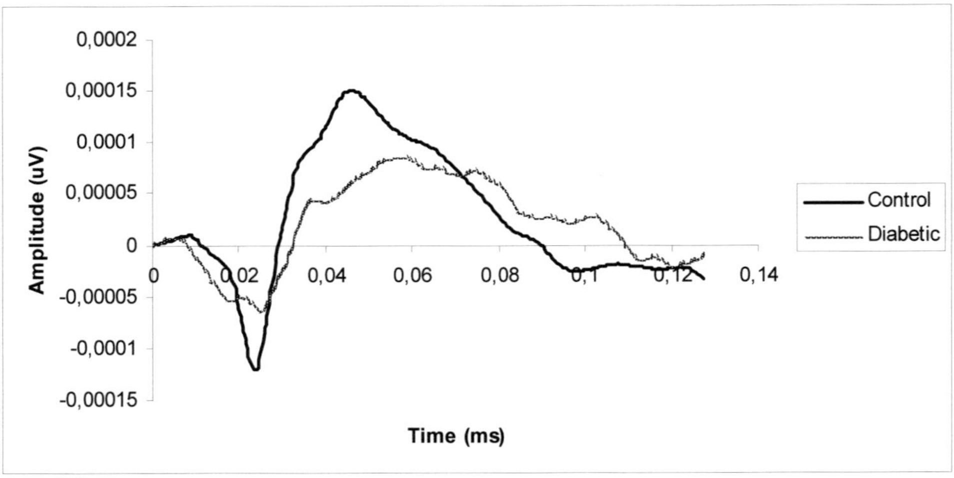

Fig. 1. Example of an electroretinogram in a control and streptozotocin-induced diabetic rat (12 weeks after the induction of diabetes).

ERG studies performed in diabetic rats have detected reduced ERG responses as early as 2 weeks after diabetes induction (Li, 2002). Experience in our lab suggest that the most consistent result is a decrease in b-wave amplitude after 1 month of streptozotocin-induced diabetes in Sprague Dawley rats and after only one week in alloxan-induced diabetic mice.

Kern et al., (2010) studied streptozotocin-induced diabetes in Lewis, Wistar and Sprague Dawley rats and observed that all strains tended to show diabetes-induced impairment of dark-adapted b-wave amplitude, but only Sprague Dawley and Lewis strains had a significant reduction in latency. The electroretinogram b-wave is generally believed to reflect mainly light-induced activity of ON-center bipolar cells and Muller cells. It has also been suggested that the b-wave of the electroretinogram is a particularly sensitive index of retinal ischemia and that, although the amount of reduction in b-wave amplitude during ischemia corresponds to the severity of the insult, the degree of recovery of the b-wave during reperfusion depends on the duration of ischemia. In this sense the b-wave of the ERG represents a functional measure for potential therapeutic efficacy of drugs interacting with these pathophysiological processes.

It is thought that the ERG a-wave originates from photoreceptors (rods and cones), and alterations have been observed in a-wave amplitude and/or latency in diabetic animals. Although it may seem that diverse studies have presented contradictory results, it is important to point that most of the studies in experimental animals show a very early alteration in the b-wave amplitude and reductions in oscillatory potentials and the differences observed in the different studies can be due to either the different models used or the different conditions of the ERG. Most interesting results of diabetes alterations in ERG from diabetic rats are summarized in Table 1

4. Clinical and laboratory findings about experimental therapies

The duration of diabetes and severity of hyperglycaemia are the major risk factors in diabetic retinopathy. Strict metabolic control and tight blood pressure control can significantly reduce the risk of developing retinopathy and its progression, but are difficult to achieve in clinical practice. Laser photocoagulation and vitrectomy are effective in preventing severe visual loss from sight-threatening diabetic retinopathy and its complications, but both modalities have potential side-effects. The use of pharmacological agents as monotherapy has allowed patients to recover vision faster than with previous treatment modalities, but these effects are frequently, but not always, short-lived. As sustained beneficial effects have been shown only in the treatment schedules which require frequent intravitreal injections, with the subsequent side-effects derived such as increase in intraocular pressure, develop of secondary glaucoma, retinal detachment, cataract formation and endophthalmitis. Due to the limitations of current treatment, new pharmacological therapies are being developed. The latter target underlying biochemical mechanisms that cause DR through involvement of protein kinase C (PKC) activation, oxidative stress, the angiogenesis pathway, and the glycation and sorbitol pathway. These treatments aim to prevent diabetes-induced damage to the retinal microvasculature.

Relatively new research on neurodegeneration is expanding our views of the pathogenesis of DR because it is becoming increasingly clear that neuronal cells of the retina are also affected by diabetes, resulting in dysfunction and even degeneration of some neuronal cells. Several experimental therapies have been used to minimize neural changes in retina of different animal models of diabetes (Table 2). Most of them have focused on the inhibition of RGC apoptosis though we do not know yet metabolic pathways causing this apoptotic response. Other agents like anti-inflammatory drugs, aldose reductase inhibitors, growth factors, erythropoietin, have also been tested with positive results.

Model	Duration	Observation	Reference
Male Sprague-Dawley STZ rats	3 months	Decreased a- and b-wave amplitudes	Ma et al., 2009
Sprague-Dawley STZ rats	1, 3 months	Reduced b-wave amplitudes and OPs with the progress of diabetes	Zhang et al., 2009
Alloxan Swiss mice	3 weeks	Reduced b-wave amplitude	Johnsen-Soriano et al., 2008
Sprague-Dawley STZ rats	4, 8 and 11 weeks	Unaffected a- and b-wave. Reduced OPs by 8 weeks.	Kohzaki et al., 2008
Male Wistar STZ rats	3, 6, 9 and 12 weeks	Reduction in the amplitude and increase in the peak time of all waves	Layton et al., 2007
Female Long Evans STZ rats	12 weeks	No differences in the amplitude of the a- or b-wave, differences in the pattern of OPs	Ramsey et al, 2006
Spontaneously Diabetic Torii rat	44 week	Prolongation of the peak latencies	Sasase et al., 2006
Sprague-Dawley STZ rats	12 weeks	Decreased amplitudes of the photoreceptor response	Phipps et al., 2006
Alloxan Swiss mice	1 week	Latency and implicit times were not affected	Miranda et al., 2006
Alloxan Swiss mice	1 week	Decreased b-wave amplitude	Miranda et al., 2004
Long-Evans male STZ rats	12 weeks	Small but significant delay in a-wave, no change in b-wave timing, sensitivity of b-wave reduced and a-wave not changed	Hancock et al., 2004
Brown-Norway STZ rats	1 month	Reduction in the amplitudes of a- and b-waves	Aizu et al., 2002
Male albino STZ rats	2 weeks	Reduced a- and b-amplitude, b-wave more affected than a-wave	Li et al., 2002
Male Wistar STZ rats	1, 2 months	Abnormal increase in latency and reduction of amplitude of ERG and VEP waves	Biró et al., 1998
Male Sprague-Dawley STZ rats	6 to 20 weeks	Reduced amplitudes of OP 1 and OP 2	Ishikawa et al., 1996
Male Sprague-Dawley STZ rats	1 month	Prolongation of the peak latency of oscillatory potentials in the b-wave of the erg	Hotta et al., 1995
Alloxan-induced diabetic rats	1, 2 months	After 1 month, 20% reduction in amplitudes, after 2 months this decrease was about 60%	Doly et al., 1992
Rats with STZ fructose-induced diabetes	4, 8 and 12 weeks	Prolonged peak latencies and intervals and reduced amplitudes	Funada et al., 1987
STZ pigmented rat	2, 4, and 19 weeks	No effect on the b-wave at 2- and 4-week; at 19 weeks reduced amplitude. c-wave reduced in amplitude at 2-week	Pautler et al., 1980

(STZ: streptozotocin, OP: oscillatory potentials, GC: ganglion cells, VEP: visual evoked potential)

Table 1. Changes in electroretinogram in different animal models of diabetes.

Drug	Type of drug	Model	Effect	Reference
Aminoguanidine	Aldose reductase inhibitor	Wistar albino STZ rats	Prevented the impairment in retrograde axonal transport and neuroaxonal changes	Zhang et al., 2008
Baicalein	Antiinflammatory	STZ rats	Reduced ganglion cell loss	Yang et al., 2009
Cannabidiol	Nonpsychotropic cannabinoid	Male Sprague-Dawley STZ rats	Reduced oxidative stress; decreased levels of TNF-α, VEGF, and ICAM-1; and prevented retinal cell death. Inhibited p38 MAP kinase	El-Remessy et al., 2006
des(1-3)IGF-1	Insulin-like growth factor (IGF)-1 analog	Male Sprague-Dawley STZ rats	Decreased IGF receptor and protein phospho-Akt (Thr 308) immunoreactivity in GCL	Kummer et al, 2003
DHA	Omega-3 fatty acid	Male Wistar STZ rats	Decreased TUNEL and caspase-3 positive cells in GCL	Arnal et al., 2009
Erythropoietin	Hormone	Sprague-Dawley STZ rats	Improves abnormalities of ERG, GC with swollen mitochondria, increased retinal glutamate and EPO-R in the retinas	Zhu et al., 2008
FeTTPS	Peroxynitrite decomposition catalyst	Male Sprague-Dawley STZ rats	Prevented tyrosine nitration, restored NGF survival signal, and prevented neuronal death	Ali et al., 2008
Insulin-like growth factor (IGF-1)	Growth factor	Male Sprague-Dawley STZ rats	Reduced the number of TUNEL and p-Akt, Caspase-3 and BAD immunoreactive	Seigel et al., 2006
KIOM-79	Mixture of extracts obtained from Puerariae lobata, Magnolia officinalis, Glycyrrhiza uralensis and Euphorbia pekinensis	db/db mice	Prevented apoptotic cell death and AGEs accumulation	Sohn et al., 2009
Latanoprost	Prostaglandin F2alpha analogue	Male Sprague-Dawley STZ rats	Rescued retinal neuro-glial cells from apoptosis inhibiting caspase-3, increased phosphorylated to total protein ratio of p44/p42 MAPK, but not of Akt	Nakanishi et al., 2006
Lutein	Carotenoid	Male Wistar STZ rats	Decreased TUNEL and caspase-3 positive cells in GCL	Arnal et al., 2009

Drug	Type of drug	Model	Effect	Reference
Memantine	Glutamate NMDA receptor antagonist	STZ Brown Norway rats	Improved amplitudes of a- and b-waves GC loss	Kusari et al., 2007
Minocycline	Antiinflammatory	Sprague-Dawley STZ rats	Repressed cytokine production, reduced release of cytotoxins from activated microglia, and reduced caspase-3 activity	Krady et al., 2005
Nepafenac (topical)	Non-steroidal cycloxygenase inhibitor	Male Lewis STZ rats	No effect on diabetes-induced loss of cells in GCL. Inhibited development of OP delays	Kern et al., 2007
Nerve growth factor	Growth factor	Male wistar STZ rats	Prevented both early PCD in RGC and Muller cells	Hammes et al., 1995
Nipradilol	Beta-adrenoceptor blocking agent	Male Sprague-Dawley STZ rats	Antiapoptotic, removal of the NO moiety from nipradilol blocked these effects	Tatsumi et al., 2008
(+)-pentazocine	Sigma receptor 1 ligand	Spontaneous diabetic Ins2(Akita/+)	Preservation of retinal architecture, reduced nitrotyrosine and HNE	Smith et al., 2008
Rottlerin	PKC delta inhibitor	Otsuka Long-Evans Tokushima fatty (OLETF)	Inhibit protein kinase C-delta and neuronal apoptosis	Kim et al., 2008
Salicylates (aspirin, sodium salicylate, sulfasalazine)	anti-inflammatory, unlike aspirin, sodium salicylate and sulfasalazine can not inhibit COX at therapeutic doses.	Male Lewis STZ rats	Inhibited translocation of NF-KB to the nucleus, prevented RGC loss	Zheng et al., 2007
Sorbinil	Aldose reductase inhibitors	Male Sprague-Dawley STZ rats	Regulated retinal homeostasis and protected neurons against damage	Asnaghi et al., 2003

(TNF-α: tumor necrosis factor-α; ICAM-1: intercellular adhesion molecule-1; GCL: ganglion cell layer; DHA: docosahexaenoic acid; ONL: outer nuclear layer; ERG: electroretinogram; NGF: nerve growth factor; AGE: advanced glycation endproduct; OP: oscillatory potentials; PCD: programmed cell death; RGC: retinal ganglion cell; HNE: hidroxynonenal).

Table 2. Experimental therapies resulting in preservation of retinal neurons in diabetes.

We will focus on oxidative stress. It has been repeatedly suggested that oxidative stress is involved in the pathogenesis of late diabetes complications (Baynes & Thorpe, 1993), though it is not definitely demonstrated if this is the cause or the consequence of these complications. It is clear that the elevated glucose levels present in diabetes and the existence of oxidative stress are inseparable. Hyperglycemia reduces antioxidant levels and concomitantly increases the production of free radicals. These effects contribute to tissue damage in diabetes mellitus, leading to alterations in the redox potential of the cell with subsequent activation of redox-sensitive genes (Bonnefont-Rousselot, 2002). The retina is the neurosensorial tissue of the eye and is extremely rich in polyunsaturated lipid membranes. This feature makes it specially sensitive to oxygen- and/or nitrogen activated species and lipid peroxidation.

Oxidative stress is linked to early apoptosis in diabetic retinopathy both at the microvasculature and neuronal cells of the retina but oxidative stress appears to be highly interrelated with other biochemical imbalances that lead to structural and functional changes.

Among the proposed pathogenic mechanisms, the polyol pathway model has received the most scrutiny. Aldose reductase (AR) is the first enzyme in the polyol pathway, converting excess glucose to sorbitol, which is then metabolized to fructose by sorbitol dehydrogenase. According to several studies, AR is correlated with the early events in the pathogenesis of diabetic retinopathy, leading to a cascade of retinal lesions including blood retinal barrier breakdown, loss of pericytes, neuroretinal apoptosis, glial reactivation, and neovascularization. Increased AR activity has been shown to contribute to increased oxidative stress by promoting nonenzymatic glycation and the activation of PKC (Stitt and Curtis, 2005). It has been demonstrated that AR inhibition counteracts diabetes induced oxidative and nitrosative stress and prevents vascular endothelial growth factor (VEGF) overexpression, basal membrane thickening, pericyte loss, and microaneurysms in retinal capillaries (Obrosova et al., 2003). Increased expression of VEGF and apoptosis and proliferation of blood vessels have been shown to be less prominent in diabetes rats than in diabetic AR-deficient animals (Obrosva et al., 2005).

A recent clinical study has substantiated the concept of "hyperglycemic memory" in the pathogenesis of diabetic retinopathy. The Diabetes Control and Complications Trial-Epidemiology of Diabetes Interventions and Complications Research, has revealed that the reduction in the risk of progressive retinopathy resulting from intensive therapy in patients with type 1 diabetes persisted for at least several years after the DCCT trial, despite increasing hyperglycemia. The process of formation and accumulation of advanced glycation end products (AGEs) and their mode of action are most compatible with the "hyperglycemic memory" theory. Advanced glycation end products are formed by nonenzymatic reactions between reducing sugars and free amino groups of proteins or lipids. AGEs have been detected within retinal vasculature and neurosensory tissue of diabetic eyes. Multiple consequences of AGE accumulation in the retina have been demonstrated, including upregulation of VEGF, upregulation of NF-κB, and increased leukocyte adhesion in retinal microvascular endothelial cells (Moore et al., 2003). In a 5-year study in diabetic dogs, administration of aminoguanidine (an inhibitor of AGE formation) prevented retinopathy (Kern et al., 2001). AGEs exert cell-mediated effects via RAGE, a multiligand signal-transduction receptor of the immunoglobulin superfamily (Schmidt et al., 1992). Consequences of ligand-RAGE interaction include increased expression of vascular cell adhesion molecule (VCAM)-1, vascular enhanced permeability, enhanced thrombogenicity, induction of oxidant stress and abnormal expression of eNOS (Schmidt et al., 1995). Recently, it has been shown that after RAGE activation NADPH oxidase is activated by phospholipase C-mediated activation of Ca(2+)-dependent PKC and that this may lead to an increase in ROS that could be associated with the initial stages of macular

edema and diabetic retinopathy (Warboys et al., 2005). Studies in models of retinopathy show that increases in oxidative stress and signs of vascular inflammation are correlated with increases in arginase activity and arginase expression, and that decreasing arginase expression or inhibiting its activity blocks these effects, and that the induction of arginase during retinopathy is blocked by inhibiting NADPH oxidase activity (Caldwell et al., 2010). Finally it has been also demonstrated that AGEs can induce glial reaction and neuronal degeneration in retinal explants (Lecleire-Collet et al., 2005).
Different antioxidants (ebselen, lutein and DHA) have been used in our lab in different animal models of diabetes, and all of them have shown good results in improving the decrease of b-wave amplitude ERG observed in these animals.
Alterations associated with oxidative stress offer many potential therapeutic targets making this an area of great interest for the development of safe and effective treatments for diabetic retinopathy. Animal models of diabetic retinopathy have shown beneficial effects of antioxidants on the development of retinopathy, but clinical trials (though very limited in number) have provided somewhat ambiguous results. Although antioxidants are being used for other chronic diseases, controlled clinical trials are warranted to investigate potential benefitial effects of antioxidants in the development of retinopathy in diabetic patients.

5. Acknowledgments

This work was supported in part by Funds from Ministerio de Ciencia e Innovación (SAF 2010-21317) and Copernicus-Santander (PRCEU-UCH/ COP(01)10/11) programme of the Universidad CEU- Cardenal Herrera

6. References

Aizu, Y.; Oyanagi, K.; Hu, J. & Nakagawa, H. (2002). Degeneration of retinal neuronal processes and pigment epithelium in the early stage of the streptozotocin-diabetic rats. *Neuropathology*, Vol. 22, No. 3 (September, 2002), pp. 161-170. ISSN 1440-1789.

Ali, T.K.; Matragoon, S.; Pillai, B.A.; Liou, G.I.; El-Remessy, A.B. (2008). Peroxynitrite mediates retinal neurodegeneration by inhibiting nerve growth factor survival signaling in experimental and human diabetes. *Diabetes*, Vol. 57, No. 4 (April, 2008), pp. 889-898. ISSN 0012-1797.

Arnal, E.; Miranda, M.; Johnsen-Soriano, S.; Alvarez-Nölting, R.; Díaz-Llopis, M.; Araiz, J.; Cervera, E.; Bosch-Morell, F. & Romero, F.J. (2009). Beneficial effect of docosahexaenoic acid and lutein on retinal structural, metabolic and functional abnormalities in diabetic rats. *Current Eye Research*, Vol.34, No.11, (November, 2009), pp. 928-938, ISSN 1460-2202.

Asnaghi, V.; Gerhardinger, C.; Hoehn, T.; Adeboje, A. & Lorenzi, M. (2003). A role for the polyol pathway in the early neuroretinal apoptosis and glial changes induced by diabetes in the rat. Barber, A.J.; Lieth, E.; Khin, S.A.; Antonetti, D.A.; Buchanan, A.G. & Gardner, T.W. (1998). Neural apoptosis in the retina during experimental and human diabetes: early onset and effect of insulin. *Journal of Clinical Investigation*, Vol. 102, No4 (August, 1998), pp. 783–791. ISSN 00219738.

Baynes, J.W. & Thorpe, S.R. (1996). The role of oxidative stress in diabetic complications. *Current Opinion in Endocrinology*, Vol. 3, pp. 277-284. ISSN 1068-3097.

Bierhaus, A.; Hofmann, M.A.: Ziegler, R. & Nawroth, P.P. (1998). AGEs and their interaction with AGE-receptors in vascular disease and diabetes mellitus. I. The AGE concept. *Cardiovascular Reseach*, Vol. 37, No. 3; (March 1998), pp. 586-600, ISSN 1755-3245.

Bíró, K.; Pálhalmi, J.; Tóth, A.J.; Kukorelli, T. & Juhász, G. (1998). Bimoclomol improves early electrophysiological signs of retinopathy in diabetic rats. *Neuroreport*, Vol. 22, No. 9 (September, 1998), pp. 2029-2033. ISSN 0959-4965.

Bonnefont-Rousselot, D. (2002). Glucose and reactive oxygen species. *Current Opinion in Clinical Nutrition and Metabolism Care*, Vol. 5, No. 5 (September, 2002), pp. 561-568. ISSN 1363-1950.

Bresnick, G.H. & Palta, M. (1987). Predicting progression to severe proliferative diabetic retinopathy. *Archives of Ophthalmology*, Vol. 105, No. 6 (June, 1987), pp. 810-814. ISSN 0012-186X.

Brownlee, M. (2001). Biochemistry and molecular cell biology of diabetic complications. *Nature*, Vol. 414; No. 6865 (December, 2001), pp. 813-820, ISSN 0028-0836.

Caldwell, R.B.; Zhang, W.; Romero, M.J.; Caldwell, R.W. (2010). Vascular dysfunction in retinopathy-an emerging role for arginase. *Brain Research Bulletin*, Vol. 81, No. 2-3 (February, 2010), pp. 303-309. ISSN 0361-9230.

Coupland, S.G. (1987). A comparison of oscillatory potential and pattern electroretinogram measures in diabetic retinopathy. *Documenta Ophthalmologica*, Vol. 66, No. 3 (June, 1987), pp. 207-18. ISSN 0012-4486.

Doly, M.; Droy-Lefaix, M.T. & Braquet, P. (1992). Oxidative stress in diabetic retina. EXS, Vol. 62, pp. 299-307. ISSN 1023-294X.

Dong, C.J.; Agey, P. & Hare, W.A. (2004) Origins of the electroretinogram oscillatory potentials in the rabbit retina. *Visual Neuroscience*, Vol. 21 , No. 4 (July-August, 2004), pp. 533-543. ISSN 0952-5238.

El-Remessy, A.B.; Al-Shabrawey, M.; Califa, Y:; Tsai, N.T.; Caldwell, R.B. & Liou, G.I. (2006). Neuroprotective and blood-retinal barrier-preserving effects of cannabidiol in experimental diabetes. *The American Journal of Pathology*, Vol. 68, No. 1 (January, 2006), pp. 235-244. ISSN 00029440.

Engerman, R.L.; Kern, T.S. & Garment, M.B. (1993). Capillary basement membrane in retina, kidney, and muscle of diabetic dogs and galactosemic dogs and its response to 5 years aldose reductase inhibition. *Journal of Diabetes and its Complications*, Vol. 7, No. 4, (October-December 1993), pp. 241-245, ISSN 1056-8727.

Frost-Larsen, K.; Sandahl Christiansen, J. & Parving, H-H. (1983). The effect of strict short-term metabolic control on retinal nervous system abnormalities in newly diagnosed type 1 (insulin-dependent) diabetic patients. *Diabetologia*, Vol. 24, No. 3 (March, 2003), pp. 207–209. ISSN 0012-186X.

Funada, M.; Okamoto, I.; Fujinaga, Y. & Yamana, T. (1987). Effects of aldose reductase inhibitor (M79175) on ERG oscillatory potential abnormalities in streptozotocin fructose-induced diabetes in rats. *Japanese Journal of Ophthalmology*, Vol. 31, No. 2, pp. 305-314. ISSN 1613-2246.

Ghirlanda,G.; Di Leo, M.A.; Caputo, S.; Falsini, B.; Porciatti, V.; Marietti, G. & Greco, A.V. (1991). Detection of inner retina dysfunction by steady-state focal electroretinogram pattern and flicker in early IDDM. *Diabetes*, Vol. 40, No. 9 (September, 1991), pp. 1122-1127. ISSN 0012-1797.

Hammes, H-P.; Federoff, H.J. & Brownlee, M. (1995). Nerve growth factor prevents both neuroretinal programmed cell death and capillary pathology in experimental diabetes. *Molecular Medicine*, Vol. 1, No. 5, (July, 1995), pp. 527-534. ISSN 1541-7786.

Hancock, H.A. & Kraft, T.W. (2004). Oscillatory potential analysis and ERGs of normal and diabetic rats. *Investigative Ophthalmology & Visual Science,* Vol. 45, No. 4 (March, 2004), pp. 1002-1008. ISSN 1552-5783.

Hardy, K.J.; Fisher, C.; Heath, P.; Foster, D.H. & Scarpello, J.H. (1995). Comparison of colour discrimination and electroretinography in evaluation of visual pathway dysfunction in aretinopathic IDDM patients. *The British Journal of Ophthalmology,* Vol. 79, No. 1 (January, 1995), pp. 35-37. ISSN 00071161.

Hotta, N.; Koh, N.; Sakakibara, F.; Nakamura, J.; Hamada, Y.; Hara, T.; Takeuchi, N.; Inukai, S.; Kasama, N.; Fukasawa, H. & Kakuta, H. (1995). An aldose reductase inhibitor, TAT, prevents electroretinographic abnormalities and ADP-induced hyperaggregability in streptozotocin-induced diabetic rats. *European Journal of Clinical Investigation,* Vol. 25, No. 12 (December, 1995), pp. 948-954. ISSN 1365-2362.

Ido, Y.; Kilo, C. & Williamson, J.R. (1997). Cytosolic NADH/NAD+, free radicals and vascular dysfunction in early diabetes mellitus. *Diabetologia,* Vol. 40, No. Suppl. 2, (July, 1997), pp. S115-S117, ISSN 0012-186X.

Ino-Ue, M.; Zhang, L.; Naka, H.; Kuriyama, H. & Yamamoto, M. (2000). Polyol metabolism of retrograde axonal transport in diabetic rat large optic nerve fiber. *Investigative Ophthalmology & Visual Science,* Vol. 41, No. 13 (December, 2000), pp. 4055-4058. ISSN 1552-5783.

Ishikawa, A.; Ishiguro, S. & Tamai, M. (1996). Changes in GABA metabolism in streptozotocin-induced diabetic rat retinas. *Current Eye Research,* Vol. 15, No. 1 (January, 1996), pp. 63-71. ISSN 0014-4835.

Johnsen-Soriano, S.; Garcia-Pous, M.; Arnal, E.; Sancho-Tello, M.; Garcia-Delpech, S.; Miranda, M.; Bosch-Morell, F.; Diaz-Llopis, M.; Navea, A. & Romero, F.J. (2008). Early lipoic acid intake protects retina of diabetic mice. *Free Radical Research,* Vol. 42, No. 7, (July, 2008), pp. 613-617. ISSN 1071-5762.

Kern, T.S.; Miller, C.M.; Du, Y.; Zheng, L.; Mohr, S.; Ball, S.L.; Kim, M.; Jamison, J.A. & Bingaman, D.P. (2007). Topical administration of nepafenac inhibits diabetes-induced retinal microvascular disease and underlying abnormalities of retinal metabolism and physiology. *Diabetes,* Vol. 56, No. 2 (February, 2007), pp. 373-379. ISSN 0012-1797.

Kern, T.S. & Barber, A.J. (2008). Retinal ganglion cells in diabetes. *The Journal of Physiology,* Vol. 586, No.18 (August, 2008), pp. 4401-4408. ISSN 0022-3751.

Kern, T.S.; Miller, C.M.; Tang, J.; Du, Y.; Ball, S.L.; Berti-Matera, L. (2010). Comparison of three strains of diabetic rats with respect to the rate at which retinopathy and tactile allodynia develop. *Molecular Vision,* Vol. 16 (August 2010), pp. 1629-39. ISSN 1090-0535.

Kim, Y.H.; Kim, Y.S.; Park, C.H.; Chung, I.Y.; Yoo, J.M.; Kim, J.G.; Lee, B.J.; Kang, S.S.; Cho, G.J. & Choi, W.S. (2008). Protein kinase C-delta mediates neuronal apoptosis in the retinas of diabetic rats via the Akt signaling pathway. *Diabetes,* Vol. 57, No. 8 (August, 2008), pp. 2181-2190. ISSN 0012-1797.

Koya, D. & King, G.L. (1998). Protein kinase C activation and the development of diabetic complications. *Diabetes,* Vol. 47, No. 6 (June, 1998), pp. 859-866. ISSN 0012-1797.

Krady, J.K.; Basu, A.; Allen, C.M.; Xu, Y.; LaNoue, K.F.; Gardner, T.W. & Levison S.W. (2005). Minocycline reduces proinflammatory cytokine expression, microglial activation, and caspase-3 activation in a rodent model of diabetic retinopathy. *Diabetes*, Vol. 54, No. 5 (May, 2005), pp. 1559-1565. ISSN 0012-1797.

Kohzaki, K.; Vingrys, A.J. & Bui, B.V. (2008). Early inner retinal dysfunction in streptozotocin-induced diabetic rats. *Investigative Ophthalmology & Visual Science*, Vol. 49, No. 8 (August, 2008), pp. 3595-3604. ISSN 1552-5783.

Kummer, A.; Pulford, B.E.; Ishii, D.N. & Seigel, G.M. (2003). Des(1-3)IGF-1 treatment normalizes type 1 IGF receptor and phospho-Akt (Thr 308) immunoreactivity in predegenerative retina of diabetic rats. *International Journal of Experimental Diabesity Research*, Vol. 4, No. 1 (January-March, 2003), pp. 45-57. ISSN 1560-4284.

Kusari, J.; Zhou, S.; Padillo, E.; Clarke, K.G. & Gil, D.W. (2007). Effect of memantine on neuroretinal function and retinal vascular changes of streptozotocin-induced diabetic rats. *Investigative Ophthalmology & Visual Science*, Vol. 48, No. 11 (November, 2007), pp. 5152-5159. ISSN 1552-5783.

Kusner, L.L.; Sarthy, V.P. & Mohr, S. (2004). Nuclear translocation of glyceraldehyde-3-phosphate dehydrogenase: a role in high glucose-induced apoptosis in retinal Muller cells. *Investigative Ophthalmology & Visual Science*, Vol. 45, No. 5 (May, 2004), pp. 1553-1561. ISSN 1552-5783.

Layton, C.J.; Safa, R. & Osborne, N.N. (2007). Oscillatory potentials and the b-Wave: partial masking and interdependence in dark adaptation and diabetes in the rat. *Graefe's Archive for Clinical and Experimental Ophthalmology*, Vol. 245, No. 9 (September, 2007), pp. 1335-1345. ISSN 0721-832X.

Layton, C.J.; Chidlow, G.; Casson, R.J.; Wood, J.P.; Graham, M. & Osborne, N.N. (2005). Monocarboxylate transporter expression remains unchanged during thedevelopment of diabetic retinal neuropathy in the rat. *Investigative Ophthalmology & Visual Science*, Vol. 46, No. 8 (August, 2005), pp. 2878-2885. ISSN 1552-5783.

Lecleire-Collet, A.; Tessier, L.H.; Massin, P.; Forster, V.; Brasseur, G.; Sahel, J.A. & Picaud, S. (2005). Advanced glycation end products can induce glial reaction and neuronal degeneration in retinal explants. *The British Journal of Ophthalmology*, Vol. 89, No. 12 (December, 2005), pp. 1631-1633. ISSN 00071161.

Li, Q. & Puro, D.G. (2002). Diabetes-induced dysfunction of the glutamate transporter in retinal Muller cells. *Investigative Ophthalmology & Visual Science*, Vol. 43, No. 9 (September, 2002), pp. 3109-3116. ISSN 1552-5783.

Li, Q.; Zemel, E.; Miller, B. & Perlman, I. (2002). Early retinal damage in experimental diabetes: electroretinographical and morphological observations. *Experimental Eye Research*, Vol. 74, No. 5 (May, 2002), pp. 615-625. ISSN 0014-4835.

Lieth, E.; Barber, A.J.; Xu, B.; Dice, C.; Ratz, M.J.; Tanase, D.; Strother, J.M. & the Penn State Retina Research Group. (1998). Glial reactivity and impaired glutamate metabolism in short-term experimental diabetic retinopathy. *Diabetes*, Vol. 47, No.5 (May, 1998), pp. 815-820. ISSN 0012-1797.

Luu, C.D.; Szental, J.A.; Lee, S.Y.; Lavanya, R. & Wong TY. (2010). Correlation between retinal oscillatory potentials and retinal vascular calibre in type 2 diabetes. *Investigative Ophthalmology & Visual Science*, Vol. 51, No. 1 (January, 2010), pp. 482-486. ISSN 1552-5783.

Ma, P.; Luo, Y.; Zhu, X.; Ma, H.; Hu, J. & Tang, S. (2009). Phosphomannopentaose sulfate (PI-88) inhibits retinal leukostasis in diabetic rat. *Biochemical and Biophysical Research Communication*, Vol. 380, No. 2 (March, 2009), pp. 402-406. ISSN 0006-291X.

Martin, P.M.; Roon, P.; Van Ells, T.K.; Ganapathy, V. & Smith, S.B. (2004). Death of retinal neurons in streptozotocin-induced diabetic mice. *Investigative Ophthalmology & Visual Science Science*, Vol. 45, No. 9 (September, 2009), pp. 3330-3336. ISSN 1552-5783.

Miranda, M.; Muriach, M.; Roma, J.; Bosch-Morell, F.; Genovés, J.M.; Barcia, J.; Araiz, J.; Díaz-Llopis, M. & Romero, F.J. (2006). Oxidative stress in a model of experimental diabetic retinopathy: the utility of peroxinytrite scavengers. *Archivos de la Sociedad Española de Oftalmología*, Vol. 81, No. 1 (January, 2006), pp. 27-32. ISSN 0365-6691.

Miranda, M.; Muriach, M.; Johnsen, S.; Bosch-Morell, F.; Araiz, J.; Romá, J. & Romero, F.J. (2004). Oxidative stress in a model for experimental diabetic retinopathy: treatment with antioxidants. *Archivos de la Sociedad Española de Oftalmolgía*, Vol. 79, No. 6 (June, 2004), pp. 289-294. ISSN 0365-6691.

Moore, T.C.; Moore, J.E.; Kaji, Y., Frizzell, N.; Usui, T.; Poulaki, V.; Campbell, I.L., Stitt, A.W.; Gardiner, T.A.; Archer, D.B. & Adamis, A.P. (2003). The role of advanced glycation end products in retinal microvascular leukostasis. *Investigative Ophthalmology & Visual Science Science*, Vol. 44, No. 10 (October, 2003), pp. 4457-4464. ISSN 1552-5783.

Nakanishi, Y.; Nakamura, M.; Mukuno, H.; Kanamori, A.; Seigel, G.M. & Negi, A. (2008). Latanoprost rescues retinal neuro-glial cells from apoptosis by inhibiting caspase-3, which is mediated by p44/p42 mitogen-activated protein kinase. *Experimental Eye Research*, Vol. 83, No. 5 (November, 2008), pp. 1108-1117. ISSN 0014-4835.

Obrosova, I.G.; Minchenko, A.G.; Vasupuram, R.; White L.; Abatan, O.I. & Kumagai, A.K. (2003). Aldose reductase inhibitor fidarestat prevents retinal oxidative stress and vascular endothelial growth factor overexpression in streptozotocin-diabetic rats. *Diabetes*, Vol. 52, No. 3 (March, 2003), pp. 864-871. ISSN 0012-1797.

Obrosova, I.G.; Pacher, P.; Szabo, C.; Zsengeller, Z.; Hirooka, H. & Stevens M.J. (2005). Aldose reductase inhibition counteracts oxidative/nitrosative stress and poly(ADPribose) polymerase activation in tissue sites for diabetes complications. *Diabetes*, Vol. 54, No. 3 (March, 2005), pp. 234-242. ISSN 0012-1797.

Oshitari, T.; Yamamoto, S.; Hata, N. & Roy, S. Mitochondria- and caspase-dependent cell death pathway involved in neuronal degeneration in diabetic retinopathy. *The British Journal of Ophthalmology*, Vol. 92; No. 4 (April, 2008), pp. 552-556. ISSN 00071161.

Park, S.H.; Park, J.W.; Park, S.J.; Kim, K.Y.; Chung, J.W.; Chun, M.H. & Oh, S.J. (2003). Apoptotic death of photoreceptors in the streptozotocin-induced diabetic rat retina. *Diabetologia*, Vol. 46, No. 9 (September, 2003), pp 1260-1268. ISSN 0012-186X.

Pautler, E.L. & Ennis, S.R. (1980). The effect of induced diabetes on the electroretinogram components of the pigmented rat. *Investigative Ophthalmology & Visual Science*, Vol. 19, No. 6 (June, 1980), pp. 702-705. ISSN 1552-5783.

Phipps, J.A.; Yee, P.; Fletcher, E.L. & Vingrys, A.J. (2006). Rod photoreceptor dysfunction in diabetes: activation, deactivation, and dark adaptation. *Investigative Ophthalmology & Visual Science*, Vol. 47, No. 7 (July, 2006), pp. 3187-3194. ISSN 1552-5783.

Ramsey, D.J.; Ripps, H. & Qian, H. (2006). An electrophysiological study of retinal function in the diabetic female rat. *Investigative Ophthalmology & Visual Science,* Vol. 47, No. 11 (September, 2006), pp. 5116-5124. ISSN 1552-5783.

Roy, M.; Gunkel, R. & Podgor, M.(1986). Color vision defects in early diabetic retinopathy. *Archives of Ophthalmology,* Vol. 104 , No. 2 (February, 1986), pp. 225-228. ISSN 0003-9950.

Sasase, T.; Ohta, T.; Ogawa, N.; Miyajima, K.; Ito, M.; Yamamoto, H.; Morinaga, H. & Matsushita, M. (2006). Preventive effects of glycaemic control on ocular complications of Spontaneously Diabetic Torii rat. *Diabetes Obesity & Metabolism,* Vol. 8, No. 5 (September, 2006), pp. 501-507. ISSN 1463-1326.

Seigel, G.M.; Lupien, S.B.; Campbell, L.M. & Ishii, D.N. (2006). Systemic IGF-I treatment inhibits cell death in diabetic rat retina. *Journal of Diabetes Complications,* Vol. 20, No. 3 (May-June, 2006), pp. 196-204. ISSN 1056-8727.

Seki, M.; Tanaka, T.; Nawa, H.; Usui, T.; Fukuchi, T.; Ikeda, K.; Abe, H. & Takei, N. (2004). Involvement of brain-derived neurotrophic factor in early retinal neuropathy of streptozotocin-induced diabetes in rats: therapeutic potential of brain-derived neurotrophic factor for dopaminergic amacrine cells. *Diabetes,* Vol. 53, No. 9 (September, 2004), pp. 2412-2419. ISSN 0012-1797.

Schmidt, A.,M.; Vianna, M.; Gerlach, M.; Brett J.; Ryan, J.; Kao, J.; Hegarty, H.; Hurley, W. & Clauss, M. (1992). Isolation and characterization of two binding proteins for advanced glycosylation end products from bovine lung which are present on the endothelial cell surface. *The Journal of Biological chemistry,* Vol. 267, No. 21 (July, 1992), pp. 14987-14997. ISSN 0021-9258.

Schmidt, A.M.; Hori, O.; Chen, J.X.; Li, J.F.; Crandall, J.; Zhang, J, Cao, R.; Yan, S.D.; Brett, J. & Stern, D. (1995). Advanced glycation end products interacting with their endothelial receptor induce expression of vascular cell adhesion molecule-1 (VCAM-1) in cultured human endothelial cells and in mice: a potential mechanism for the accelerated vasculopathy of diabetes. *Journal of Clinical Investigation,* Vol. 96, No. 3 (September, 1995), pp. 1395-1403. ISSN 0021-9258.

Smith, S.B.; Duplantier, J.; Dun Y.; Mysona, B.; Roon, P.; Martin, P.M. & Ganapathy, V. (2008). In vivo protection against retinal neurodegeneration by sigma receptor 1 ligand (+)-pentazocine. *Investigative Ophthalmology & Visual Science,* Vol. 49, No. 9 (September, 2008), pp. 4154-4161. ISSN 1552-5783.

Sohn, E.J.; Kim, Y.S.; Kim, C.S.; Lee, Y.M.; Kim, J.S. (2009). KIOM-79 prevents apoptotic cell death and AGEs accumulation in retinas of diabetic db/db mice. *Journal of Ethnopharmacology,* Vol. 121, No. 1 (January, 2009), pp. 171-174. ISSN 0378-8741.

Stitt, A.W. & Curtis, T.M. (2005). Advanced glycation and retinal pathology during diabetes. *Pharmacological Reports,* Vol. 57, pp. 156-168. ISSN 1734-1140.

Tatsumi, Y.; Kanamori, A.; Nagai-Kusuhara A.; Nakanishi Y.; Agarwal, N.; Negi. A. & Nakamura. M. (2008). Nipradilol protects rat retinal ganglion cells from apoptosis induced by serum deprivation in vitro and by diabetes in vivo. *Current Eye Research,* Vol.33, No. 8 (August, 2008), pp. 683-692, ISSN 1460-2202.

Yang, L.P.; Sun, H.L.; Wu, L.M.; Guo, X.J.; Dou, H.L.; Tso, M.O.; Zhao, L. & Li, S.M. (2009). Baicalein reduces inflammatory process in a rodent model of diabetic retinopathy. *Investigative Ophthalmology & Visual Science,* Vol. 50, No. 5 (May, 2009), pp. 2319-2327. ISSN 1552-5783.

Warboys, C.M.; Toh, H.B. & Fraser, P.A. (2005). Role of NADPH oxidase in retinal microvascular permeability increase by RAGE activation. *The British Journal of Ophthalmology*, Vol. 89, No. 3 (March, 2005), pp. 1631-1633. ISSN 00071161.

Zhang, Y.; Wang, Q.; Zhang, J.; Lei, X.; Xu, G.T. & Ye, W. (2009). Protection of exendin-4 analogue in early experimental diabetic retinopathy. *Graefe's Archive for Clinical and Experimental Ophthalmology*, Vol. 247, No. 5 (May, 2009), pp. 699-706. ISSN 0721-832X.

Zhang, J.; Wu, Y.; Jin, Y.; Ji, F.; Sinclair, S.H.; Luo, Y.; Xu, G.; Lu, L.; Dai, W.; Yanoff, M.; Li, W. & Xu, G.T. (2008). Intravitreal injection of erythropoietin protects both retinal vascular and neuronal cells in early diabetes. *Investigative Ophthalmology & Visual Science*, Vol. 49, No. 2 (February, 2008), pp. 732-742. ISSN 1552-5783.

Zheng, L.; Howell, S.J.; Hatala, D.A.; Huang, K. & Kern, T.S. (2007). Salicylate-based anti-inflammatory drugs inhibit the early lesion of diabetic retinopathy. *Diabetes*, Vol. 56, No.2 (February, 2007), pp. 337-345. ISSN 0012-1797.

Zhu, B.; Wang, W.; Gu, Q. & Xu, X. (2008). Erythropoietin protects retinal neurons and glial cells in early-stage streptozotocin-induced diabetic rats. *Experimental Eye Research*, Vol. 86, No. 2 (February, 2008), pp. 375-382. ISSN 0014-4835.

Part 3

ERG in Animal Models

9

Electroretinographic Recordings from the Isolated and Superfused Murine Retina

Alnawaiseh Maged, Albanna Walid, Banat Mohammed,
Abumuaileq Ramzi, Hescheler Jürgen and Schneider Toni
University of Cologne
Institute of Neurophysiology & Center for Molecular Medicine Cologne (CMMC)
Germany

1. Introduction

Vertebrate retina has routinely been isolated from bovine [1-4] or rat eyes [5]. However, many animal models for disturbances in neuronal signalling rely on gene inactivation or transgenes in mice. To get access to the isolated retina from these model systems to investigate neuronal processing, the technique of retina isolation and recording in a closed chamber was transferred from the bovine to the murine eye.

The ERG recordings of the isolated and superfused retina from bovine eye were most successfully performed in a closed recording chamber, in which a defined and controlled oxygen concentration can be achieved. Under these conditions, repetitive ERG recordings (interval time 5 min) can be performed up to 10 hours [4]. For rat and murine ERG recordings an open system was introduced recently, in which oxygen may escape easier, and stable recordings were shortened to about 90 min [6]. Therefore, we tried to optimize murine ERG recordings in the same closed system as it was introduced for frog and bovine retina [7;8].

2. Optimization of murine ERG recordings and applications

In the first section the history to optimize murine ERG recordings will be described for the last six years, in which initially an incomplete ERG was recorded, which was mainly dominated by the a-wave. After changes for the retina isolation as well as for the recording conditions, a full ERG was obtained, which even could be subdivided for the b-wave response into at least two different fractions [9].

Finally, two important topics will be covered for successful ERG recordings. (i) Using still the bovine retina, it will be analysed that a trace metal free solution can be achieved by using a tricine-based buffer system, which chelates heavy metal divalent cations selectively. Such a buffering may be very helpful for ERG recordings in the presence of submicromolar copper ion concentrations, which may be as important as investigations with the artificial Ni^{2+}-ions [3;10] or the native occurring Zn^{2+}-ions [11]. (ii) Flashes of high light intensity will be used to trigger repetitive ERG responses and to test the stability of the optimized murine ERG recording conditions.

2.1 Development of methods to record full murine ERGs for basal and reciprocal signalling

The diameter of a murine eye (male, 10 – 15 weeks of age) is about 10-fold smaller than the diameter of the bovine eye (age of 9 – 12 month). Therefore, an optimal isolation procedure is critical for subsequent successful and stable ERG recordings from the isolated murine retina.

In the following three chapters, we introduce three different procedures, which were used in our laboratory to realize and to improve the reproducible ERG recording from the murine retina.

The first procedure, the retina isolation by a rotating razor blade, was used to mimic the way of working as done with the bovine retina. Instead of using a knife to open up the eye bulb, we added a razor blade to a rotator, which cut the murine eye bulb laying in the stator very harsh, as we noted later. Under these conditions, the ERG recordings were dominated by the a-wave.

The second and the third procedure used a more gentle way to open up the eye bulb. The access to the retina was achieved by opening up the eye bulb at the level of the cornea. Consecutively, the lens was removed, and the eye cup was gently cut apart. The second and the third procedure differ with respect to the waiting time, after which ERG recordings were started. Initially (second procedure), we realized that a full ERG was better achieved by incubating the retina in nutrient solution for four hours in darkness. One may assume that it recovered from the ischemic conditions during the isolation procedure. Although basic signalling recovered during these 4 hours, reciprocal signalling obviously vanished. Therefore, we omitted preincubation, and started immediately (third procedure).

The main focus of our research was directed to understand the mechanisms of reciprocal signalling via voltage-gated Ca^{2+} channels, sensitive to heavy metal cations (Ni^{2+}, Zn^{2+}, Cu^{2+}). It was started first by using $NiCl_2$, an often used non-selective Ca^{2+}-channel blocker with some preference for $Ca_v2.3$/R-type and for $Ca_v3.2$/T-type Ca^{2+} channels, which have IC_{50} values at 10 μM. Therefore, an optimal recording of only basal retinal signal transduction was not sufficient, and we had to pay attention to more favourable conditions for ERG recording, preserving also signalling via feedback from amacrine cells to bipolar neurons.

2.1.1 Retina isolation by a rotating razor blade

Initial preparations of the murine retina followed the idea that the eye bulb should be opened up in a similar way as for the bovine retina by cutting the eye bulb at the ora serrata region. Therefore, a rotating razor blade was used, which led fast and reproducibly to a nearly full sized retina, isolated from the proximal cup of the remaining eye bulb. Under these conditions, it was possible to record photoreceptor responses reliably for at least 90 min [12]. Interestingly, from the incomplete ERG, which was characterized by a large a-wave (**Fig. 1A – 1C**), the photoreceptor response was sensitive towards low concentrations of dihydropyridines (25 nM racemic isradipine). Under similar recording conditions, the bovine photoreceptor response was insensitive even towards 2 μM isradipine [12].

Detailed analysis of the mechanism for dihydropyridine sensitivity of the murine photoreceptor response (a-wave) led to the detection that preincubation of the murine retina in 1 – 10 mM D-aspartate, a well known antagonist of transsynaptic signalling [13], eliminated the sensitivity towards this classical L-type Ca^{2+} channel antagonist. Similarly, also the sensitivity of the a-wave towards the T-type Ca^{2+} channel antagonist mibefradil (1 -

10 μM) was reversibly occluded by D-aspartate preincubation leading to the conclusion that minor transsynaptic signal transduction was present before aspartate application [12]. Such a very minor b-wave component could be deduced from our recordings by subtracting the mean values of murine ERGs in the presence of aspartate (1 mM) from those ERGs initially recorded before applying aspartate (**Fig. 1D**).

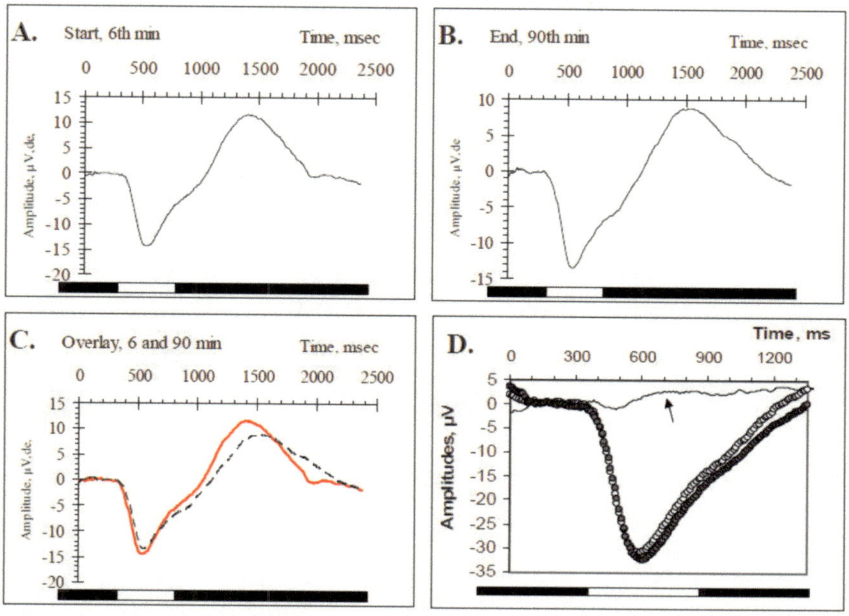

Fig. 1. Murine ERGs from isolated retinas of "razor-blade" isolated retina. The retina was dark-adapted and the electroretinogram was elicited by a single white flash at intervals of 3 min. The flash intensity was initially set to 6.3 lx (Fig. 1 and procedure 1) at the retinal surface using calibrated neutral density filters with light stimulation lasting 500 ms (see bar under the ERG traces), controlled by a timer operating a mechanical shutter system. Later (procedure 2 and 3) the flash intensity was raised to 63 mlx. During all conditions, the ERG was recorded by using two silver/silver-chloride electrodes, which are on both sides of the recording chamber. The ERG was amplified and bandpass limited between 1 and 300 Hz. The signal was AD converted and stored using a PC-based signal acquisition and analysis system. Temperature was 30°C (procedure 1), and 27.5°C (procedure 2 and 3). Flow rate for nutrient solution (Sickel solution) was 1 ml/min (procedure 1), and 2 ml/min (procedure 2 and 3). A. ERG recorded 6 min after begin of superfusion of nutrient solution. B. ERG recorded 90 min after begin of superfusion of nutrient solution. C. Superposition of traces from panel A. and B. The dashed line represents the ERG trace after 90 min of superfusion. Panel A. - C. represents data from the same experiment. D. ERG traces before (open circles) and after superfusion of 1 mM D-aspartate for 30 min (filled circles). The difference between both traces was calculated (thin line).

Overall, under the conditions of razor-blade isolated retina it was impossible to record a full ERG with a "healthy" b-wave component, as it was routinely observed for the isolated bovine retina in the same setup system. Therefore, the isolation protocol was changed completely.

2.1.2 Retina isolation under more gentle conditions followed by a preincubation period

The isolation of the murine retina was changed in a way that mechanical stress was reduced. In a well documented approach, the murine retina was isolated by opening up the eye bulb from the anterior side by dissecting the cornea, and by explanting the eye lens first [14]. We assume that the rotating razor blade in the former procedure may have introduced too much mechanical tension on the retina leading to a trauma and a loss of full transretinal signalling capacity. The new isolation procedure can be followed up in a detailed animation, which is available in the internet as a supplement [14]. In short, enucleated murine eyes **(Fig. 2)**

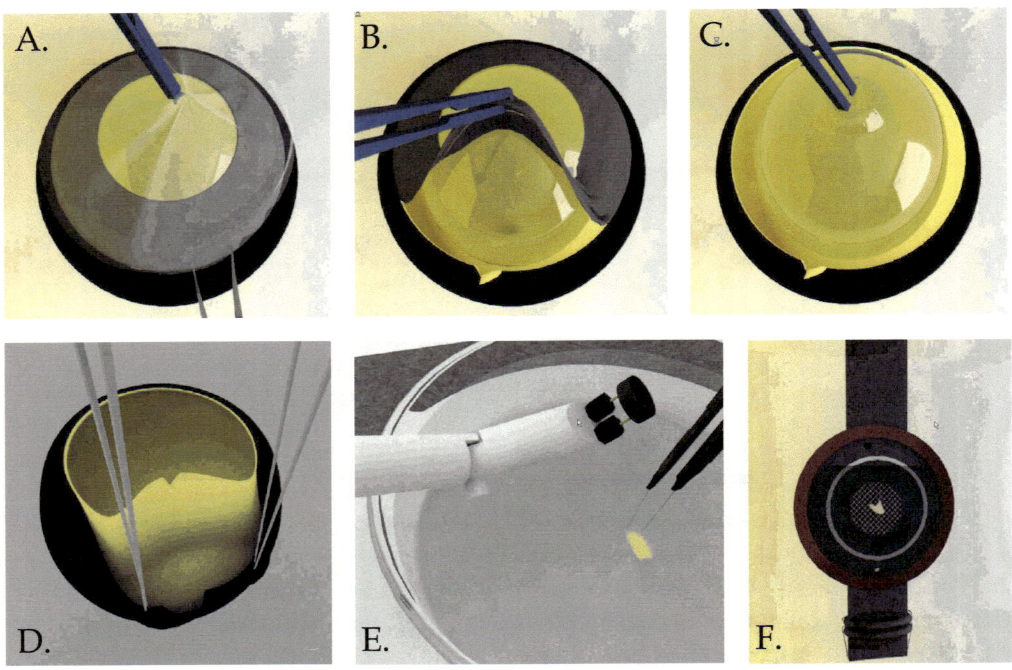

Fig. 2. Isolation of murine retina segments for ERG-recordings by opening up the eye bulb from the front side of the eye. The pictures are taken from a detailed animation (generated by Nadeen Albanna), which can be watched in the supplement of the related publication [14].A. The extirpated eye cup was initially treated with a 27 gauge needle from the front side to relief the tension. The cornea is used to hold the eye cup by fixing it via a lancette. The cornea will be partially separated. B. A triangled cut is incised into the sclera, reaching down to the ora serrata region. A forceps is moved through the triangle cut to remove the iris (for details of the used tools refer to [14]). C. After removing the iris, the lens will be taken off, and the opened eye is gently moved within the nutrient solution to tear off gently the retina from the underlying pigment epithelium. D. Next, two forceps are used to open up the sclera layers by tearing it apart at the site of initial incision. The retina usually stays intact, and can be cut into up to 4 - 6 pieces. E. The white supporting lever arm is connected with a 3 mm in diameter facing ring, to which the retina can be attached. It is held by surface tension to the ring and covers the central hole of 1 mm diameter. F. The retina-loaded support system is moved to the recording chamber, and docked into the central hole of the gasket. The recording chamber is closed by rubber rings, glas plates and interconnecting metal rings.

were placed into nutrient solution, fixed by a lancette and opened from the front side first by punching a tiny hole through the cornea to relieve the aqueous humour from the anterior and posterior chamber of the eye, and thus, to reduce the tension (**Fig. 2A**). Thereafter, the cornea was removed, and the iris disconnected, and a tiny triangle shaped incision was made into the sclera (**Fig. 2B**) for an easier separation later of the proximal eye cup, and for the immediate introduction of a small forceps. Finally, the lens was carefully removed (**Fig. 2C**). Consecutively, the opened eye-cup was held and separated apart by a forceps in order to detach the retina from the pigment epithelium by repetitive moving in the nutrient solution (**Fig. 2D**). The successive separation of the retina from the pigment epithelium has to be performed gently, and is supported by the cutting of the sclera layers from the outside. Finally, the isolated retina may be divided into 4 - 6 segments.

One of the posterior retina segments was finally mounted on a plastic mesh occupying the centre of the perfusing chamber by using a supporting tool (**Fig. 2E**). The ring, fixed by the submerged lever tool, is loaded with a retina segment, which was stored floating in the oxygenized nutrient solution. It is touched with the forceps at the region where formally the fibres of the N. opticus had left the eye cup. The retina segment adheres by itself and the supporting lever is turned upside down to move the retina loaded ring into the holder of the recording chamber (**Fig. 2F**). The view from the underlying nylon mesh further visualizes one of the two silver/silver-chloride electrodes, which are on both sides of the recording chamber. After closing the chamber by two gaskets and two glasses, the nutrient solution is perfused over the front and the rear side (**Fig. 2F**) of the recording chamber.

Based on the more gentle isolation procedure, full ERG recordings could be achieved, and optimal conditions for the recordings for mice were summarized and published [14]. For example, light intensity for scotopic ERG recordings was as low as 6.3 mlx for the bovine retina but 10-fold higher for the murine retina.

ERG recordings even in the presence of low $NiCl_2$ concentrations (up to 50 µM) could be easily followed up for several hours without loosing a full b-wave response (**Fig. 3B**).

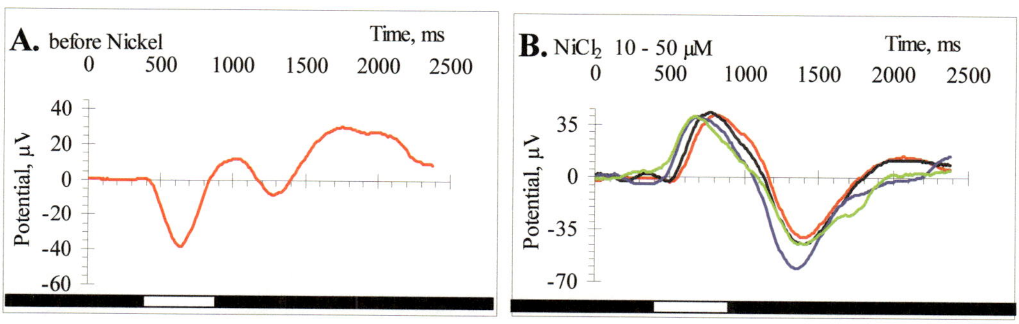

Fig. 3. Murine ERGs, which were recorded after gentle retina isolation and a 4 hour preincubation period. Light flashes were given at 63 mlx for 0.5 sec (see bar under the ERGs). Temperature was 27.5 °C. Flow rate for nutrient solution (Sickel solution) was 2 ml/min. A. Early registration of ERG in the absence of $NiCl_2$. Recording was started 30 min after loading the recording chamber. B. Full ERGs after $NiCl_2$ superfusion. Superposition of ERG traces after 60 min (red line, 10 µM $NiCl_2$), 86 min (black line, 15 µM $NiCl_2$), 150 min (blue line, 50 µM $NiCl_2$), and 215 min (green line, 50 µM $NiCl_2$).

Usually, the murine retina needed a while before a full ERG was seen. Early ERGs **(Fig. 3A)** were characterized a dominant a-wave, and the b-wave developed during the next 30 min [14]. The superimposed traces in **Fig. 3B** reveal that over time (60 – 215 min) the amplitude did not decrease much, but the implicit time got shorter and the shape of the b-wave changed indicating that the transretinal signalling varied (compare to later results with the different mouse mutants, especially the ERGs from $Ca_v2.3$-deficient mice, which are lacking the later fraction of the b-wave [9]).

The major goal for murine ERG-recording was the demonstration of an increase of the b-wave amplitude after the superfusion of low $NiCl_2$ (10 – 30 μM). Under these conditions (15 μM $NiCl_2$) the ERG b-wave amplitude of the isolated bovine retina was increased up to 1.5-fold [3]. For the bovine retina it was concluded that the pharmacoresistant Ca^{2+} channel $Ca_v2.3$ may trigger the GABA release necessary for reciprocal signalling backwards to the bipolar neurons [10]. This conclusion should be validated or disproven in mouse models with selective Ca^{2+} channel inactivation, either lacking $Ca_v2.3$ or $Ca_v3.2$ or even both subunits of voltage-gated Ca^{2+} channels. Therefore, the murine retina had to be isolated in a way that not only the basal signal transduction but also the reciprocal signalling would be conserved over time. Under these conditions, retinas from $Ca_v2.3$-competent and $Ca_v2.3$-deficient mice were isolated and their sensitivity towards $NiCl_2$ (15 and 30 μM) was analysed and compared between different genotypes [14]. For the ERGs from $Ca_v2.3$-competent mice, the data for 30 μM $NiCl_2$ are summarized (**Tab. 1**).

Exp. #	Before $NiCl_2$: Amplitude, μV	After NiCl2, 30 μM: Amplitude, μV	Washout: Amplitude, μV	**Ratio 1:** under $NiCl_2$ / before $NiCl_2$	**Ratio 2:** under $NiCl_2$ / after Washout
1	6,15	11,18	6,87	1,82	1,63
2	14,88	16,63	11,58	1,12	1,44
3	4,97	7,63	4,65	1,54	1,64
4	9,70	16,2	9,28	1,67	1,75
5	5,90	9,0	6,23	1,53	1,44
6	9,82	13,91	10,85	1,42	1,28
7	6,55	8,39	7,44	1,28	1,13
8	24,98	20,27	22,72	0,81	0,89
9	98,30	142,8	111,2	1,45	1,23
			Mean:	1,40	1,38
			Stdev	0,3	0,28
			SEM	0,1	0,09

Table 1. Development of b-wave amplitude after a 4 hour preincubation period for $Ca_v2.3$-competent mice by superfusing nutrient solution (= before $NiCl_2$), 30 μM $NiCl_2$ for 30 min (= after $NiCl_2$), and by washing out the $NiCl_2$ (= washout). Note, such a reversible increase of the b-wave amplitude, as shown for 9 experiments, was not always observed. In nearly the same number of experiments, no significant increase was detected, which may be attributed to the 4 hour preincubation period, during which reciprocal signalling was partially reduced or completely lost for unknown reasons.

As the full ERG-response with "healthy" b-waves was only achieved after a prolonged incubation period of 4 hours, we were afraid and realized that the capacity for maximal reciprocal signalling was partially or fully lost during such a preincubation. The consecutive large scatter for Ni^{2+}-mediated stimulation of the b-wave amplitude led us to conclusion to modify the recording procedure for a more stable transretinal signalling.

2.1.3 Retina isolation under gentle conditions without a preincubation period

To overcome any variable loss of reciprocal signalling, the murine retina was isolated again by the more gentle procedure as outlined before [14]. The adaptation period however was skipped to avoid any loss of reciprocal signalling. Early ERG recordings, which were still dominated by the photoreceptor response, were digitalized and stored, and mean values were calculated for the response before adding any $NiCl_2$. Thereafter, $NiCl_2$ superfusion (15 µM) was initiated within the first 15 - 20 min after introducing the retina segments into the recording chamber. The $NiCl_2$ application routinely lasts for 30 min, a time, after which a new equilibrium was reached and stable full ERG responses were recorded. From those ERG traces a mean trace curve was calculated and the mean ERG trace without $NiCl_2$ superfusion was subtracted from the mean trace under $NiCl_2$. Such difference-ERG traces were normalized and compared between different genotypes [9].

To our surprise, even the photoreceptor response differed between the two mouse lines either lacking $Ca_v3.2$ (including the double knockout) and the $Ca_v2.3$-competent or -deficient mouse line. The larger hyperpolarization at the beginning of each experiment for $Ca_v3.2$-deficient mice or double knockout mice was the reason that the amplitude of the difference-ERG was much larger than in retinas from $Ca_v2.3$-competent or –deficient mice. Most interesting, however, was the result deduced from implicit times of the normalized difference-ERGs. Obviously, $Ca_v2.3$ / R-type and $Ca_v3.2$ / T-type Ca^{2+} channels may contribute to different fractions of the signal transduction in the retinal network. In $Ca_v2.3$-deficient mice, the implicit time for the apparent b-wave is significantly shorter (346 ± 12 ms; n = 8 retinas) than in $Ca_v2.3$-competent mice (474 ± 27 ms; n = 5 retinas; $p < 0.001$), which implies that the later b-wave fraction, which is missing in the $Ca_v2.3$-deficient mice, would be carried in $Ca_v2.3$-compentent mice by the pharmacoresistant R-type channel triggering synaptic neurotransmitter release. This interpretation is in line with the assumption [10] that $Ca_v2.3$ may act in the synapse of a third order neuron, e.g. after the bipolar - amacrine synapse, while $Ca_v3.2$ may rather be responsible for a T-type triggered neurotransmitter release in the bipolar - amacrine synapse. T-type Ca^{2+} currents were routinely identified in these bipolar neurons [15-17].

The inactivation of Ca^{2+} channel genes could also disturb the overall retinal organisation. However, at least the inactivation of $Ca_v2.3$ does not disturb macroscopic structures in the retina as evaluated by histochemical staining (**Fig. 4**). Visual inspection and quantification of the thickness for retinal layers confirmed that no massive loss of neurons has occurred, which may also be true for the other knockout models.

2.2 Tricine-containing nutrient solution to chelate traces of divalent heavy metals

The use of Ni^{2+} as Ca^{2+} channel antagonist for R- and T-type Ca^{2+}-channels has a long tradition [18;19]. Only recently zinc and copper ions have been recognized as important endogenous modulators of neuronal excitability [20], and the most Ni^{2+}-sensitive Ca^{2+} channels were also characterized for its capability to be blocked by these native heavy metal cations [21-24]. The disturbance of their homoeostasis may be responsible for several neurological diseases as for example Morbus Alzheimer [25;26]. Much more is known for the physiological role of Zn^{2+} than for Cu^{2+}, which proves to be effective (submicromolar) even in lower concentrations than Zn^{2+}.

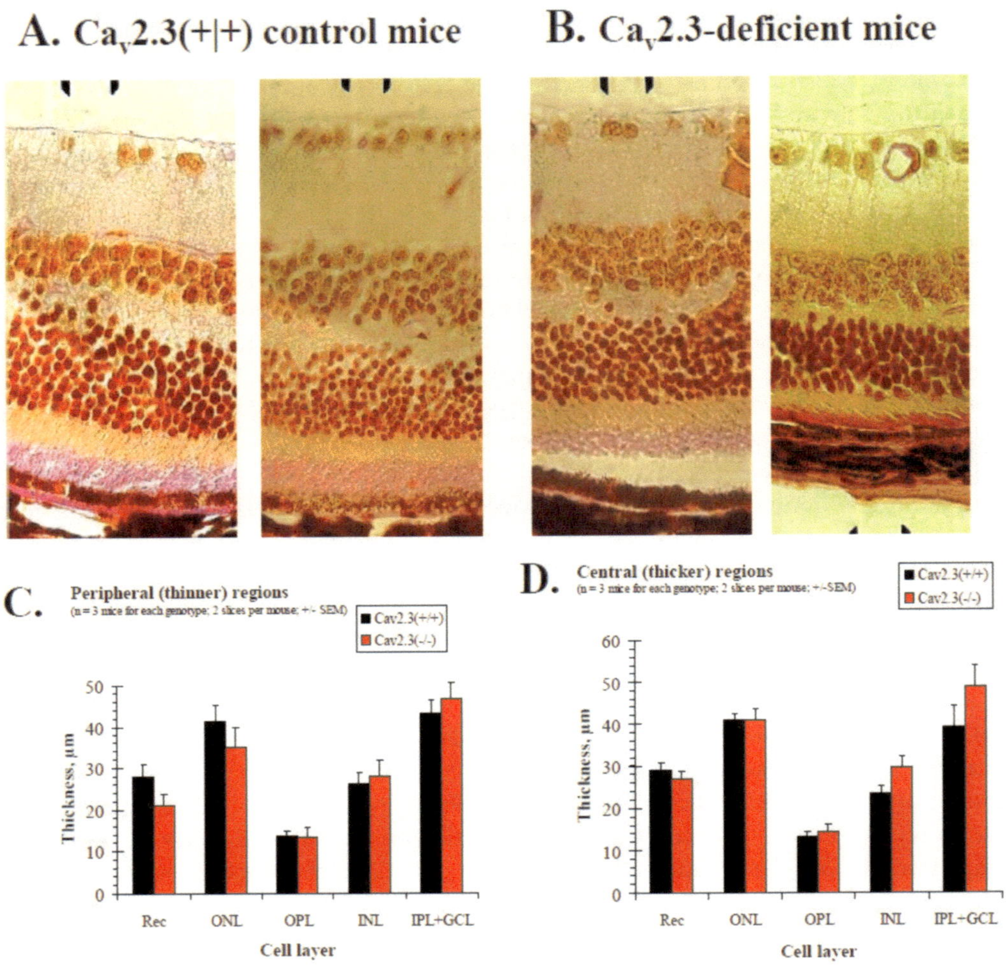

Fig. 4. Comparison of thicknesses in retinal cross sections obtained from control and $Ca_v2.3$-deficient mice. Light micrographs were taken from thicker (more central) regions and from thinner (more peripheral) regions away from the optical nerve head. Each layer is identified by its abbreviations (Rec = photoreceptors; ONL = outer nuclear layer; OPL = outer plexiform layer; INL = inner nuclear layer; IPL + GCL: inner plexiform layer and granular cell layer were summarized for quantification; data were produced by Mehran Maghsoodian and Petra Müller). A. Retinal sections from control female mice at the age of 34 month. B. Retinal sections from $Ca_v2.3$-deficient female mice at the same age of 34 month. C & D.: Quantification of thicknesses for individual retinal layers for controls and KO's.

The effect of $ZnCl_2$ (10 - 15 µM) on transretinal signalling resembles the effect of $NiCl_2$, which was investigated in detail for the isolated bovine retina [11].

The second most abundant trace element in the human body is represented by Zn^{2+}. In total it reaches up to two grams in adult humans. Most Zn^{2+} in the body is located intracellularily. But as only a small labile portion in the liver may be available during Zn^{2+} deficiency, a regular dietary supply of Zn^{2+} during growth and aging is needed [27].

After Zn^{2+} deficiency, the multitude of physiological roles for Zn^{2+} are best seen, which include anorexia, retarded growth, weight loss, impaired immune function, delayed sexual maturation, testicular atrophy, epidermal hyperkeratinization, alopecia, hypogeuisa, and night blindness [27;28]. In ocular tissues, the concentration of Zn^{2+} is unusually high when compared to other tissues. Zn^{2+} was localized in retina, chorioid, ciliary body, iris, optic nerve, sclera, cornea, and lens [27;29].

As soon as the function of Cu^{2+} would also be investigated, contaminations of submicromolar heavy metal cations may count for the validity of experiments in the future. To test a well known buffer system, which can be used to calibrate the desired cation concentration, tricine was added in various amounts (15 mM, 10 mM, and 5 mM) to the normally used nutrient solution. The bovine retina was used in these experiments. While 15 and 10 mM inhibited the b-wave response, no substantial change was observed at 5 mM tricine. Sometimes we observed a slight decrease of the b-wave amplitude, which may be attributed to heavy metal contaminations in the nutrient solution. After a chelation of traces by tricine, the effect of $NiCl_2$ (15 µM) was analysed leading to a similar and transient increase of the b-wave response **(Fig. 5)**.

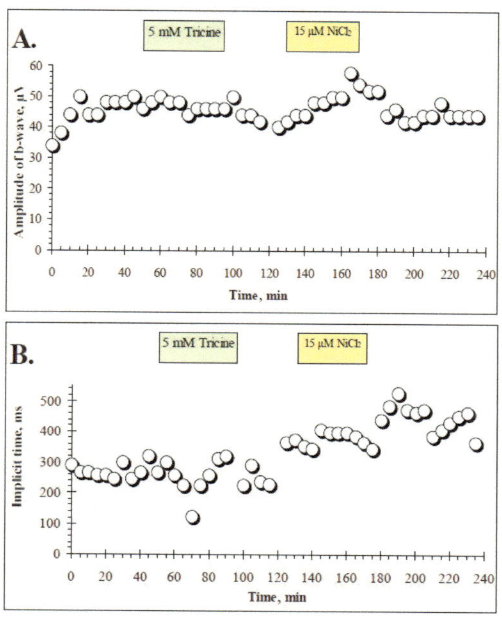

Fig. 5. ERG recordings from the isolated bovine retina. After isolation of a standard retina segment, the retina was equilibrated for at least 30 min. A. During the superfusion of 5 mM tricine buffer added to the normal nutrient solution, no lasting change of b-wave response was observed. Tricine was washed and exchanged to normal nutrient solution including $NiCl_2$ (15 µM), leading to a transient increase of the b-wave response. B. Implicit times increase mostly after superfusion with $NiCl_2$.

2.3 Stability testing for murine ERG responses under high intensity light conditions

So far, murine ERGs were recorded under low light intensity (63 mlx for 0.5 sec). But the testing of higher light intensities may be needed, because reciprocal signalling should be more pronounced at elevated light intensities, if the reciprocal signalling participates in light/dark adaptation. Therefore, we analysed the effect of increasing light intensities on the photoreceptor response of the isolated murine retina (**Fig. 6**).

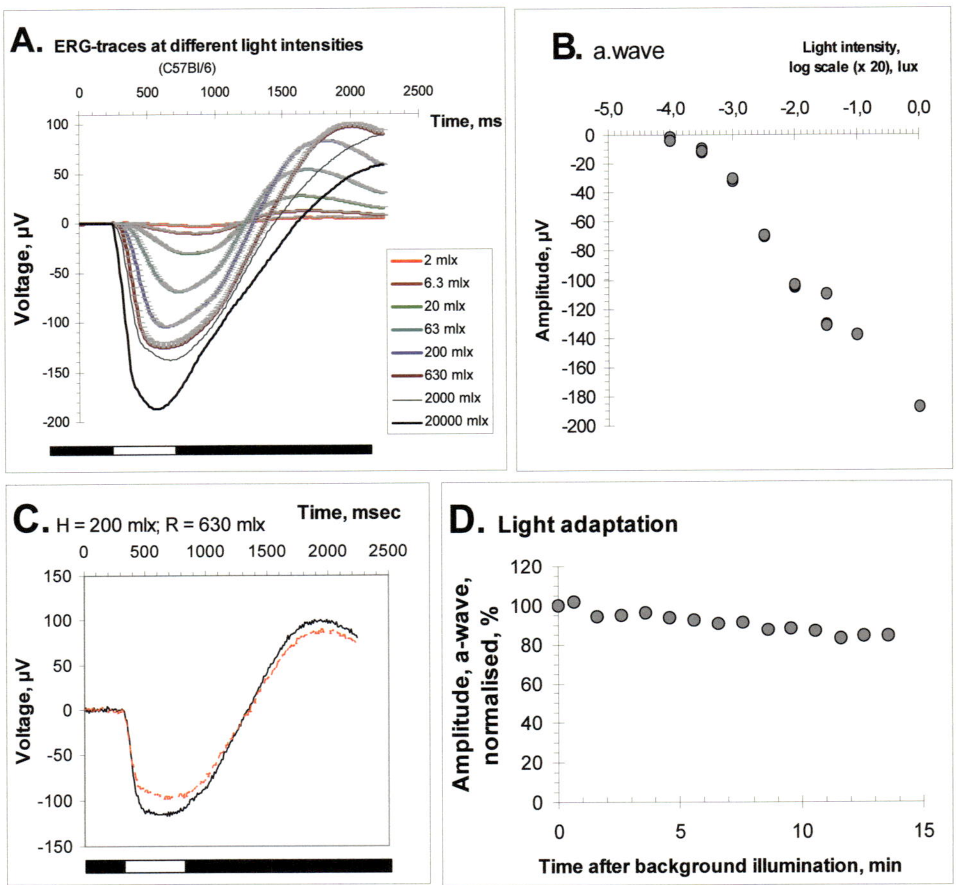

Fig. 6. Murine ERGs were recorded after gentle retina isolation without a preincubation period. Light flashes were given in 3 min intervals interrupted by darkness. Light stimuli were at various light intensities for 0.5 sec (light bar at the bottom of each figure). Temperature was 27.5 °C. In some panels the background light intensity (= H), and the stimulus intensity (= R) is given. A. Early registration of ERGs in the absence of $NiCl_2$. Recording was started within 30 min after loading the recording chamber. B. Light intensity - response curve for the apparent a-wave amplitude (data taken from the ERG records in panel A). The semi-logarithmic plot shows a linear increase up to the highest light intensity tested (2 mlx - 20 lx). C. Superposition of ERG traces before (solid black line) and 15 min after light adaptation (fine dashed red line) under continuous light (200 mlx). Stimulus light intensity was 630 mlx. Note the minor reduction of the apparent a-wave may be attributed to a slowly increasing b-wave, which gets more pronounced after $NiCl_2$ application (see Fig. 7). D. Time course of light adaptation under the conditions as described in panel C.

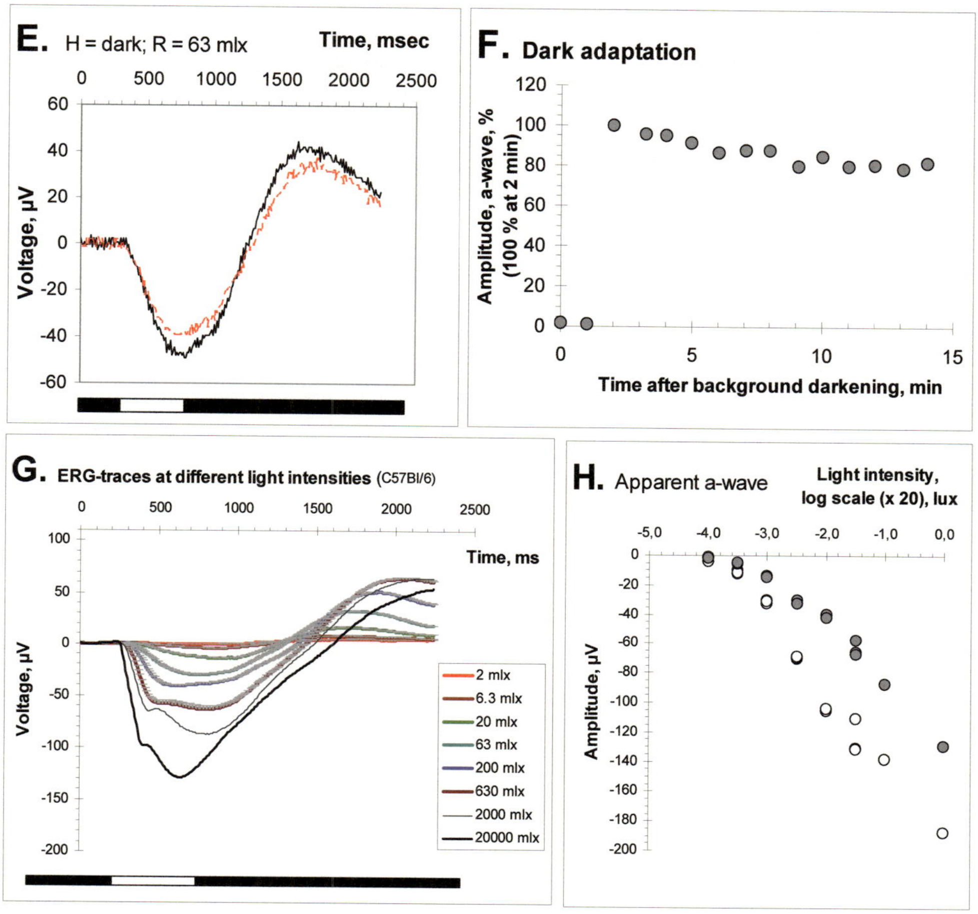

Fig. 6 (continued). E. After the light adaptation for 15 min (see panel D), dark adaption was tested for the stability of the photoreceptor response. Superposition of ERG traces 6 min (solid black line) and 15 min after dark adaptation (fine dashed red line). Stimulus light intensity was 63 mlx. Again, a minor reduction of the apparent a-wave may be attributed to a slowly increasing b-wave, which gets more pronounced after $NiCl_2$ application (see Fig. 7). Note the stimulus light intensity under scotopic conditions was 1/10th of that during light adaptation in panel D. F. Time course of the photoreceptor response during 15 min dark adaptation using a stimulus light intensity of 6.3 mlx (at 0 and 3 min) and of 63 mlx for the remaining light flashes. Note the flash light intensity during the first 6 min was reduced to ensure dark adaptation to start fast. G. Superposition of ERG responses (dominated by a-wave) from different light intensities (2 mlx - 20 lx). Especially during higher light intensities (200 mlx - 20 lx) a small b-wave gets visible. H. Light intensity - response curve for the apparent a-wave amplitude (filled circles; data taken from the ERG records in panel G). The semi-logarithmic plot shows a near linear increase up to the highest light intensity tested (2 mlx - 20 lx), which reveals lower apparent a-wave amplitudes as during the first regime (open circles; data are identical to panel B). Threshold values for light intensities are similar in both regimes.

During an experimental regime of early dose-response (Fig. 6A, 6B), light (Fig. 6C, 6D) and dark adaptation (Fig. 6E, 6F), and late dose-response (Fig. 6G, 6H), it gets obvious that the isolated murine retina yields rather stable photoreceptor responses, which are only slightly reduced by the slowly growing b-wave. A faster development of the b-wave response can be achieved by adding $NiCl_2$. The superfusion of 15 µM $NiCl_2$ leads within 30 min to a fast increase of the developing b-wave. The ERG traces before and after $NiCl_2$ superfusion indicate that during this period b-wave gets maximally increased (**Fig. 7**), as reported recently [9].

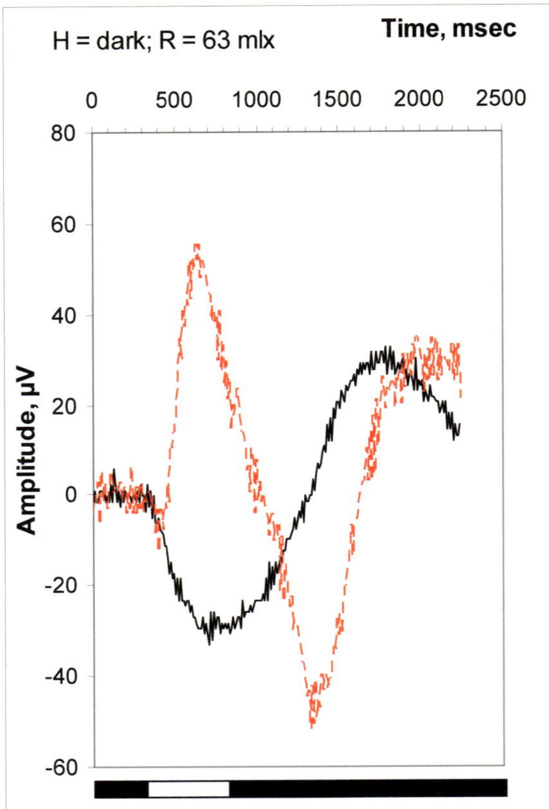

Fig. 7. Development of b-wave by $NiCl_2$ application. Superposition of ERG traces before (black solid line) and after $NiCl_2$ superfusion (15 µM; red dashed line). The increase is still half-maximal within 6 min of $NiCl_2$ superfusion. Note, after full development of b-wave, it superimposes nearly completely the a-wave response, as it is expected for a light intensity of 63 mlx (compare [14]). H = background in darkness in between each light flash. R = stimulus intensity.

To test the stability of the isolated murine retina for its transretinal signalling capability (**Fig. 8**), the b-wave amplitude was recorded and used as the readout during similar experiments as it was performed for photoreceptor responses. The light induced stress was even increased by recording the light intensity - response curve under continuous background light first at 630 mlx (not shown) and thereafter at 2000 mlx (**Fig. 8E, 8F**).

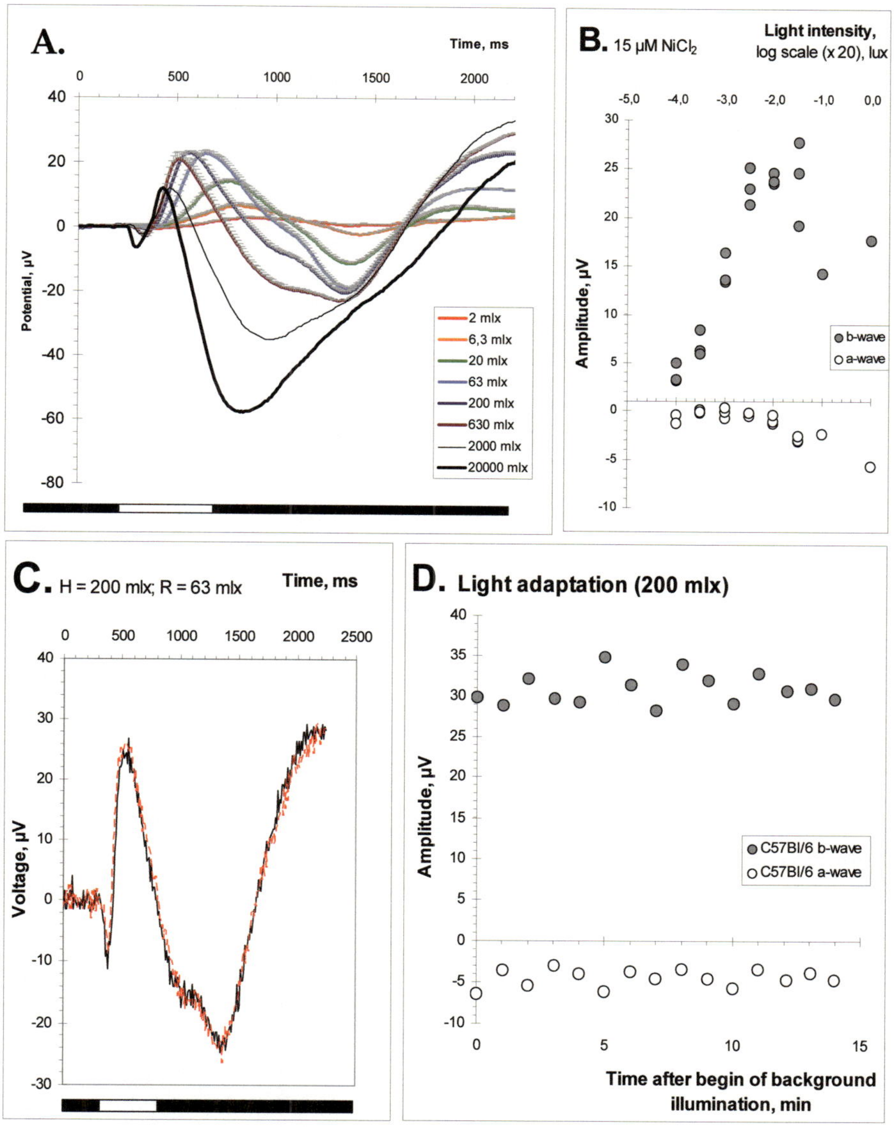

Fig. 8. Murine ERGs were recorded after gentle retina isolation without a preincubation period in the presence of 15 µM $NiCl_2$. Light flashes were given after 3 min at various light intensities for 0.5 sec. Background illumination as indicated in each panel. Temperature was 27.5 °C. A. Recording was continued without delay after the b-wave was reached (Fig. 7). Superposition of individual ERG traces at the indicated light intensities. Background was in darkness. B. Light intensity - response curve for the b-wave amplitude (data taken from the ERG records in panel A). The semi-logarithmic plot shows an optimum of the b-wave response between 63 and 630 mlx. C. Superposition of ERG traces recorded at 63 mlx stimulus light before (solid black line) and 15 min of light adaptation (fine dashed red line) under continuous light (200 mlx). Stimulus light intensity was 63 mlx. Note the ERG traces are nearly identical at both time points. D. Time course of light adaptation for apparent a- and b-wave under the conditions as described in panel C.

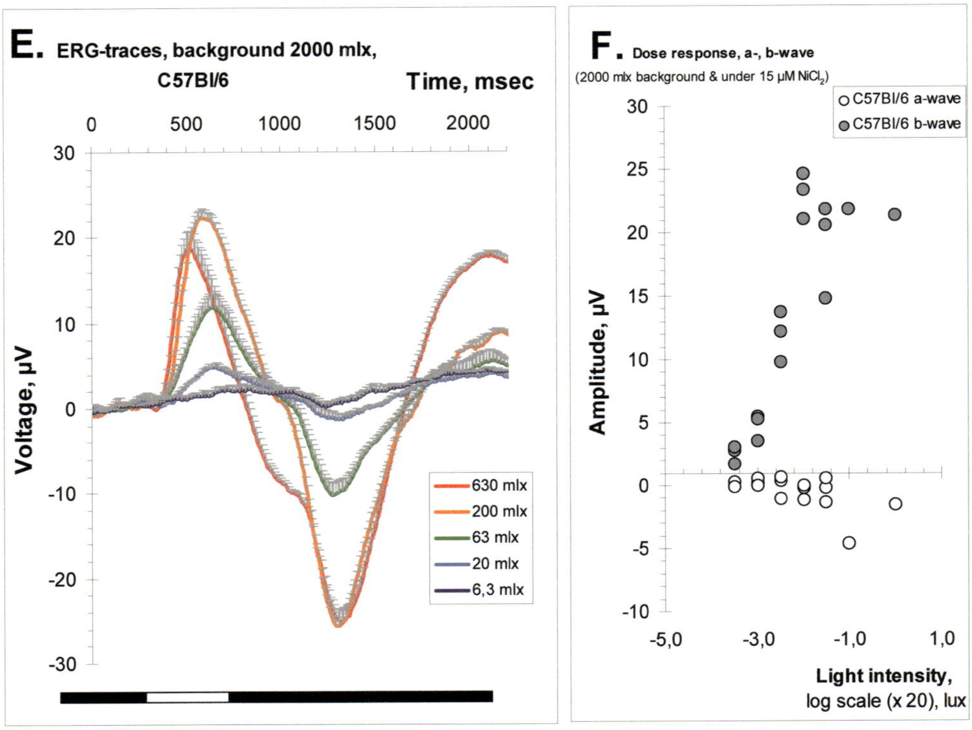

Fig. 8 (continued). E. After the light adaptation for 15 min, the light intensity-response was recorded first with 630 mlx background light (not shown) and next with 2000 mlx background light. Superposition of ERG traces for the stimulus light intensities as indicated. F. Light intensity – response curve for the b-wave amplitude (data taken from the ERG records in panel E). The semi-logarithmic plot shows an optimum of the b-wave response at 200 mlx.

Increasing the light intensity beyond 63 to 630 mlx caused a reduction of the b-wave amplitude as reported in the literature, and reflecting the process of light adaptation. Consecutively, the apparent a-wave amplitude gets increased **(Fig. 8B)**. For the b-wave, the implicit time gets shorter during increased light intensities. Interestingly, under these conditions of 15 min continuous background light (200 mlx), the stability of the b-wave response is remarkable. Even more astonishing is the observation that under 630 and 2000 mlx background light, the b-wave responses continue to be very pronounced tolerating the increased light intensity at the recording chamber.

3. Conclusion

The transfer of the ERG recording technique from the bovine retina model to the various murine knockout models is possible, and the higher sensitivity of the murine retina towards ischemia maybe overcome by a more gentle preparation technique as outlined in detail [14]. Future investigations of the murine retina from different mouse models may benefit from such an isolation procedure.

Besides ERG recordings additional electrophysiological recording techniques (e.g. patch clamp registration) will be needed to characterize signalling through retinal circuits.

4. Acknowledgment

We thank Priv.-Doz. Dr. Matthias Lüke, Dr. Siarhei A. Siapich for their excellent and permanent assistance during the work with the bovine retina, which is an important prerequisite for the transfer to the murine retina. The authors would also like to thank Nadeen Albanna (animation), Renate Clemens (genotyping and breeding of mice), Mehran Maghsoodian and Petra Müller (retinal IHC) for their support, as well as the animal keepers of the central facility for their excellent and permanent assistance. This work was financially supported by the Köln Fortune Programme of the Faculty of Medicine, University of Cologne (to MA, WA and MB) and by the Center for Molecular Medicine Cologne (CMMC, to TS and JH, Faculty of Medicine, University of Cologne).

5. References

[1] Walter P & Sickel W: Identification of fast spurts of pyridine nucleotide oxidation evoked by light stimulation in the isolated perfused vertebrate retina. Graefes Arch Clin. Exp. Ophthalmol. 1994;232: 318-323.

[2] Lüke C, Walter P, Bartz-Schmidt KU, Brunner R, Heimann K & Sickel W: Effects of Antiviral Agents on Retinal Function in Vertebrate Retina. Adv. Ocul. Tox. 1997;13: 107-112.

[3] Lüke M, Henry M, Lingohr T, Maghsoodian M, Hescheler J, Sickel W & Schneider T: A Ni^{2+}-sensitive component of the ERG-b-wave from the isolated bovine retina is related to E-type voltage-gated Ca^{2+} channels. Graefes Arch. Clin. Exp. Ophthalmol. 2005;243: 933-941.

[4] Lüke M, Weiergräber M, Brand C, Siapich SA, Banat M, Hescheler J, Lüke C & Schneider T: The isolated perfused bovine retina - a sensitive tool for pharmacological research on retinal function. Brain Res. Brain Res. Protoc. 2005;16: 27-36.

[5] Green DG & Kapousta-Bruneau NV: Electrophysiological properties of a new isolated rat retina preparation. Vision Res. 1999;39: 2165-2177.

[6] Green DG, Guo H & Pillers DA: Normal photoresponses and altered b-wave responses to APB in the mdx(Cv3) mouse isolated retina ERG supports role for dystrophin in synaptic transmission. Vis. Neurosci 2004;21: 739-747.

[7] Sickel W: Respiratory and electrical responses to light stimulation in the retina of the frog. Science 1965;148: 648-651.

[8] Sickel W. (1972) Retinal Metabolism in Dark and Light. In *Handbook of Sensory Physiology* (Autrum,H., Jung,R., Loewenstein,W.R., MacKay,D.M. & Teuber,H.L., eds), pp. 667-727. Springer-Verlag, Berlin, Heidelberg, New York.

[9] Alnawaiseh M, Albanna W, Chen C-C, Campbell KP, Hescheler J, Lüke M & Schneider T: Two separate Ni^{2+} sensitive voltage-gated Ca^{2+} channels modulate transretinal signalling in the isolated murine retina. Acta Ophthalmologica 2011; in press.

[10] Siapich SA, Banat M, Albanna W, Hescheler J, Lüke M & Schneider T: Antagonists of ionotropic gamma-aminobutyric acid receptors impair the NiCl2-mediated stimulation of the electroretinogramm b-wave amplitude from the isolated superfused vertebrate retina. Acta Ophthalmol. 2009;87: 854-865.

[11] Siapich SA, Wrubel H, Albanna W, Hescheler J, Weiergräber M, Lüke M & Schneider T: Effect of ZnCl2 and chelation of zinc ions by N,N-diethyldithiocarbamate (DEDTC) on the ERG b-wave amplitude from the isolated and superfused vertebrate retina. Curr. Eye Res. 2010;35: 322-334.

[12] Banat M, Lüke M, Siapich SA, Hescheler J, Weiergräber M & Schneider T: The dihydropyridine isradipine inhibits the murine but not the bovine A-wave response of the electroretinogram. Acta Ophthalmol. 2008;86: 676-682.

[13] Hanawa I & Tateishi T: The effect of aspartate on the electroretinogram of the vertebrate retina. Experientia 1970;26: 1311-1312.

[14] Albanna W, Banat M, Albanna N, Alnawaiseh M, Siapich SA, Igelmund P, Weiergraber M, Luke M & Schneider T: Longer lasting electroretinographic recordings from the isolated and superfused murine retina. Graefes Arch. Clin. Exp. Ophthalmol. 2009;247: 1339-1352.

[15] Pan ZH: Differential expression of high- and two types of low-voltage-activated calcium currents in rod and cone bipolar cells of the rat retina. J. Neurophysiol. 2000;83: 513-527.

[16] Pan ZH, Hu HJ, Perring P & Andrade R: T-type Ca(2+) channels mediate neurotransmitter release in retinal bipolar cells. Neuron 2001;32: 89-98.

[17] Hu C, Bi A & Pan ZH: Differential expression of three T-type calcium channels in retinal bipolar cells in rats. Vis. Neurosci. 2009;26: 177-187.

[18] Kostyuk PG: Calcium channels in the neuronal membrane. Biochim. Biophys. Acta 1981;650: 128-150.

[19] Lacinova L: Voltage-dependent calcium channels. Gen. Physiol Biophys. 2005;24 Suppl 1: 1-78.

[20] Mathie A, Sutton GL, Clarke CE & Veale EL: Zinc and copper: pharmacological probes and endogenous modulators of neuronal excitability. Pharmacol. Ther. 2006;111: 567-583.

[21] Castelli L, Tanzi F, Taglietti V & Magistretti J: Cu2+, Co2+, and Mn2+ modify the gating kinetics of high-voltage-activated Ca2+ channels in rat palaeocortical neurons. J. Membr. Biol. 2003;195: 121-136.

[22] Magistretti J, Castelli L, Taglietti V & Tanzi F: Dual effect of Zn2+ on multiple types of voltage-dependent Ca2+ currents in rat palaeocortical neurons. Neuroscience 2003;117: 249-264.

[23] Kang HW, Park JY, Jeong SW, Kim JA, Moon HJ, Perez-Reyes E & Lee JH: A molecular determinant of nickel inhibition in Cav3.2 T-type calcium channels. J. Biol. Chem. 2006;281: 4823-4830.

[24] Kang HW, Vitko I, Lee SS, Perez-Reyes E & Lee JH: Structural determinants of the high affinity extracellular zinc binding site on Cav3.2 T-type calcium channels. J. Biol. Chem. 2010;285: 3271-3281.

[25] Lovell MA: A potential role for alterations of zinc and zinc transport proteins in the progression of Alzheimer's disease. J. Alzheimers. Dis. 2009;16: 471-483.

[26] Jomova K, Vondrakova D, Lawson M & Valko M: Metals, oxidative stress and neurodegenerative disorders. Mol. Cell Biochem. 2010;345: 91-104.

[27] Grahn BH, Paterson PG, Gottschall-Pass KT & Zhang Z: Zinc and the eye. J. Am. Coll. Nutr. 2001;20: 106-118.

[28] Aggett PJ & Comerford JG: Zinc and human health. Nutr. Rev. 1995;53: S16-S22.

[29] Karcioglu ZA: Zinc in the eye. Surv. Ophthalmol. 1982;27: 114-122.

10

Comparison of Rat Cone ERG Elicited by a Pulse Flicker and Sine-Wave Modulated Light Stimuli

Haohua Qian[1] and Manthan R. Shah[2]
[1]*National Eye Institute, Bethesda, MD*
[2]*Departments of Ophthalmology and Visual Sciences*
University of Illinois at Chicago, Chicago, IL
USA

1. Introduction

The electroretinogram (ERG) affords a quantitative, objective, and noninvasive method by which to examine light-evoked neuronal activity, and is commonly used to study the functional integrity of normal and diseased retinas (Fishman, 2001; Frishman, 2006; Peachey and Ball, 2003). ERG elicited by a periodic stimulus (flicker ERG) is a useful tool to investigate temporal property of retinal circuitry, especially cone pathway in the retina (Alexander et al., 2005; Burns et al., 1992; Kondo and Sieving, 2001; Qian et al., 2010; Qian et al., 2008). Two kinds of light stimuli are commonly used for flicker ERG recordings: sine-wave modulated light and a pulse light flickers. Sine-wave modulated light, due to its simplicity in spectrum component, is often used to characterize frequency-response relationship of ERG (Alexander et al., 2003; Burns et al., 1992; Kondo and Sieving, 2001; Krishna et al., 2002; Qian et al., 2008; Viswanathan et al., 2002). On the other hand, pulse light flicker can easily be implemented technically, and has long been applied for clinical use (Audo et al., 2008; Garry et al., 2010; Jacobs et al., 1996). Indeed, 30 Hz pulse flicker under light-adapted condition is recommended by the International Society for Clinical Electrophysiology of Vision (ISCEV) for evaluating activity of the cone system in human patients (Marmor et al., 2009).

For a pulse train consisting of a series of flashes with intensity I, duration d, and period P, the Fourier transform in the frequency domain is given by the expression:

$$x(t) = I[k + \frac{2}{\pi}(\sin k\pi \cos \omega t + \frac{1}{2}\sin 2k\pi \cos 2\omega t + ... + \frac{1}{n}\sin nk\pi \cos n\omega t + ...)]$$

where k = d/P and ω = 2π/P. When the duration of each flash is very brief (i.e. d is small compared to P, such as is with a xenon flash), k is small and $\sin(nk\pi)$ approaches nkπ. Under such condition, the Fourier transform of a pulse flicker reduces to:

$$x(t) = I[k + 2k(\cos \omega t + \cos 2\omega t + ... + \cos n\omega t + ...)]$$

Therefore, for a flickering stimulus comprised of a series of brief pulses, the frequency domain consists of a series of harmonics, each with equal energy. In other words, pulse flicker can be viewed as a mixture of sine-wave flicker at fundamental and harmonic frequencies. Consequently, for a linear system, the frequency-response relation derived from harmonic components of the ERG response to one pulse train flicker should be similar as those derived with a series of sine-wave modulated light stimuli. In this study, we recorded rat cone flicker ERG elicited by these two light stimuli from the same animals and compared the response in the frequency domain derived from Fourier analysis (Bach and Meigen, 1999).

Our results indicate that, for response frequencies less than 30 Hz, frequency-response relationship derived with a single pulse flicker stimulus has similar shape as the one derived from the fundamental responses to a series of sine-wave light stimuli. Therefore, pulse flicker ERG can be used as an alternative method to probe the frequency-response relationship of flicker ERG at low response frequencies.

On the other hand, the high frequency harmonic responses derived from a pulse flicker ERG consistently contained higher peaks than the fundamental response of sine-wave flickers. In this study, we investigated two potential mechanisms for these high harmonic components: a nonlinear response to harmonic components in a pulse flicker and ERG oscillatory potentials.

Oscillatory potentials (OPs) are wavelets that superimposed on the rising phase of the ERG b-wave. OPs have been shown to arise within the proximal retina (Wachtmeister and Dowling, 1978), and the individual peaks have different retinal depth profiles, suggestive of distinct cellular origins (Wachtmeister, 1980). The specific retinal cells that are responsible for the OPs are still being debated, but there is strong evidence that GABAergic neurons, and their synaptic interactions, are key elements in the generation of the response (Wachtmeister, 1980). Bicuculline, an inhibitor for $GABA_A$ receptor activity in the retina, reduces OP in flash ERG (Wachtmeister, 1980). In this study, we used bicuculline to probe the contribution of OPs in high harmonic responses of ERG elicited by pulse flicker stimulus.

In a non-linear system, response to a mixture of two sine-wave stimuli will not only include fundamental responses at each stimulus frequencies, it also includes components (beats) at both the difference and the sum of these two stimulus frequencies and their multiples. These beats responses have been used to investigate nonlinearities in human flicker ERG (Alexander et al., 2001; Burns et al., 1992; Wu et al., 1995). In this study, we used a beat response to measure the non-linearity in rat flicker ERG response. Our results indicate that nonlinearity of retinal signal processing mechanisms in rat eye also has a large contribution to the high harmonic responses observed with ERG responses elicited by pulse light stimuli.

2. Methods

2.1 Animals and anesthesia

Adult pigmented (Long Evans) rats (both sexes, weight 250-500g) were used for this study. Animals were housed in the Biological Resources Laboratory (BRL) of the University of Illinois at Chicago in a 14/10-hour light/dark cycle, the standard lighting regimen of the BRL. Rats were anesthetized with ketamine (100 mg/kg) and xylazine (6 mg/kg), and the pupils were dilated with topical phenylephrine (2.5%) and tropicamide (1%). Topical proparacaine (0.5%) was used to anesthetize cornea. Body temperature was maintained at ~37°C with a heating pad. All experimental procedures conformed to the statement on animal care of the Association for Research in Vision and Ophthalmology.

2.2 ERG recording and light stimulation

Instrumentation and recording procedures have described in our previous publication (Qian et al., 2008). Light stimuli were delivered by multiple light-emitting diodes (LEDs) with a peak wavelength of 505 nm (Nichia NSPE590S, Tokushima, Japan) mounted in a small integrating sphere (Oriel 70500, Newport Corp., Stratford, CT) to provide a full-field stimulus. The current driving the LEDs was pulse-width modulated at 1 MHz under computer control. Pulse flickers were composed of ≤4 ms flashes delivered at various temporal frequencies (2 to 12 Hz). In most experiments, the peak luminance of each pulse was 690 cd/m^2 unless otherwise specified. A background light (5 cd/m^2) was used to saturate the rod pathway (Xu et al., 2003). Eyes were adapted to background luminance before ERG recording. Sine-wave modulated light stimuli had a mean luminance of 100 cd/m^2 and Michelson contrast of 90%. Each stimulus was about 10s long, and contained an even number of cycles (or pulses). For mixture sine-wave stimulus, light intensity was modulated by sum of two sine-waves, each has a contrast of 45% and period of 56 ms (18 Hz) and 42 ms (24 Hz), respectively. ERG responses were recorded from a chlorided silver wire electrode placed in the centre of the cornea and connected to the input stage of a Grass AC amplifier (Model P511, with a bandwidth of 0.3 to 300 Hz and without a 60 Hz notch filter) and a sampling frequency of 2 kHz.

2.3 Intravitreal injection

Bicuculline methcloride (Sigma-Aldrich, St. Louis, MO) was dissolved in mammalian saline solution and delivered to the anesthetized rat eye by intravitreal injection through a glass capillary needle introduced into the vitreous cavity by piercing the sclera 3 mm posterior to the temporal limbus at approximately a 45-degree angle to the optical axis. The injection site was monitored under a dissecting microscope and a 3-μl aliquot of a solution containing 1 mM bicuculline was injected into each eye. The final vitreal concentration (~80 μM) was derived by assuming complete mixing in the rat vitreous with an estimated volume of 38 μl (Xu et al., 2003).

2.4 Data analysis

The amplitudes of each harmonic component were derived from discrete Fourier transforms using the Matlab Signal Processing Toolbox (The Mathworks, Boston, MA). For each 10s recordings of ERG waveform, about 500 ms of data at the beginning and end of the recording were omitted. The exact length that was omitted depended on the stimulus period and was an even number of cycles or pulses. As a result, Fourier analyses of ERG were based on approximately 9-s segments of continuous data, consisting of an even number of cycles or pulses. We adopted a criterion for harmonic component responses as greater than 3 times the noise level at neighboring frequencies, which exceeds the 5% significant level (Meigen and Bach, 1999). A digital zero-phase band-pass filter (40-200 Hz) was used to isolate the OP components from flash ERG (Ramsey et al., 2006). Data analysis tools in Microsoft Excel were used to calculate statistical significance (two-tail *t*-test analysis).

3. Results

3.1 Frequency-response relationship for sine-wave flicker ERG and pulse flicker ERG

Fig. 1A illustrates flicker ERG responses elicited from a rat eye by sine-wave modulated light stimuli at selected temporal frequencies with 90% contrast. For clear presentation, the traces on right side (responses to high frequency stimuli) are magnified 5 times more than those on the left side (responses to low frequency stimuli) of the figure. [Examples of rat flicker ERG responses elicited by sine-wave stimuli plotted on the same magnitude scale can be find in Figure 1 of (Qian et al., 2008)]. For presentation purpose, each waveform shown in the figure represents an averaged 500-ms segment over 10-s recorded responses. The top panel of Fig. 1B shows an example of flicker ERG response elicited from the same rat eye by a 6-Hz pulse flicker light. The trace represents an averaged 1-s segment over 10-s recorded responses, and is plotted with the same scale as those shown on the left side traces of Fig. 1A. Fourier spectrum of the entire 9-s ERG waveform is shown in the bottom panel of Fig. 1B. It is clear that, in addition to fundamental response at 6 Hz, there are prominent harmonic components in rat pulse flicker ERG response.

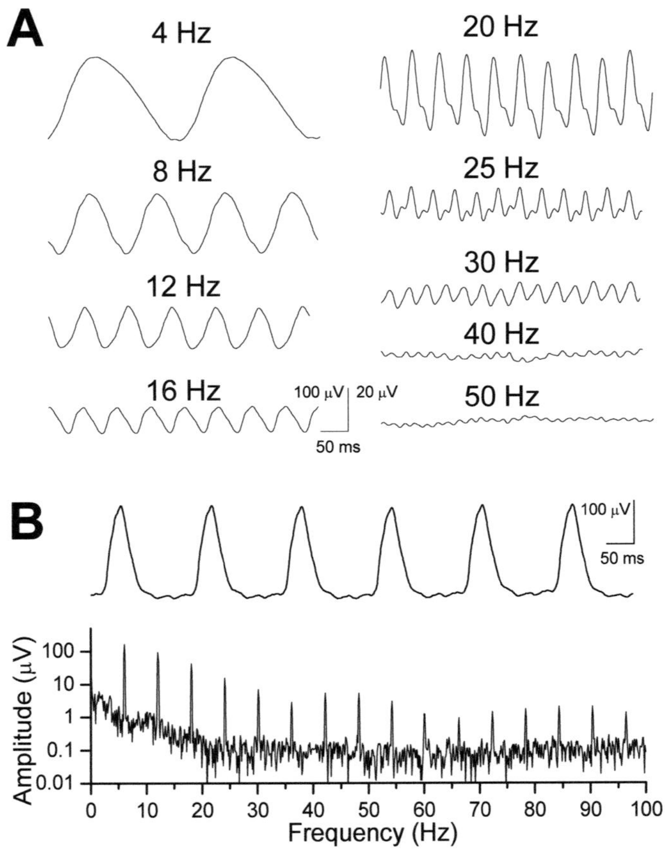

Fig. 1. Examples of typical ERG waveforms elicited from a rat eye. **A**. ERG waveforms elicited by sinusoidally modulated light stimuli at 90% contrast presented as selected temporal frequencies indicated above each traces. Each trace represents the average of eighteen 500-ms segments from a 10-s recording. Please note the traces on right side were plotted with 5 x more amplification than those on the left. **B**. Top, ERG waveform elicited by 6 Hz pulse flicker from the same eye as in **A**. An averaged 1-s segment was shown for clarity. Bottom, Fourier spectrum of the 9-s ERG trace of pulse flicker ERG. In addition to fundamental response at 6 Hz, other harmonics are clearly evident.

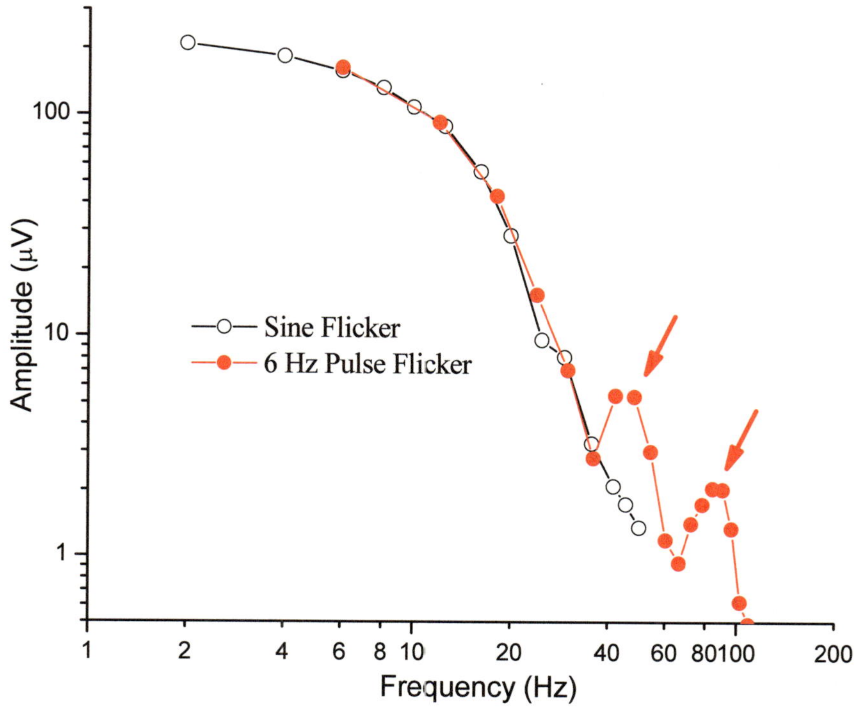

Fig. 2. Frequency-response relationship of rat ERG elicited by sine-wave flickers and pulse flickers. The amplitudes of the harmonic components of pulse flicker at 6 Hz and the fundamental responses of sine-wave flicker at various temporal frequencies are plotted. For response frequencies <30 Hz, frequency-response relation for pulse flicker ERG exhibits a shape similar to that derived for sine-wave flicker ERG. For response frequencies >30 Hz, larger peaks are observed in pulse flicker ERG than sine-wave ERG responses (arrows).

Fig. 2 shows frequency-response relationship of rat cone ERG derived by Fourier analysis of the waveforms shown in Fig. 1. For the response elicited by sine-wave modulated light stimuli, the amplitudes of the fundamental responses at each respective stimulus frequency are plotted. In agreement with our previous report (Qian et al., 2008), the amplitude of the fundamental response to sine-wave flicker exhibited a monotonic low-pass pattern. Response elicited by a 6 Hz pulse flicker is plotted as the amplitudes of fundamental and harmonic components. For response frequencies <30 Hz, the amplitudes of fundamental and harmonic responses to pulse flicker exhibit similar values as the fundamental response to sine-wave modulated light stimulus at respective temporal frequency. At high response frequencies, however, the amplitudes of harmonic responses to pulse flicker stimulus exhibit larger peaks than the fundamental response derived from sine-wave stimulus (arrows).

These high frequency harmonic components are common in rat cone ERG elicited with pulse flickers. Figure 3 shows averaged data from 12 eyes of the responses elicited by pulse flickers at frequency range from 2 to 12 Hz (open circles), and in comparison with the responses elicited by sine-wave flickers from the same animals (solid circles). The response amplitudes elicited by pulse flicker were smaller for lower temporal frequency stimulus than those elicited by higher temporal frequency stimulus, indicating the dependence of response on stimulus energy since high frequency pulse flickers contain more energy for each harmonic component than low frequency stimulus. In all cases, a peak in the high harmonic component is evident at all flash frequencies tested (2-12 Hz, arrows). However, location of this high frequency component varied with the pulse stimulus frequency, i.e. the component appeared at higher response frequency with higher pulse flicker frequency.

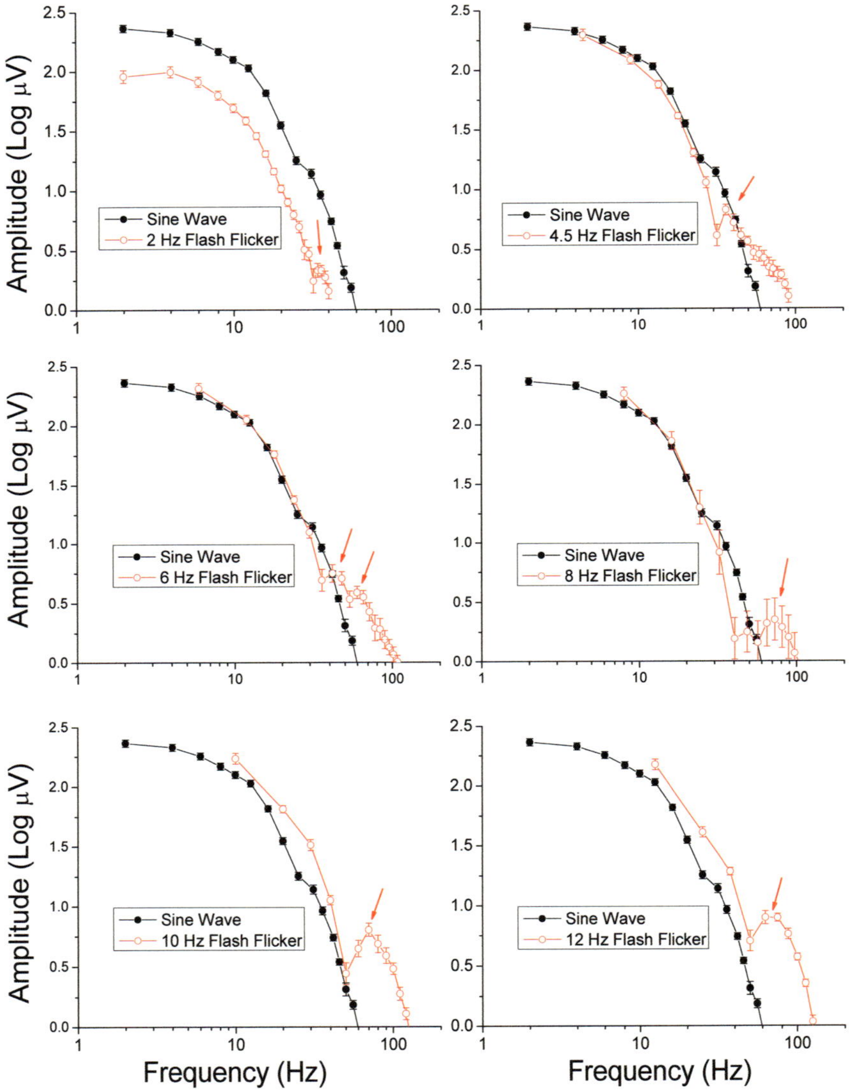

Fig. 3. Comparison of the mean frequency-response relationship elicited by sine-wave flicker ERG and with harmonic responses to pulse flicker ERG at various temporal frequencies. For all ERG responses elicited by pulse flickers, a peak in the high harmonic component is evident at all flash frequencies tested (2-12 Hz, arrows). Date was averaged from 12 eyes and presented as mean + SEM.

3.2 Effects of flash intensity on pulse flicker ERG

We examined the effects of flash intensity on frequency-response relationship of pulse flicker ERG elicited from rat eyes. Fig. 4 shows the results, averaged from 8 rat eyes, of frequency spectrum of ERG responses elicited with 6-Hz pulse flickers when the flash intensity varied from 50 cd/m^2 to 690 cd/m^2. In all flash luminosities tested, humps in high harmonic components were observed in pulse flicker ERG responses. It has been reported that, for sine-wave flicker ERG, responses elicited from rat eyes exhibit two distinct processes at low and high temporal frequencies (Qian et al., 2008). In particular, the contrast-response relation is linear when tested with a low-frequency (6 Hz) stimulus, but saturated in response to a high-frequency (20 Hz) stimulus. We tested if these two distinct retinal processes could also be revealed with pulse flicker stimulus. Fig. 5 plotted intensity-response relationship of 6-Hz pulse flicker for fundamental response (6 Hz) and fourth harmonic (24 Hz). Data were normalized to response elicited with maximal flash intensity (690 cd/m^2). Similar as observed with sine-wave stimulus, low frequency response (6 Hz) exhibited relative linear relationship in intensity-response function, whereas high frequency response (24 Hz) showed saturating behaviour. These results indicate that pulse flicker ERG can also be used to distinguish two retinal processes in rat eyes.

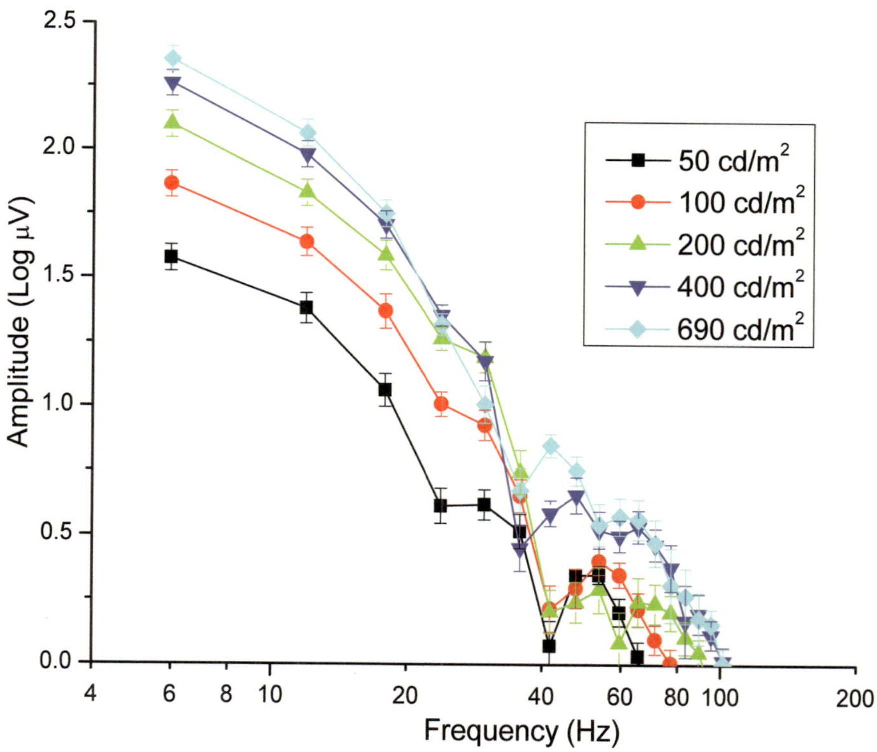

Fig. 4. Effects of flash intensity on the frequency-response relationship of rat pulse flicker ERG. Responses were elicited with 6-Hz pulse flickers. Flash intensity was varied from 50 cd/m^2 to 690 cd/m^2. Peaks in high harmonic components were observed at all flash intensities. Data was averaged from 8 rat eyes.

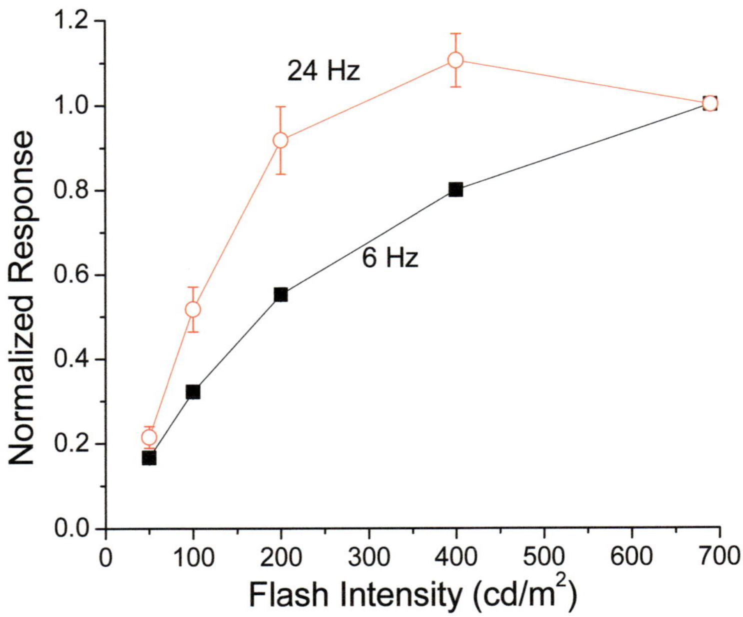

Fig. 5. Intensity-response relationship for fundamental (6 Hz) and fourth harmonic (24 Hz) of a 6 Hz pulse flicker ERG. Whereas the low frequency (6 Hz) response exhibited relative linear relation with the flash intensity, the high frequency response (24 Hz) reached saturation around 200 cd/m^2. Date were derived from those shown in Fig. 4.

3.3 Potential mechanisms for high frequency components in pulse flicker ERG

To examine retinal mechanism of the high frequency components in rat pulse flicker ERG, we isolated high frequency response waveform using a digital filter. An example is shown in Fig. 6. The top panel illustrates original response waveform for a 4.5 Hz pulse flicker ERG. The high frequency component isolated by a 40 Hz high-pass filter is shown at the bottom. It is clear that the high frequency components in pulse flicker ERG from rat eye mainly occurs at the rising phase of flicker ERG.

It is well know that oscillatory potentials (OPs) appear as the wavelets on the rising phase of flash ERG b-wave (Wachtmeister, 1980; Wachtmeister and Dowling, 1978). Therefore, it is possible that the high frequency components of rat pulse flicker ERG are mediated by OPs. OPs are generated in the inner retina by GABAnergic neurons, most likely amacrine cells, and these ERG wavelets can be reduced by inhibiting $GABA_A$ receptor activity in the retina (Wachtmeister, 2001). We examined the effect of intravitreal injection of bicuculline, a $GABA_A$ receptor antagonist, on OPs of dark-adapted rat ERG elicited by a flash of light. Fig. 7 shows an example of the waveforms of flash ERG recorded from a saline injected and a bicuculline (80 μM) inject rat eye. The flash ERG waveforms are shown on top raw, and bottom panel illustrates OPs isolated by a digital filter with bandwidth of 40 - 200 Hz. It is clear that bucuculline greatly reduced OP amplitudes in the rat eye.

We examined the effects of intravitreal injection of bicuculline on high frequency components of rat pulse flicker ERG, and results are shown in the left panel of bar graph in

Fig. 8. The high frequency components were derived by sum of harmonic components with frequencies higher than 40 Hz, and were normalized to the total flicker ERG response. When compared with responses elicited from saline injected eyes, the high frequency components from bicuculline-injected eyes were reduced by about 42% (n=8, $p<0.05$).

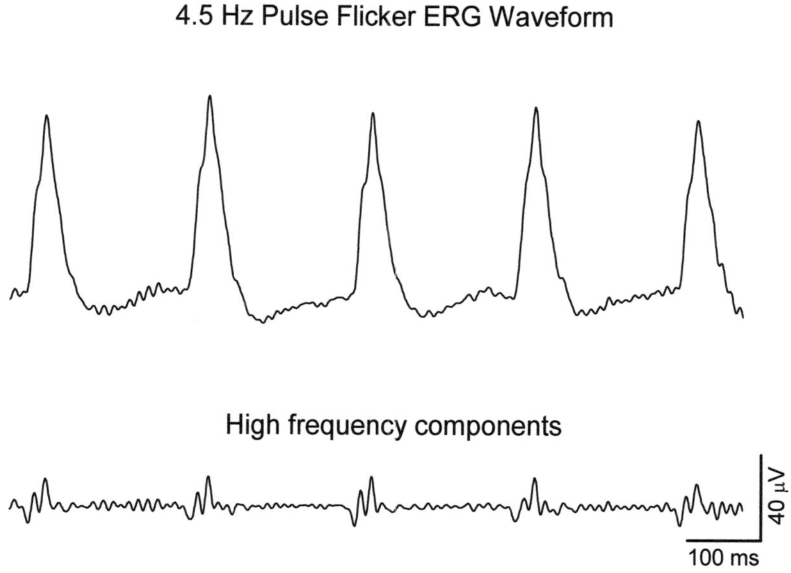

Fig. 6. Waveform of ERG elicited by 4.5-Hz pulse flicker. The original response waveform is shown at the top panel. The high frequency component (>40 Hz) of the response, derived with a high-pass digital filter, is shown at the low panel. The high frequency components occur at the rising phase of flicker ERG.

Another possible mechanism for generating high frequency components in pulse flicker ERG is the non-linear property of rat ERG responses. As pulse flicker stimulus itself contains multiple harmonic components each with similar energy strength, a non-linear response system will be able to generate beat components at high frequencies in response to low frequency stimulus. Such non-linear mechanism could also contribute to the observed high frequency components in pulse flicker rat ERG. To test this possibility, we examined non-linear responses by monitoring beat components of rat cone flicker ERG in response to a light stimulus that is composed of a mixture of two sine-waves, with frequency at 18 and 24 Hz respectively. Fig. 9 shows an example of frequency spectrum of the ERG response elicited from a rat eye by such light stimulus. The fundamental components for two stimuli frequency are pointed by arrows and marked as F1 and F2, respectively. In addition, beat components are also prominent in the response spectrum, as pointed by dashed arrows, indicating non-linear nature of rat cone flicker ERG response. To quantitate the amount of non-linearity in the system, we measured the ratio of the response at beat frequency of F1 + F2 to the sum of fundamental responses (i.e. response at frequency F1 and at F2). The results are summarized in the right panel of bar graph of Fig. 8. The bar graph also compared the effects of intravitreal injection of bicuculline on non-linear responses of rat cone flicker ERG. Interestingly, blocking $GABA_A$ receptor in the retina with bicuculline increased non-linearity of the flicker ERG response, as measured by the beat component of harmonic components ($p<0.05$).

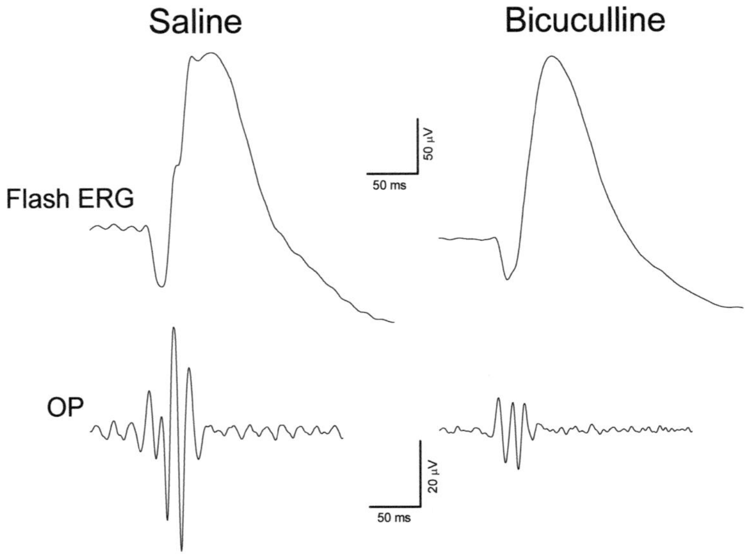

Fig. 7. Oscillatory potential (OP) in rat ERG. OPs (low panel) were isolated by a band pass filter (40-200 Hz) from the flash ERG illustrated in the top panel. Intravitreal injection of bicuculline greatly suppressed the OP amplitude with minimal effects on b-wave amplitude.

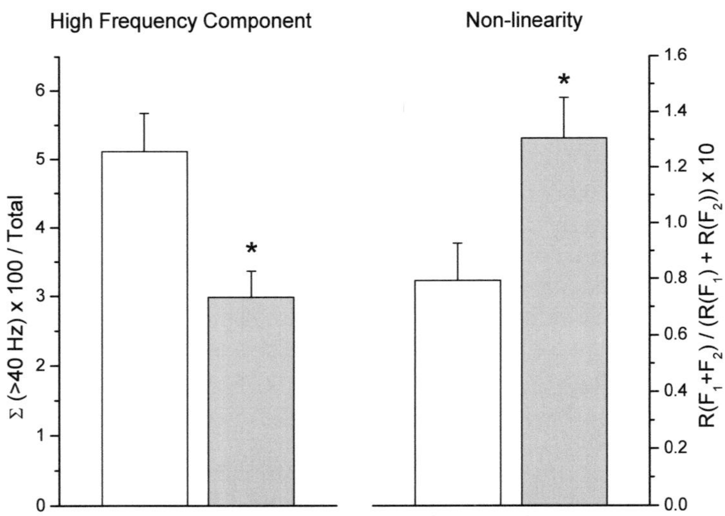

Fig. 8. Effects of bicuculline on high harmonic component and non-linearity in rat flicker ERG. A ratio of summed amplitude for harmonic responses above and below 40 Hz was used as an index for the high frequency component of pulse flicker ERG. Non-linearity was expressed as the ratio of beat response amplitude (F1 + F2) to the sum of the fundamental response to F1 (period 56 ms) and F2 (period 42 ms). Intravitreal injection of bicuculline (20 mM) significantly reduced the high frequency component in ERG elicited by pulse flicker, but enhanced the non-linearity of the response (*, $p < 0.05$). Date was averaged from 8 rats.

4. Discussion

In this study, we compared the frequency-response relationship for rat cone ERG elicited by flickering light stimuli, either to a series of flash pulses or to sinusoidally modulated light. Our results indicate that the frequency-response relationship derived from fundamental and harmonic component of pulse flicker ERG responses, with any temporal frequency range from 2 to 12 Hz, exhibited a similar shape as the fundamental response elicited by sine-wave flickers for response frequencies less than 30 Hz (Fig. 2 and 3). This is consistent with earlier observation that rat cone flicker ERG contains only small non-linear (second harmonic) components elicited with sine-wave stimulus for temporal frequency up to 16 Hz (Qian et al., 2008). Therefore, it is possible to use pulse flicker to determine low-pass character of rat cone flicker ERG. For practical purpose, a low pulse flicker will be a better choice since more harmonic components are available to provide response data points (Fig. 3). However, the exact amplitudes at each response frequency varied with the temporal frequency of pulse flicker stimulus (Fig. 3). This is large due to the fact that high frequency pulse flicker delivered more photons than low frequency stimulus, and the amplitudes of rat flicker ERG vary with flash intensity as shown in Fig. 4.

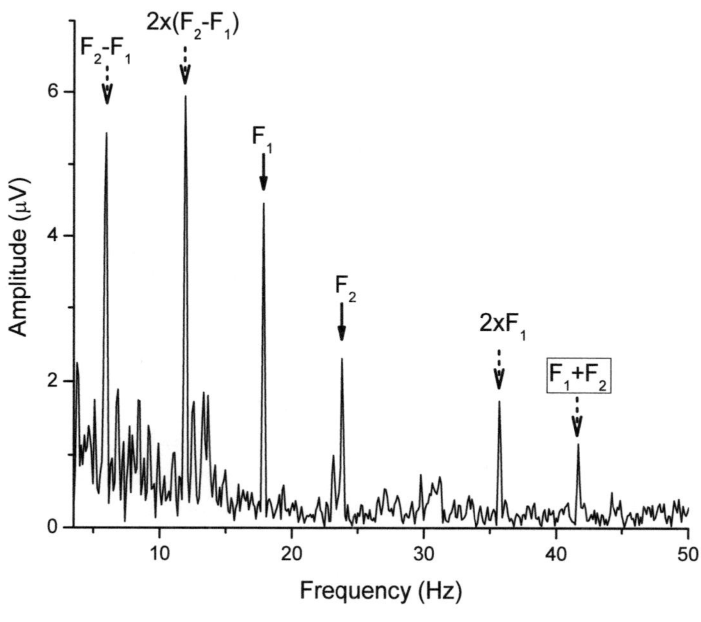

Fig. 9. Non-linearity in rat flicker ERG. Spectrum of ERG elicited by a mixture of two sine-wave modulated light stimuli with periods of 56 ms (18 Hz, F1) and 42 ms (24 Hz, F2), respectively. Fundamental responses to F1 and F2 are marked by arrows, beat components are marked by dashed arrows, and the beat response to (F1 + F2) used as an index for non-linearity in rat flicker ERG was marked by a box.

On the other hand, it has been reported that primate photopic 32-Hz ERG for Sine-, square-, and pulsed stimuli were largely different, perhaps due to non-linear interactions among retinal signal pathways (Kondo and Sieving, 2002). It should be noted that rodent photopic ERG exhibit a number of difference from primates and diurnal animals (Alexander et al.,

2005; Ekesten et al., 1998; Hare and Ton, 2002; Qian et al., 2010; Rosolen et al., 2005; Shah et al., 2010). The ERG protocol developed for rodent eye may not be applicable to study of human ERG responses.

Using frequency-response relationship derived from harmonic analysis of pulse flicker ERG, we can also differentiate two distinct retinal processing mechanisms at low and high response frequencies (Fig. 4 and 5). Similar as responses elicited by sine-wave flickers (Qian et al., 2008), low frequency responses (fundamental response to 6 Hz pulse flicker stimulus) were relatively linear in relation with stimulus light intensity (Fig. 5), whereas high frequency responses (fourth harmonic responses to 6 Hz stimulus) have a relatively higher gain to low stimulus light intensity and responses become saturated with intensity above 200 cd/m^2. Therefore, pulse flicker stimulus will be particular valuable in cases that long-term recordings are hard to obtain, such as single cell recordings of retinal neurons. Instead of requiring multiple episodes of sine-wave modulated light stimuli, the responses elicited by a single pulse flicker stimulus will be enough to provide valuable information about frequency-response relationship for rodent eye with response frequency less than 30 Hz.

It should be noted that pulse flicker ERG does not capture all the features revealed by sine-wave flicker, which examines responses one temporal frequency at a time. For example, it is clear from response waveform shown in Fig. 1A that the flicker ERG elicited from this rat eye contained period-doubling for 20 Hz sine-wave frequency stimulus (Shah et al., 2010). However, this feature is not captured on frequency-response relationship derived from pulse flicker ERG (Fig. 1 and 2).

For response frequencies over 30 Hz, there were larger high harmonic components in pulse flicker ERG compared with the fundamental response elicited by sine-wave stimulus at corresponding frequency (Fig. 2 – 4). These high harmonic components in pulse flicker ERG were present for all flash frequencies tested (2-12 Hz) (Fig. 3), and persisted with the flash luminance varied from 50 cd/m^2 to 690 cd/m^2 (Fig. 4). To investigate the origin of these high harmonic components, we tested two possibilities: oscillatory potentials and non-linearity of the ERG response. The waveform of high frequency components is mainly located on the rising phase of the flicker ERG response (Fig. 6), a feature similar as oscillatory potentials of dark-adapted flash ERG. Intravitreal injection of a $GABA_A$ receptor antagonist, bicuculline, both reduced oscillatory potentials in flash ERG and the high frequency components in pulse flicker ERG response (Fig. 7 and 8), indicating mechanisms similar as OP generators are contributing, at least in part, to the high harmonic components observed in pulse flicker ERG. To investigate the contribution of non-linearity in rat flicker ERG, we used a sum of two sine-wave modulate light at frequency of 18 and 24 Hz as stimulus, and measured beat response at frequency of 42 Hz, i.e. sum of 18 and 24 Hz. Our results indicate that non-linearity is a prominent component of rat cone flicker ERG in this region of response frequency (Fig. 9). Interestingly, eyes injected with bicuculline exhibited higher non-linearity compared with those of saline-injected eyes. The mechanisms of this action of $GABA_A$ receptor antagonist are yet to be determined.

5. Conclusion

Pulsed light stimulus is commonly used to elicit flicker ERG, whereas sine-wave modulated light provides better characterization of frequency-response relation. In this study, we compared rat cone flicker ERG elicited by these two stimuli in frequency domain, and investigated the mechanism for the higher harmonic responses. Our results indicate that a single pulse light stimulus can be used as an alternative method to probe the frequency-response relationship of flicker ERG for response frequencies less than 30 Hz. We also demonstrated that pulse light stimuli are useful to distinct two retinal processes revealed by sine-wave stimuli (Qian et al., 2008). In addition, pulse flicker ERG contains high harmonic components which have contributions from retinal generators of oscillatory potentials and non-linear interactions of retinal signal pathways. Pulse flicker stimulus could also be used as a tool to investigate retinal mechanisms of these two processes.

6. Acknowledgment

This study is supported in part by a grant from Illinois Society for the Prevention of Blindness.

7. References

Alexander, K.R., Barnes, C.S., Fishman, G.A., 2001. Origin of deficits in the flicker electroretinogram of the cone system in X-linked retinoschisis as derived from response nonlinearities. J Opt Soc Am A Opt Image Sci Vis 18, 747-754.

Alexander, K.R., Barnes, C.S., Fishman, G.A., 2003. ON-pathway dysfunction and timing properties of the flicker ERG in carriers of X-linked retinitis pigmentosa. Invest Ophthalmol Vis Sci 44, 4017-4025.

Alexander, K.R., Levine, M.W., Super, B.J., 2005. Characteristics of period doubling in the human cone flicker electroretinogram. Vis Neurosci 22, 817-824.

Audo, I., Michaelides, M., Robson, A.G., Hawlina, M., Vaclavik, V., Sandbach, J.M., Neveu, M.M., Hogg, C.R., Hunt, D.M., Moore, A.T., Bird, A.C., Webster, A.R., Holder, G.E., 2008. Phenotypic variation in enhanced S-cone syndrome. Invest Ophthalmol Vis Sci 49, 2082-2093.

Bach, M., Meigen, T., 1999. Do's and don'ts in Fourier analysis of steady-state potentials. Doc Ophthalmol 99, 69-82.

Burns, S.A., Elsner, A.E., Kreitz, M.R., 1992. Analysis of nonlinearities in the flicker ERG. Optom Vis Sci 69, 95-105.

Ekesten, B., Gouras, P., Moschos, M., 1998. Cone properties of the light-adapted murine ERG. Doc Ophthalmol 97, 23-31.

Fishman, G.A., 2001. Electrophysiologic testing in disorders of the retina, optic nerve, and visual pathway, 2nd ed. Foundation of the American Academy of Ophthalmology, San Francisco, CA.

Frishman, L.J., 2006. Origins of the electroretinogram, in: Heckenlively, J.R., Arden, G.B. (Eds.), Principles and practive of clinical electrophysiology of vision, Second ed. The MIT Press, Cambridge, Massachusetts, pp. 139-183.

Garry, D., Hansen, R.M., Moskowitz, A., Elias, E.R., Irons, M., Fulton, A.B., 2010. Cone ERG responses in patients with Smith-Lemli-Opitz Syndrome (SLOS). Doc Ophthalmol 121, 85-91.

Hare, W.A., Ton, H., 2002. Effects of APB, PDA, and TTX on ERG responses recorded using both multifocal and conventional methods in monkey. Effects of APB, PDA, and TTX on monkey ERG responses. Doc Ophthalmol 105, 189-222.

Jacobs, G.H., Neitz, J., Krogh, K., 1996. Electroretinogram flicker photometry and its applications. J Opt Soc Am A Opt Image Sci Vis 13, 641-648.

Kondo, M., Sieving, P.A., 2001. Primate photopic sine-wave flicker ERG: vector modeling analysis of component origins using glutamate analogs. Invest Ophthalmol Vis Sci 42, 305-312.

Kondo, M., Sieving, P.A., 2002. Post-photoreceptoral activity dominates primate photopic 32-Hz ERG for sine-, square-, and pulsed stimuli. Invest Ophthalmol Vis Sci 43, 2500-2507.

Krishna, V.R., Alexander, K.R., Peachey, N.S., 2002. Temporal properties of the mouse cone electroretinogram. J Neurophysiol 87, 42-48.

Marmor, M.F., Fulton, A.B., Holder, G.E., Miyake, Y., Brigell, M., Bach, M., 2009. ISCEV Standard for full-field clinical electroretinography (2008 update). Doc Ophthalmol 118, 69-77.

Meigen, T., Bach, M., 1999. On the statistical significance of electrophysiological steady-state responses. Doc Ophthalmol 98, 207-232.

Peachey, N.S., Ball, S.L., 2003. Electrophysiological analysis of visual function in mutant mice. Doc Ophthalmol 107, 13-36.

Qian, H., Alexander, K.R., Ripps, H., 2010. Harmonic analysis of the cone flicker ERG of rabbit. Experimental eye research 91, 811-817.

Qian, H., Shah, M.R., Alexander, K.R., Ripps, H., 2008. Two distinct processes are evident in rat cone flicker ERG responses at low and high temporal frequencies. Experimental eye research 87, 71-75.

Ramsey, D.J., Ripps, H., Qian, H., 2006. An electrophysiological study of retinal function in the diabetic female rat. Invest Ophthalmol Vis Sci 47, 5116-5124.

Rosolen, S.G., Rigaudiere, F., Le Gargasson, J.F., Brigell, M.G., 2005. Recommendations for a toxicological screening ERG procedure in laboratory animals. Doc Ophthalmol 110, 57-66.

Shah, M.R., Alexander, K.R., Ripps, H., Qian, H., 2010. Characteristics of period doubling in the rat cone flicker ERG. Experimental eye research 90, 196-202.

Viswanathan, S., Frishman, L.J., Robson, J.G., 2002. Inner-retinal contributions to the photopic sinusoidal flicker electroretinogram of macaques. Macaque photopic sinusoidal flicker ERG. Doc Ophthalmol 105, 223-242.

Wachtmeister, L., 1980. Further studies of the chemical sensitivity of the oscillatory potentials of the electroretinogram (ERG) I. GABA- and glycine antagonists. Acta Ophthalmol (Copenh) 58, 712-725.

Wachtmeister, L., 2001. Some aspects of the oscillatory response of the retina. Prog Brain Res 131, 465-474.

Wachtmeister, L., Dowling, J.E., 1978. The oscillatory potentials of the mudpuppy retina. Invest Ophthalmol Vis Sci 17, 1176-1188.

Wu, S., Burns, S.A., Elsner, A.E., 1995. Effects of flicker adaptation and temporal gain control on the flicker ERG. Vision Res 35, 2943-2953.

Xu, L., Ball, S.L., Alexander, K.R., Peachey, N.S., 2003. Pharmacological analysis of the rat cone electroretinogram. Vis Neurosci 20, 297-306.

11

Electroretinogram Assessment of Dark Adaptation and Rod Phototransduction from the Central Retina of Japanese Macaques with Dominantly Inherited Drusen

Brett G Jeffrey[1,4], Catherine W Morgans[2,5], Robert M Duvoisin[3,5] and Martha Neuringer[2,4,5]
[1]*Ophthalmic Genetics and Visual Function Branch National Eye Institute, Bethesda, MD*
[2]*Casey Eye Institute*
[3]*Department of Physiology and Pharmacology*
[4]*Oregon National Primate Research Center*
[5]*Oregon Health and Science University, Portland Oregon USA*

1. Introduction

The central retina of humans, apes and monkeys is uniquely characterized amongst mammals by the presence of the macula, a distinct and specialized area 6 mm in diameter (≈22 degrees of visual angle) centered on the fovea (Curcio et al., 2000). The fovea which measures just 0.8 mm and contains the highest photoreceptor and RPE densities in the retina, enables the high visual acuities achieved by primates. A defining characteristic of the macula includes the presence of the xanthophyll pigments, lutein and zeaxanthin, which give the macula its distinctive yellow color (Snodderly et al., 1984). Within the macula, rods outnumber cones by 9:1, lower than the 20:1 rod to cone ratio found for the retina as a whole (Curcio et al., 2000). Therefore, while the macula is cone enriched compared with the peripheral retina, rods are the predominant photoreceptor. In primates, the macula is surrounded by the "rod ring", an area with a radius of approximately 10 to 25 degrees, which contains the highest rod density within the retina (Curcio et al., 1990; Packer et al., 1989; Wikler et al., 1990). For the purposes of the present paper, the central retina is taken to be the area covering 40 degrees of visual angle which encompasses the macula and much of the surrounding rod ring.

With increasing age, changes in retinal morphology include an overall thinning of the retina, accumulation of lipofuscin within the retinal pigment epithelium, thickening of Bruch's membrane, accumulation of basal deposits on and within Bruch's membrane, and accumulation of drusen, the extracellular deposits below the retinal pigment epithelium (Bonilha 2008). The number of photoreceptors within the central and peripheral retina are differentially affected by age. Within the central retina, rod density decreases by 30% between 20 and 90 years of age, while cone density remains constant at the fovea and across the central retina (Curcio et al., 1993; Gao & Hollyfield 1992). In contrast, cone density in the peripheral retina decreases by 20% between 20 and 90 years of age, while the number of peripheral rods remains constant after 35 years of age (Curcio et al., 1993; Gao & Hollyfield 1992).

Age-related changes in retinal function largely correlate with the morphological changes that occur within the retina with increasing age. Psychophysical studies have documented approximately 35% slowing in the rate of dark adaptation and a 3-fold rise in absolute rod threshold between 20 and 90 years (Jackson et al., 1999). Age-related changes in cone mediated function include reduced contrast sensitivity, lower critical flicker/fusion frequency, poorer color discrimination and lower hyperacuities (Haegerstrom-Portnoy 2005; Wang 2001).

With increasing age, changes observed in both rod and cone ERGs include delays in ERG implicit times, and decreases in ERG a- and b-wave amplitudes (Berrow et al., 2010; Gerth 2009). Aged related changes in phototransduction, measured from the bright flash ERG a-wave, include lower rod sensitivity and slowing of rod inactivation kinetics (Jackson et al., 2006). The changes in psychophysical and ERG functional measures with increasing age cannot be accounted for by changes in optical media properties alone and are therefore, attributable to functional/morphological changes in the retina and/or central nervous system (Morrison, & McGrath 1985; Spear 1993).

Age-related macular degeneration (AMD) is the most common cause of legal blindness in the elderly in the developed world. AMD is a heterogeneous disorder affecting the retinal pigment epithelium/Bruch's membrane complex which results in photoreceptor dysfunction and loss. Early AMD is associated with changes in pigmentation of the retinal pigment epithelium and the presence of soft or confluent drusen in the macula. Signs of advanced AMD include development of geographic atrophy of the retinal pigment epithelium and choroidal neovascularization. AMD is associated with the same changes in retina and retinal pigment epithelium observed with normal aging but in AMD these changes are more marked, progressive and may result in severe visual loss (Bonilha 2008). In AMD, both rod and cone photoreceptors are lost, and photoreceptor density decreases by 30-40% relative to age-matched controls within 0.5 - 3 mm from the fovea (Curcio et al., 1996). Thus the loss of photoreceptors in the paramacular of AMD patients occurs over the same area of maximal rod loss seen in non-pathological aging. Rod death precedes that of cones and there is a greater loss of rods in most AMD patients (Curcio et al., 1996). A recent study, however, reported earlier and more extensive aberrant distribution of opsin immunolabeling compared with rhodopsin in AMD eyes (Shelley et al., 2009). These results suggest that sub-clinical pathological changes may occur earlier in cone photoreceptors than in the rods of AMD eyes.

Psychophysical studies largely support the histopathological evidence of rod and cone photoreceptor loss in early AMD. Cone mediated functions, including flicker and s-cone sensitivities, color vision, temporal contrast, and light adaptation recovery kinetics, are altered in early AMD (Hogg, & Chakravarthy 2006; Neelam et al., 2009; Phipps et al., 2003). Longitudinal studies indicate that some of these parameters alone or in combination may predict those eyes that will progress to more advanced AMD with good specificity and sensitivity (Neelam et al., 2009). Psychophysical studies also support histopathological evidence for greater dysfunction and loss of rods over cones in the parafovea (two to four degrees from the fovea) in early AMD (Neelam et al., 2009). Losses in rod sensitivity precede associated losses in photopic sensitivity and in 87% of AMD patients, the degree of rod sensitivity loss is greater than for cone sensitivity (Jackson et al., 2002). The time constant of dark adaptation is also markedly delayed in AMD patients (Eisner et al., 1992; Haimovici et al., 2002; Owsley et al., 2001). These disturbances of psychophysical function in AMD patients are not limited to the macula but extend across the central retinal area at radii up to 25 to 40 degrees from the fovea, for rod and cone adaptation respectively (Neelam et al., 2009).

ERG assessment of central retinal function in aging and AMD have largely focused on the recording of cone-mediated responses from photopic multifocal (mfERG), focal (fERG) and pattern (pERG) ERGs [Reviewed in (Berrow et al., 2010)]. AMD is associated with delayed implicit times and/or reduction in ERG amplitudes in at least one of the response components of each of these ERG modalities. Drusen are associated with slight delays in mfERG implicit times, although changes are not limited to areas with drusen (Berrow et al., 2010). Correlations between the amplitude of the focal ERG and severity of non-exudative AMD have been reported (Falsini et al., 1999). A focal ERG implementation of the photo stress test also found a significantly slower recovery of bleach cone response in ARM patients (Binns, & Margrain 2007).

Many studies have documented that rhesus macaques develop age related changes in the macula including the formation of drusen and pigmentary changes within the retinal pigment epithelium that are the hallmark of early human AMD (e.g. (Dawson et al., 2008; Gouras et al., 2008)). Like humans, the prevalence and severity of drusen increase with age in rhesus macaques, while some 30% of macaques do not develop drusen at any age (Gouras et al., 2008; Hope et al., 1992) . Drusen do develop earlier in macaques than human and drusen may be observed in up to 53 % of macaques by 10 years of age (Hope et al., 1992), approximately equivalent to 30 human years. Early- and late-onset macular disease has also been reported in a closely related species, the cynomologus macaque (Macaca fascicularis) (Umeda et al., 2005a). Drusen from both macaque species have been confirmed by histopathology to closely resemble human drusen (Gouras et al., 2008). Furthermore, immunohistochemistry and proteonomic studies of isolated drusen from macaques have identified many of the compounds present in human drusen, including apolipoprotein E, complement component C5, membrane cofactor protein and vitronectin (Umeda et al., 2005b). Lastly, rhesus and cynomologus macaques share genetic and nutritional risk factors with human AMD (Francis et al., 2008; Singh et al., 2009; Umeda et al., 2003, Umeda et al., 2005b)

We have identified a distinct retinal disease syndrome that is characterized by dominant inheritance and the early onset of pan-retinal drusen in Japanese macaques (Macaca fuscata) at our Oregon National Primate Research Center (Neuringer M, et al. IOVS 2011;52:ARVO E-Abstract 4008). In a survey of retinal status of 160 of these animals, 42 (26%) showed this disease phenotype. These Japanese macaques are also closely related to the rhesus macaque and we wanted to determine whether the drusen observed in these monkeys were associated with changes in retinal function. Further, given the nature of the photoreceptor changes seen in human AMD, we sought to determine whether central retinal function was selectively altered in these Japanese macaques, particularly as a function of age.

While psychophysical measures of visual function are possible in non-human primates, our experience is that the time involved in training is substantial. Depending of the complexity of the psychophysical task, training may take 6 months to 2 years per animal, making detailed functional examination of a large number of animals prohibitively costly. The widely used full field-electroretinogram (ERG), provides an objective, quick and detailed assessment of retinal function in non-human primates (e.g (Jeffrey et al., 2002)). However, full field ERG is relatively insensitive to the local structural and functional changes that occur in the central retina in maculopathies such as AMD. Given that rods comprise 90% of macular photoreceptors and that dysfunction and degeneration of rods may precede that of cones with age and in AMD, there is a need for a robust ERG measure of central rod function. Several methods have been used to measure a rod focal ERG for areas ranging from 5 to 40 degrees of the central retina (reviewed in (Binns, & Margrain 2006). The basis of all methods used for obtaining a focal rod ERG is the elimination of the scattered light component generated from the peripheral retina. Sandberg et al (1996) used a subtraction technique to eliminate the stray light component of the double peaked focal flash response. Sandberg's method was extremely time consuming as it required recording full-field ERGs of varying intensity until a response was found that exactly matched amplitude and temporal characteristics of the scattered light response of the focal ERG. The focal response was calculated by subtracting the scattered light response from the original double peaked ERG b-wave response. Other methods used for recording a focal rod-ERG include suppressing the peripheral rods using a dim background, or using a using a very small five degree dim stimulus that produced no recordable scattered light component (Binns, & Margrain 2006; Choshi et al., 2003; Hood et al., 1998). While rod-isolated focal ERG responses can be obtained by these methods, the b-wave responses recorded are extremely small (<10 μV).

Nusinowitz et al (1995) described a method for deriving focal rod-isolated ERG a-waves from a 40 degree field centered on the macula. The technique used bright paired flashes. The first bright flash triggers a response from local rods and cones in the central 40 degree field, as well as from peripheral photoreceptors due to scattered light. The second flash, given while central rods are still saturated from the first flash, triggers a response from cones and peripheral rods, but not central, rods. The rod-isolated ERG response from the central 40 degree field, is obtained by subtracting the second flash response from the that of the first. Relatively large focal rod ERG a-waves, with peak a-wave amplitude of some 40 μV were obtained using this paired flash method. Nusinowitz et al (1995) was also able to fit a P3 model to these central rod a-waves, thereby providing a quantitative description of central rod phototransduction. However, to achieve the alignment necessary for their technique, Nusinowitz et al (1995) used Maxwellian view projection, a method not amenable to use with anesthetized animals.

Here we adapt the method described by Nusinowitz et al (1995) to enable measurement of rod phototransduction from the central retina of the anesthetized monkey using a standard Ganzfeld stimulus. The results demonstrate a selective reduction in central rod function that worsens with age in a group of Japanese macaques with dominant drusen. By comparison there was no effect of drusen in these macaques on the kinetics of dark adaptation measured with the full field bright flash ERG.

2. Experimental methods and results

2.1 Animals

All experiments were reviewed and approved by the Institutional Animal Care and Use Committee of the Oregon National Primate Research Center and were conducted in accordance with the ARVO statement for the Use of Animals in Ophthalmic and Vision Research.

Color retinal fundus photography was used to screen for retinal phenotypes in a troop of Japanese macaques (Macaca fuscata) resident at the Oregon National Primate Research Center since 1964. Selected macaques were also assessed by fluorescein angiography. We identified a distinct retinal disease syndrome in these macaques that is characterized by dominant inheritance and the early onset of pan-retinal drusen (Neuringer M, et al. IOVS 2011;52:ARVO E-Abstract 4008). Electroretinograms (ERGs) were recorded from eight of these Japanese macaques that were aged between 6 and 27 years at the time of testing. Four monkeys had no evidence of drusen, while the other 4 monkeys had severe drusen noted on retinal fundus photographs and fluroscein angiograms.

2.2 Animal preparation

In preparation for ERG recording, monkeys were anesthetized with intramuscular injection of ketamine (10 mg/kg), xylazine (1.0 mg/kg) and atropine (0.4 mg/kg). Anesthesia was maintained with ketamine (5 mg/kg), xylazine (0.5 mg/kg) and atropine (0.4 mg/kg) at 30- to 50-minute intervals as required. Ketamine and atropine were administered at least five minutes before xylazine injection. Supplemental oxygen was delivered via nasal canula at 0.5 liters/minute, and both the heart rate and oxygen saturation were monitored by pulse oximetry. Core body temperature was maintained between 37.0°C and 38.5°C by using water-circulated heated pads placed either side of the animal. After completion of the ERG studies, a triple antibiotic (Vetropolycin; Dechra Pharmaceuticals, Overland Park, KS) was placed on the eyes and an analgesic (ketaprofen, 20 mg/kg) given intramuscularly. Animals were recovered in a darkened room before being returned to their holding cage.

Before ERG recording, pupils were dilated to approximately 8 mm with phenylephrine (2.5%) and tropicamide (1%). The cornea was anesthetized with proparacaine (1%) and lubricated with methylcellulose (1%) before insertion of a bipolar Burian-Allen contact lens electrode (Hansen Ophthalmic Development Laboratory, Iowa City, IA). A subdermal needle electrode placed in the back served as ground. With the bright flash intensities used here, we often encountered large flash artifacts during ERG recording. We found that covering the silvered speculum of the Burian-Allen electrode with black ink from a permanent marker and placing a collar made from black plastic around the top edge of the speculum minimized such flash artifacts. Animals were dark adapted for 30 minutes prior to ERG recording. ERGs were amplified (10 000) and filtered (-3dB at 0.1Hz & 1 kHz) before being sampled at 5 kHz with a 12-bit A/D converter and stored for off-line analysis.

2.3 Light stimulation

Flash stimulation was provided by two high-intensity photoflash units (2405CX and a modified 1205 CX power supplies with 205 flash units: Speedotron; Chicago, Ill) mounted on a customized 35-cm Ganzfeld. Flash intensities in candela-seconds/metre^2 (cd-s/m^2) were measured by a photometer with a scotopic filter set to integration mode for measurement of brief flashes (PR1980A-PL, Photo Research, Chatsworth CA). Retinal illuminance in scotopic trolands (sc Td-s) was calculated from the respective flash energies and pupil size (Wyszecki, & Stiles 1982).

2.4 Method for measuring full field rod phototransduction

The left columns of Figures 1 & 2 outline the paired flash protocol (Birch, & Hood 1995) used to derive full-field rod isolated ERG a-waves. Full-field ERG rod a-waves were recorded to flash intensities of 2.1 - 4.5 log sc Td-s in approximately 0.3 log unit steps. ERGs to the first (test) flash contained both rod and cone contributions (Figure 1A). Isolating the cone contributions to these ERGs required a differential approach that depended on first flash intensity. For test flash intensities greater than 3.3 log sc Td-s, rods saturate for longer

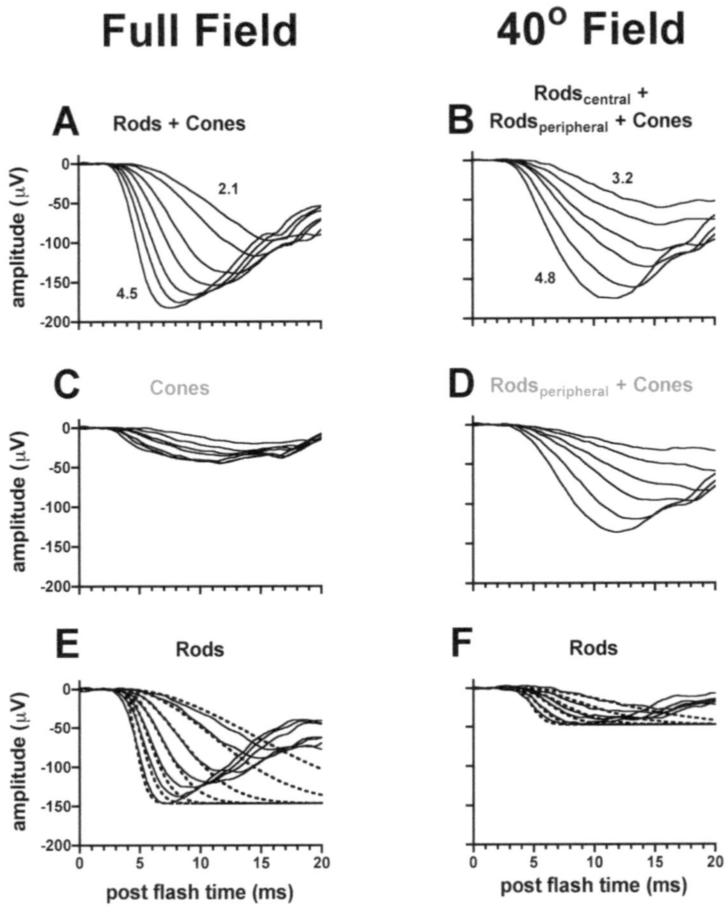

Fig. 1. Derivation of full- and restricted -field rod ERG a-waves. **Left column: A.** Mixed rod/cone ERG a-waves to a range of flash intensities (2.1 - 4.5 log sc Td-s) in response to the first flash of paired-flash paradigm. **C.** Cone ERG a-waves to the same flash intensities in response to the second of the paired flashes. **E.** Full-field rod-isolated ERG a-waves obtained by subtracting response in C from those in A. Dashed lines show the ensemble fit of the P3 model (eqn 1) to the leading edges of the ERG a-waves. For this 27 year old monkey, $Rmax_{P3}$ = -146 µV, S = (16.2 sc Td-s)$^{-1}$ s^{-2}, td = 3.6 ms. **Right column: B.** Mixed rod/cone ERG a-waves to a range of flash intensities (3.2 - 4.8 log sc Td-s) in response to an isolated flash. **D.** The cone and scattered rod contributions are calculated from the same flashes presented 2.2 sec after a 3.3 log sc Td-s conditioning flash. **F.** Rod-isolated ERG a-waves from the central 40° obtained by subtracting responses in D from those in B. Dashed lines show the ensemble fit of the P3 model (eqn 1) to the leading edges of the ERG a-waves.For this 27 year old monkey, $Rmax_{P3}$ = -47 µV, S = (5.1 sc Td-s)$^{-1}$ s^{-2}, t_d=3.5 ms

than 1.5 seconds, but cones recover in less than 400 milliseconds (unpublished data). Therefore, dark adapted cone ERGs were obtained by presenting two identical flashes separated by an interstimulus interval (ISI) of one second (Figure 2B). Thus, the second flash was presented while the rods were still saturated from the first flash. For retinal illuminances under 3.3 log scot Td-s, rods did not saturate for sufficient time to allow direct application of this paired flash method. Instead a two step process was necessary (Figure 2A). In the first step, ERGs were recorded to isolated test flashes (Figure 2A). In the second step, the ERG was then recorded to these same test flashes, presented 1 second after a 3.3 log sc Td-s conditioning flash (Figure 2A). This 1.0 sec interval ensured that the test flash occurred after complete cone recovery but before the onset of rod recovery from the conditioning flash. Figure 1C shows the full-field cone ERGs obtained using this differential approach. Rod isolated ERG a-waves (Figure 1E) were obtained by subtracting the dark-adapted cone-isolated ERGs (Figure 1C) from the mixed rod/cone responses (Figure 1A).

2.5 Method of rod phototransduction analysis

Rod phototransduction was quantified from the fit of the following P3 model to the leading edges the rod-isolated ERG a-waves (Birch et al., 1995):

$$P3\ (i,t) \cong [1 - \exp(-I \bullet S \bullet (t - t_d)^2)] \bullet Rmax_{P3} \quad t > td \tag{1}$$

where P3 is the leading edge of the a-wave at time (t) seconds, in response to a flash with a retinal illuminance of I (sc Td-s). The parameters derived to fit the model were: S ((sc Td-s)$^{-1}$ s^{-2}), the sensitivity parameter that scales retinal illuminance; t_d (secs), the delay due to the filter and finite duration of the flash; and $Rmax_{P3}$ (μV) , the maximum rod photoresponse .

The parameters of the P3 model were determined by fitting equation 1 simultaneously (ensemble fit) to the leading edges of the of the ERG a-waves for retinal illuminances from 2.4 to 4.2 log scot Td-s . The "leading edge" of the ERG a-wave for each flash intensity was determined to be all points with amplitude less than 80% of the a-wave peak. The 80% value was chosen to avoid the influence of the post-receptoral components that contribute to the a-wave near its peak (Robson et al., 2003). During fitting, $Rmax_{P3}$ was fixed at the maximal a-wave amplitude obtained and S and t_d were varied. All analysis was performed with custom written Matlab programs (David Birch, Retina Foundation of the Southwest, Dallas, TX.).

In Figure 1C, the fit of the P3 model (dotted lines) provides a good description of the rising phases to the ERG a-waves for all but the two highest intensities where rate saturation becomes a limiting factor (Breton et al., 1994; Lamb et al., 1992).

2.6 Method for measuring restricted field rod phototransduction

The right columns of Figures 1 & 2 outline the protocol used to derive rod isolated ERG a-waves from a 40 degree field centered on the macula (Nusinowitz et al., 1995). The restricted field ERG protocol also makes used of the paired flash method, but requires two recording steps (Figure 2 C). In the first step, the ERG is recorded to an isolated test flash (3.2 - 4.8 log sc Td-s) presented over a 40 degree field centered on the macula (Figure 2C). The ERG response ERG_{total} to this isolated test flash (Figure 1B), contains rod and cone components from the central 40 degree field as well as rod and cone components from the peripheral retina generated by scattered light (Nusinowitz et al., 1995).; i.e.

$$ERG_{total} = Rods_{central} + Cones_{central} + Rods_{peripheral} + Cones_{perpipheral} \tag{2a}$$

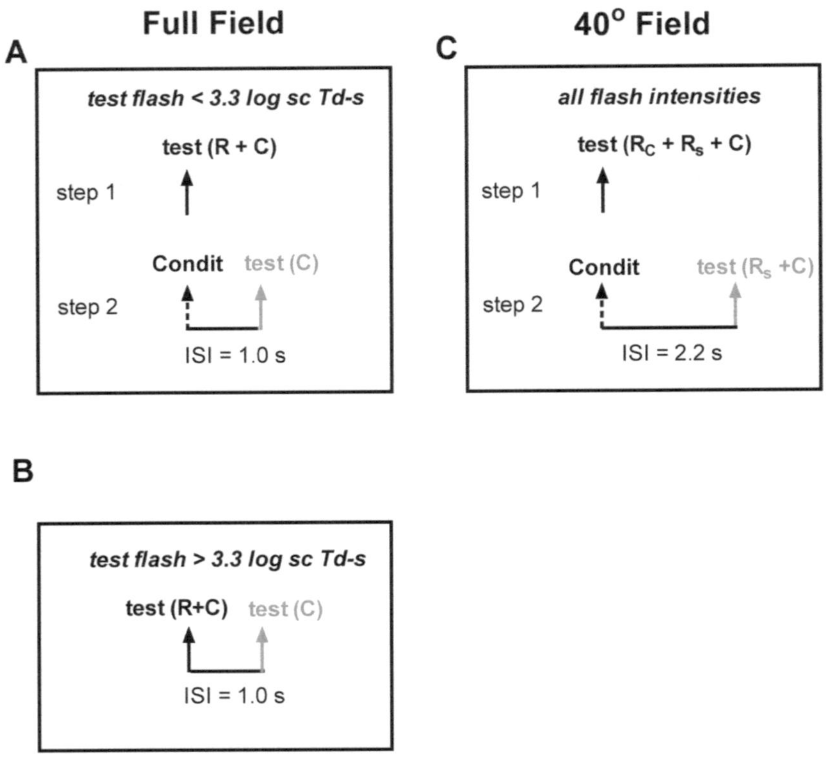

Fig. 2. Graphical representation of stimuli timing for rod phototransduction.**A.** Derivation of full-field rod-isolated ERG a-wave requires two steps for test flash intensities < 3.3 log sc Td-s. Isolated test flashes (step 1) contain both rod and cone (R+C) contributions. Step 2: The interstimulus interval (ISI) between the conditioning flash (3.3 log sc Td-s) and test flash was set to 1.0 sec. With this ISI, the ERG to the test flash contains only cone contributions. **B.** For test flash intensities above 3.3 log sc Td-s, ERGs are recorded to identical flashes separated by an ISI of 1.0 sec. **C.** Step 1: the test flashes presented in isolation in a 40° field centered on the macula contain rod and cone contributions from the central retina (R_c + C_c) and from the peripheral retina (R_p + C_p). Step 2: When presented 2.2 sec after a 4.4 log sc Td-s conditioning flash, ERG recorded to the test flashes contain central and peripheral cone contributions and peripheral rod contributions (see main text).

In the second recording step, the same test flash intensities from step 1 are each presented 2.2 sec after a 4.4 log sc Td-s conditioning flash (Figure 1C) that saturates central rods for >2.4 sec (Jeffrey et al., 2002; Jeffrey, & Neuringer 2009). Cones recover in less than 0.4 sec to this conditioning flash intensity (unpublished data). The intensity of the scattered light is estimated to be 1.5 - 2.0 log units dimmer than the conditioning flash, i.e. scattered light intensity in the peripheral retina ranges from 2.4 - 2.9 log sc Td-s (Nusinowitz et al., 1995). At theses flash intensities, rods achieve greater than 90% recovery 2.2 sec after a flash (Jeffrey, & Neuringer 2009). Therefore, ERGs recorded to the test flash presented 2.2 sec after a conditioning flash, do not contain any rod responses from the central retina. However, by 2.2 sec, the central cones and peripheral photoreceptor responses will have fully recovered.

Thus, the ERG response to a test flash presented 2.2 sec after the conditioning flash (Figure 1D) will be:

$$ERG_{test} = Cones_{central} + Rods_{peripheral} + Cones_{perpipheral} \qquad (2\,b)$$

The final step to isolating the rod ERG a-wave from the central 40 degree is to subtract the ERGs recorded in step 2 (eqn 2b) from the total ERG response recorded to the same flash intensities in step 1 (eqn 2a). i.e.

$$Rods_{central} = ERG_{total} - ERG_{test} \qquad (2c)$$

Figure 1F shows the rod-isolated ERG a-waves from a 40 degree field centered on the macula of a 27 year old monkey.

For the restricted field ERG, the P3 model was fit to the leading edges of the ERG a-waves for retinal illuminances from 3.5 to 4.8 log sc Td-s. The range of retinal illuminances for the restricted field analysis, which was higher than the intensity range used for the full-field, was necessary due to the lower sensitivity obtained from the rods in the central visual field (see section 2.7 below).

2.7 Results: full- and restricted-field phototransduction

We examined whether rod phototransduction was altered in eight Japanese macaques that either had no or only mild central drusen (n=4; mean age ± SE = 11.8 ± 2.3 years) or severe drusen (n=4; mean age ± SE = 16.3 ± 4.1 years). Rod phototransduction parameters were compared using a 2-way ANOVA for the main effects of drusen and field size. There were

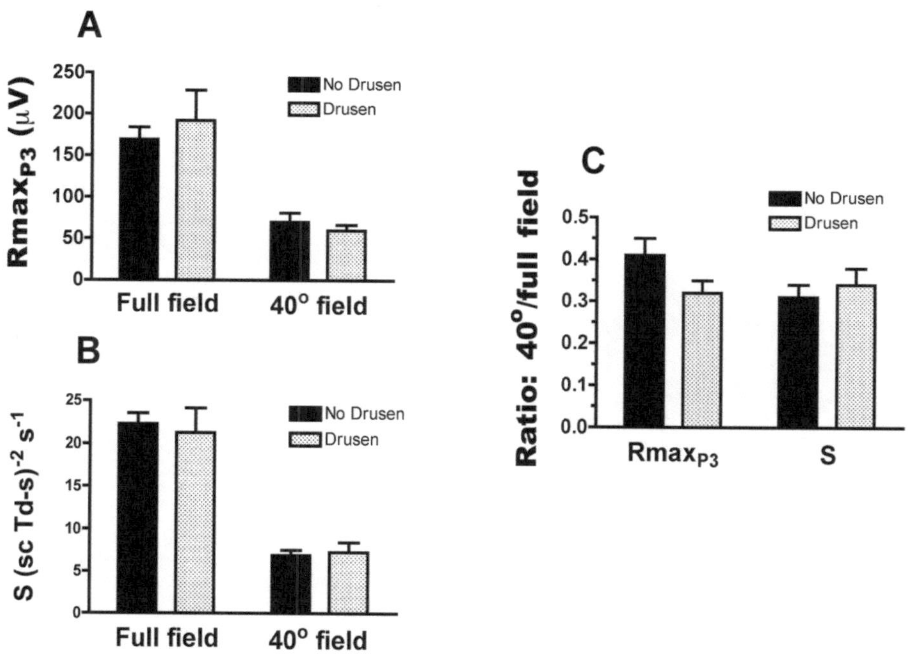

Fig. 3. Mean phototransduction parameters by drusen group. Mean rod maximal responses, $Rmax_{P3}$ (**A**) and sensitivities S (**B**) for drusen and no drusen monkeys for both full- and 40°-fields. **C**. Ratio of 40° to full field values for $Rmax_{P3}$ and S.

no significant differences between drusen and no drusen monkeys for the absolute values of maximal rod response, $Rmax_{P3}$ (Figure 3A) nor for rod sensitivity, S (Figure 3B). For both $Rmax_{P3}$ and S, there was a significant effect of field size ($p<0.0001$). For all monkeys combined, $Rmax_{P3}$ from the central 40 degree field (mean ± SE = -65.4 ± 6.7 μV) was reduced by 63 % in comparison with the mean full field value (-178.6 ± 16.7 μV). Similarly rod sensitivity from the central retina (7.1 ± 0.6 $[sc\ Td\text{-}s]^{-1}\ s^{-2}$) was reduced 68 % compared with full field values (21.8 ± 1.3 $[sc\ Td\text{-}s]^{-1}\ s^{-2}$) . Overall monkeys with severe drusen had greater variability for both full- and restricted field values of $Rmax_{P3}$ and S (Figures 3A & B).

While absolute values of rod phototransduction were not different between drusen and no drusen monkeys, we wanted to examine whether there may be selective loss of central rod function in monkeys with drusen. To this end, we calculated the ratio of the 40 deg to full field values for each of the rod phototransduction parameters. Calculating this ratio negates the inherent variability in absolute amplitude measures, and enables the central retina to be normalized with respect to the whole retina for each animal. Figure 3C shows a trend for a reduction in the 40°/full field ratio of $Rmax_{P3}$ from the drusen monkeys, although the difference did not reach significance ($p=0.13$). This reduction in the 40°/full field $Rmax_{P3}$ ratio suggests a selective loss of central rod function in drusen monkeys compared with the no drusen monkeys. There was no difference in the 40°/full field S ratio between the drusen and no drusen groups (Figure 3C).

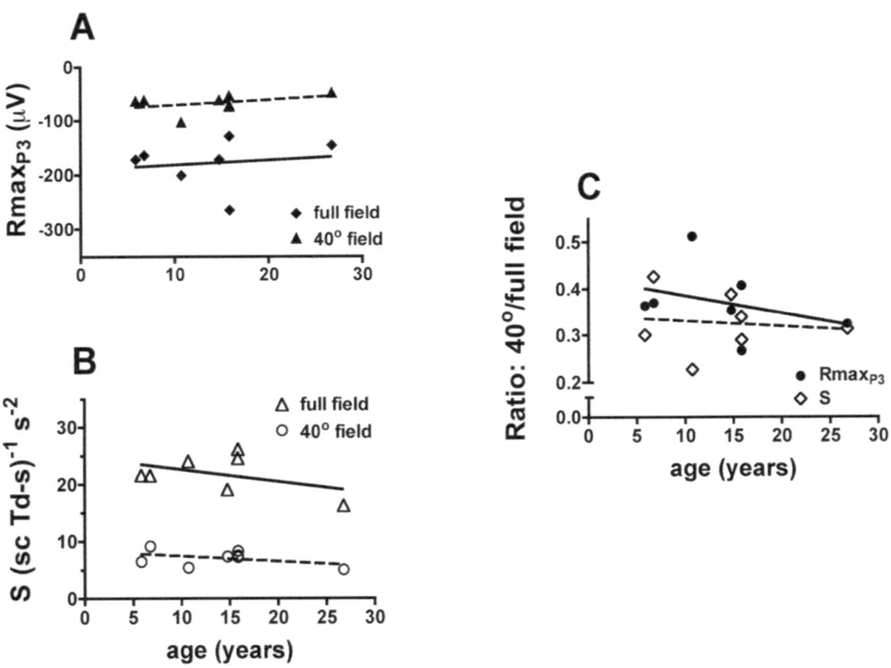

Fig. 4. Variation in phototransduction parameters with age.Rod maximal amplitude, $Rmax_{P3}$ (**A**) and rod sensitivity S (**B**) plotted as a function of age for both full- and 40°-fields. Solid lines: 40° field, dashed lines: full field. **C**. Ratio of 40° to full field values for $Rmax_{P3}$ and S plotted as a function of age. Solid line: $Rmax_{P3}$, dashed line: S.

We also examined the effect of age on rod phototransduction parameters. There were general trends for inverse relationships between both $Rmax_{P3}$ (Figure 4A) and S (Figure 4B) with age. Note that since $Rmax_{P3}$ is plotted as a negative voltage, an inverse relationship for amplitude (Figure 4A) will be in the opposite direction to the same relationship for S (Figure 4B). Figure 4C shows the plots of 40°/full field ratios for $Rmax_{P3}$, and S as a function of age. The negative slope of the 40°/full field $Rmax_{P3}$ ratio with age (Figure 4C; solid symbols, solid line) suggests a selective loss of central rod function with increasing age in these Japanese macaques.

2.8 Dark adaptation: ERG recording methods and analysis

The left column of Figure 5 outlines the paired flash protocol used to quantify the kinetics of dark adaptation as measured from the recovery of rod-isolated ERG a-wave amplitude following a bleach. In order to bleach greater than 99% of all retinal pigment, one eye of the monkey was exposed to a yellow background with retinal illuminance of 15 000 cd/m^2 for two minutes (Thomas, & Lamb 1999). To obtain the background intensity necessary for a full bleach, we built a six cm mini-ganzfeld that was connected to an incandescent light

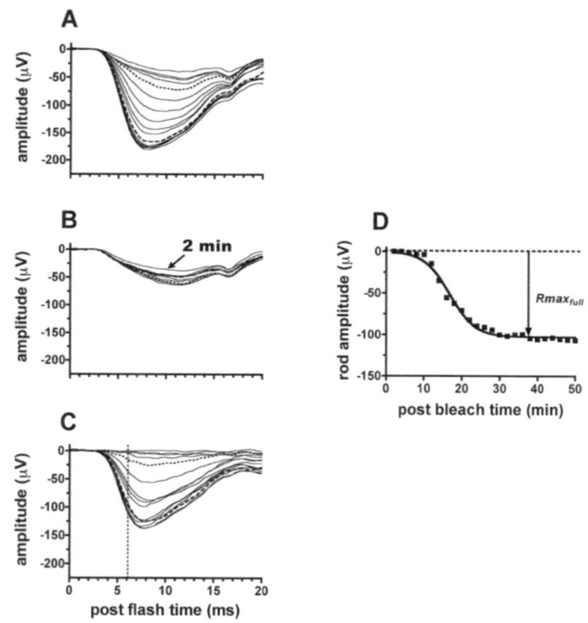

Fig. 5. Derivation of full-field dark adaptation. **A.** Recovery of ERG a-wave amplitude to a 4.4 log sc Td-s flash over a 50 minute period following a >99% bleach. All ERG's recorded over the first 20 min are shown; at longer post-bleach times, every other ERG recorded (i.e. 4 min separation) is shown. Responses at 10 and 24 min post-bleach are indicated by the dotted and dashed lines respectively. All ERGs contain mixed rod and cone contributions. **B.** Cone isolated ERG a-waves to an identical flash (4.4 log sc Td-s) for the same post bleach times shown in A. **C.** Full-field rod-isolated ERG a-waves obtained by subtracting the cone responses in B from the mixed rod/cone responses in A. Vertical dotted line indicates the time (6 ms post flash) at which rod ERG a-wave amplitude was measured. **D.** Rod isolated ERG a-wave amplitude plotted as a function of time post bleach. The solid line, shows the plot of equation 3. For this 27 year old monkey, $Rmax_{P3}$ = -103 μV, c_a = 146, τ_{DA} = 3.4 min.

source through a filter box via two fiber optic cables. Following the full bleach, scotopic full-field ERGs were recorded to paired identical flashes (4.4 log sc Td-s flash, ISI = 1.0 sec) every two minutes for 50 minutes. The technique for isolating the rod ERG a-wave is essentially identical to the method used above (Section 2.4) for assessing full field rod phototransduction. Figure 5A shows the mixed rod/cone ERG responses recorded to the first flash and Figure 5B corresponding cone isolated responses obtained from the second flash of the pair. Rod isolated ERG a-waves (Figure 5C) were then obtained by subtracting a dark-adapted cone-isolated ERGs (Figure 5B) from the mixed rod/cone responses (Figure 5A). Rod ERG a-wave amplitude was measured at 6 millisecond post flash (Figure 5C: vertical dotted line) to avoid contamination by post-receptoral components that may be present at the a-wave peak (Robson et al., 2003). Figure 5D shows the recovery of rod-isolated full-field rod ERG a-wave amplitude plotted as a function of post-bleach time. The recovery of ERG a-wave amplitude was well described by the following equation (Thomas, & Lamb 1999):

$$Rmax(T) = Rmax()/[\,1 + c_a \bullet \exp(-T/\tau_{DA})] \qquad (3)$$

where Rmax(T) is the ERG a-wave amplitude (μV) at post-bleach time T (min) and Rmax() = ERG a-wave amplitude (μV) in the fully dark adapted retina. Derived parameters were c_a (no units) which describes the degree of reduction immediately after a bleach, and τ_{DA} (minutes) is the time constant of recovery of ERG a-wave amplitude.

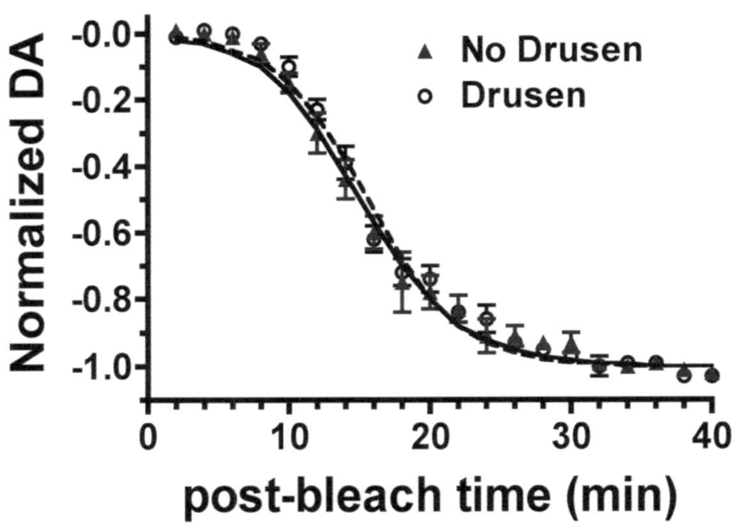

Fig. 6. Mean normalized dark adaptation by drusen group. Plot of mean normalized dark adaptation for the no drusen (solid squares) and drusen (open circles) monkeys plotted as a function of time. Solid and dashed lines show the mean fits of (eqn 3) for the no drusen and drusen groups, respectively.

Figure 5D shows that rod recovery began around 10 minutes post bleach and was almost complete by 24 minutes. The ERG responses at 10 and 24 minutes post-bleach are indicated by the dotted and dashed lines respectively in Figures 5 A-C. The cone response recorded 2

minutes post bleach (Figure 5B) was consistently smaller than all remaining cone ERGs. This was true for all monkeys in this study and indicates that cone recovery following a full bleach takes up to four minutes, similar to that reported for the human (Mahroo, & Lamb 2004) .
Figure 6 shows kinetics of dark adaptation were not different between the drusen and no drusen monkeys. For all monkeys combined, the time constant of dark adaptation was 3.1 ± 0.1 minutes (mean ± SE) and ERG a-wave amplitude had reached >97% of the full dark-adapted value within 28 minutes after a full bleach. These results in the Japanese macaque are similar to those obtained for humans using a similar ERG protocol (Thomas, & Lamb 1999).

3. Conclusion

In a unique colony of Japanese macaques at the Oregon National Primate Research Center we identified a distinct retinal disease characterized by dominant inheritance and the early onset of pan-retinal drusen syndrome (Neuringer M, et al. IOVS 2011;52:ARVO E-Abstract 4008). Although only a small number of these animals were available for functional testing, the ERG data presented in this report point to changes in the function of the central rods of these monkeys. The reduction in the 40°/full field ratio for $Rmax_{P3}$ in the drusen monkeys suggests that the drusen in these animals is associated with selective changes in their central rod function. An alternative interpretation would be that selective loss of central $Rmax_{P3}$ may purely be a function of age based on the observed inverse correlation of 40°/full field $Rmax_{P3}$ ratio with age, which was independent of drusen status. Monkeys in the drusen group were older (mean ± SE) at 16.3 ± 4.1 years than the no-drusen monkeys at 11.8 ± 2.3 years, although the difference did not reach significance. Regardless of the cause (drusen/age), the reduction in the 40°/full field ratio for $Rmax_{P3}$ strongly suggests selective dysfunction or loss of rods from central retina of these Japanese macaques. Given these two results, a larger study will be required to determine if drusen status and/or age account for the loss of rod response from the central retina of this unique group of macaques.
Apart from drusen, these animals have no other overt signs of retinal disease. Therefore, the results presented in this study highlight that restricted field ERG measure of phototransduction may provide an objective and robust means to detect early pre-clinical signs of retinal dysfunction prior to the presence of more advances stages of age-related retinal disease.
This group of Japanese macaques with early onset dominantly inherited drusen adds to and complements other large scale studies in cynomologus and rhesus macaques that have reported drusen, with similar phenotype and genotypic characteristics to those observed with human drusen/early AMD. These non-human primate models of early AMD will prove invaluable as a resource for studying both the molecular and genetic mechanisms associated with the development of early AMD. In addition non-human primate models, especially those with early onset drusen, will likely provide an invaluable resource for preclinical testing of AMD therapies. Although rodent models can provide information regarding some of the processes underlying macular degeneration in AMD, non-human primates are the only animals with a retina essentially identical to that of the human. Only monkeys, apes and humans have nearly identical retinal structure including the presence of a macula and a foveal pit with high cone density and adjacent peak RPE cell density. Lastly, rodents do not accumulate significant xanthophylls in the retina, whereas a defining characteristic of the primate macula is the presence of the xanthophylls lutein and zeaxanthin.

4. Acknowledgment

Funded in part by American Health Assistance Foundation's Macular Degeneration Research Program; The Foundation Fighting Blindness, Research to Prevent Blindness and National Institutes of Health grant RR00163. We thank David Birch PhD (Retina Foundation of the Southwest, Dallas Tx) for the Matlab routines used for fitting the P3 model to the ERG a-waves for assessment of rod phototransduction. We thank Lauren Renner BSc for assistance with ERG recording and animal care.

5. References

Berrow, E.J., Bartlett, H.E., Eperjesi, F. & Gibson, J.M., 2010, The electroretinogram: a useful tool for evaluating age-related macular disease? *Documenta ophthalmologica. Advances in ophthalmology*, 121(1), pp. 51-62.

Binns, A. & Margrain, T.H., 2006, Development of a technique for recording the focal rod ERG, *Ophthalmic & physiological optics* 26(1), pp. 71-9.

Binns, A.M. & Margrain, T.H., 2007, Evaluating retinal function in age-related maculopathy with the ERG photostress test, *Investigative ophthalmology & visual science*, 48(6), pp. 2806-13.

Birch, D.G. & Hood, D.C. 1995, Abnormal rod photoreceptor function in Retinitis Pigmentosa, in RE Anderson (ed), *Degenerative diseases of the Retina*, Plenum Press, New York, pp. 359-69.

Birch, D.G., Hood, D.C., Nusinowitz, S. & Pepperberg, D.R., 1995, Abnormal activation and inactivation mechanisms of rod transduction in patients with autosomal dominant retinitis pigmentosa and the pro-23-his mutation, *Investigative Ophthalmology and Visual Science*, 36(8), pp. 1603-14.

Bonilha, V.L., 2008, Age and disease-related structural changes in the retinal pigment epithelium, *Clinical ophthalmology* , 2(2), pp. 413-24.

Breton, M.E., Schueller, A.W., Lamb, T.D., Pugh, E.N. & Jr., 1994, Analysis of ERG a-wave amplification and kinetics in terms of the G-protein cascade of phototransduction, *Investigative Ophthalmology and Visual Science*, 35(1), pp. 295-309.

Choshi, T., Matsumoto, C.S. & Nakatsuka, K., 2003, Rod-driven focal macular electroretinogram, *Japanese journal of ophthalmology*, 47(4), pp. 356-61.

Curcio, C.A., Medeiros, N.E. & Millican, C.L., 1996, Photoreceptor loss in age-related macular degeneration, *Investigative ophthalmology & visual science*, 37(7), pp. 1236-49.

Curcio, C.A., Millican, C.L., Allen, K.A. & Kalina, R.E., 1993, Aging of the human photoreceptor mosaic: evidence for selective vulnerability of rods in central retina, *Investigative ophthalmology & visual science*, 34(12), pp. 3278-96.

Curcio, C.A., Owsley, C. & Jackson, G.R., 2000, Spare the rods, save the cones in aging and age-related maculopathy, *Investigative ophthalmology & visual science*, 41(8), pp. 2015-8.

Curcio, C.A., Sloan, K.R., Kalina, R.E. & Hendrickson, A.E., 1990, Human photoreceptor topography, *Journal of Comparative Neurology*, 292(4), pp. 497-523.

Dawson, W.W., Dawson, J.C., Lake, K.P. & Gonzalez-Martinez, J., 2008, Maculas, monkeys, models, AMD and aging, *Vision research*, 48(3), pp. 360-5.

Eisner, A., Klein, M.L., Zilis, J.D. & Watkins, M.D., 1992, Visual function and the subsequent development of exudative age-related macular degeneration, *Investigative ophthalmology & visual science*, 33(11), pp. 3091-102.

Falsini, B., Serrao, S., Fadda, A., Iarossi, G., Porrello, G., Cocco, F. & Merendino, E., 1999, Focal electroretinograms and fundus appearance in nonexudative age-related macular degeneration. Quantitative relationship between retinal morphology and function, *Graefe's archive for clinical and experimental ophthalmology*, 237(3), pp. 193-200.

Francis, P.J., Appukuttan, B., Simmons, E., Landauer, N., Stoddard, J., Hamon, S., Ott, J., Ferguson, B., Klein, M., Stout, J.T. & Neuringer, M., 2008, Rhesus monkeys and humans share common susceptibility genes for age-related macular disease, *Human molecular genetics*, 17(17), pp. 2673-80.

Gao, H. & Hollyfield, J.G., 1992, Aging of the human retina. Differential loss of neurons and retinal pigment epithelial cells, *Investigative ophthalmology & visual science*, 33(1), pp. 1-17.

Gerth, C., 2009, The role of the ERG in the diagnosis and treatment of Age-Related Macular Degeneration, *Documenta ophthalmologica. Advances in ophthalmology*, 118(1), pp. 63-8.

Gouras, P., Ivert, L., Mattison, J.A., Ingram, D.K. & Neuringer, M., 2008, Drusenoid maculopathy in rhesus monkeys: autofluorescence, lipofuscin and drusen pathogenesis, *Graefe's archive for clinical and experimental ophthalmology*, 246(10), pp. 1403-11.

Haegerstrom-Portnoy, G., 2005, The Glenn A. Fry Award Lecture 2003: Vision in elders--summary of findings of the SKI study, *Optometry and vision science* , 82(2), pp. 87-93.

Haimovici, R., Owens, S.L., Fitzke, F.W. & Bird, A.C., 2002, Dark adaptation in age-related macular degeneration: relationship to the fellow eye, *Graefe's archive for clinical and experimental ophthalmology*, 240(2), pp. 90-5.

Hogg, R.E. & Chakravarthy, U., 2006, Visual function and dysfunction in early and late age-related maculopathy, *Progress in retinal and eye research*, 25(3), pp. 249-76.

Holder, G.E., 2001, Pattern electroretinography (PERG) and an integrated approach to visual pathway diagnosis, *Progress in retinal and eye research*, 20(4), pp. 531-61.

Hood, D.C., Wladis, E.J., Shady, S., Holopigian, K., Li, J. & Seiple, W., 1998, Multifocal rod electroretinograms, *Investigative ophthalmology & visual science*, 39(7), pp. 1152-62.

Hope, G.M., Dawson, W.W., Engel, H.M., Ulshafer, R.J., Kessler, M.J. & Sherwood, M.B., 1992, A primate model for age related macular drusen, *The British journal of ophthalmology*, 76(1), pp. 11-6.

Jackson, G.R., McGwin, G., Phillips, J.M., Klein, R. & Owsley, C., 2006, Impact of aging and age-related maculopathy on inactivation of the a-wave of the rod-mediated electroretinogram, *Vision research*, 46(8-9), pp. 1422-31.

Jackson, G.R., Owsley, C. & Curcio, C.A., 2002, Photoreceptor degeneration and dysfunction in aging and age-related maculopathy, *Ageing research reviews*, 1(3), pp. 381-96.

Jackson, G.R., Owsley, C. & McGwin, G., 1999, Aging and dark adaptation, *Vision research*, 39(23), pp. 3975-82.

Jeffrey, B.G. & Neuringer, M., 2009, Age-Related Decline in Rod Phototransduction Sensitivity in Rhesus Monkeys Fed an n-3 Fatty Acid Deficient Diet, *Investigative ophthalmology & visual science*, 50(9), pp. 4360-7.

Jeffrey, B.G., Mitchell, D.C., Gibson, R.A. & Neuringer, M., 2002, n-3 fatty acid deficiency alters recovery of the rod photoresponse in rhesus monkeys, *Investigative ophthalmology & visual science*, 43(8), pp. 2806-14.

Lamb, T.D., Pugh, E.N. & Jr., 1992, A quantitative account of the activation steps involved in phototransduction in amphibian photoreceptors, *Journal of Physiology (Lond)*, 449, pp. 719-58.

Mahroo, O.A. & Lamb, T.D., 2004, Recovery of the human photopic electroretinogram after bleaching exposures: estimation of pigment regeneration kinetics, *The Journal of physiology*, 554(Pt 2), pp. 417-37.

Morrison, J.D. & McGrath, C., 1985, Assessment of the optical contributions to the age-related deterioration in vision, *Quarterly journal of experimental physiology*, 70(2), pp. 249-69.

Neelam, K., Nolan, J., Chakravarthy, U. & Beatty, S., 2009, Psychophysical function in age-related maculopathy, *Survey of ophthalmology*, 54(2), pp. 167-210.

Nusinowitz, S., Hood, D.C. & Birch, D.G., 1995, Rod transduction parameters from the a wave of local receptor populations, *Journal Optical Society America A*, 12(10), pp. 2259-66.

Owsley, C., Jackson, G.R., White, M., Feist, R. & Edwards, D., 2001, Delays in rod-mediated dark adaptation in early age-related maculopathy, *Ophthalmology*, 108(7), pp. 1196-202.

Packer, O., Hendrickson, A.E. & Curcio, C.A., 1989, Photoreceptor topography of the retina in the adult pigtail macaque (Macaca nemestrina), *Journal of Comparative Neurology*, 288(1), pp. 165-83.

Phipps, J.A., Guymer, R.H. & Vingrys, A.J., 2003, Loss of cone function in age-related maculopathy, *Investigative ophthalmology & visual science*, 44(5), pp. 2277-83.

Robson, J.G., Saszik, S.M., Ahmed, J. & Frishman, L.J., 2003, Rod and cone contributions to the a-wave of the electroretinogram of the macaque, *The Journal of physiology*, 547(Pt 2), pp. 509-30.

Sandberg, M.A., Pawlyk, B.S. & Berson, E.L., 1996, Isolation of focal rod electroretinograms from the dark-adapted human eye, *Investigative ophthalmology & visual science*, 37(5), pp. 930-4.

Shelley, E.J., Madigan, M.C., Natoli, R., Penfold, P.L. & Provis, J.M., 2009, Cone degeneration in aging and age-related macular degeneration, *Archives of ophthalmology*, 127(4), pp. 483-92.

Singh, K.K., Krawczak, M., Dawson, W.W. & Schmidtke, J., 2009, Association of HTRA1 and ARMS2 gene variation with drusen formation in rhesus macaques, *Experimental eye research*, 88(3), pp. 479-82.

Snodderly, D.M., Auran, J.D. & Delori, F.C., 1984, The macular pigment. II. Spatial distribution in primate retinas, *Investigative ophthalmology & visual science*, 25(6), pp. 674-85.

Spear, P.D., 1993, Neural bases of visual deficits during aging, *Vision research*, 33(18), pp. 2589-609.

Thomas, M.M. & Lamb, T., 1999, Light adaptation and dark adaptation of human rod photoreceptors measured from the a-wave of the human electroretinogram, *Journal of Physiology*, 518, pp. 479-96.

Umeda, S., Ayyagari, R., Suzuki, M.T., Ono, F., Iwata, F., Fujiki, K., Kanai, A., Takada, Y., Yoshikawa, Y., Tanaka, Y. & Iwata, T., 2003, Molecular cloning of ELOVL4 gene from cynomolgus monkey (Macaca fascicularis), *Experimental animals / Japanese Association for Laboratory Animal Science*, 52(2), pp. 129-35.

Umeda S, Ayyagari R, Allikmets R, Suzuki MT, Karoukis AJ, Ambasudhan R, Zernant J, Okamoto, H., Ono, F., Terao, Mizota, A Yoshikawa Y, Tanaka Y Iwata, T. K., 2005a Early-onset macular degeneration with drusen in a cynomolgus monkey (Macaca fascicularis) pedigree: exclusion of 13 candidate genes and loci. *Investigative ophthalmology & visual science* 46, pp. 683-691.

Umeda, S., Suzuki, M.T., Okamoto, H., Ono, F., Mizota, A., Terao, K., Yoshikawa, Y., Tanaka, Y. & Iwata, T., 2005b, Molecular composition of drusen and possible involvement of anti-retinal autoimmunity in two different forms of macular degeneration in cynomolgus monkey (Macaca fascicularis), *The FASEB journal*, 19(12), pp. 1683-5.

Wang, Y.-Z., 2001, Effects of aging on shape discrimination, *Optometry & Vision Science*, 78(6), pp. 447-54.

Wikler, K.C., Williams, R.W. & Rakic, P., 1990, Photoreceptor mosaic: number and distribution of rods and cones in the rhesus monkey retina, *Journal of Comparative Neurology*, 297(4), pp. 499-508.

Wyszecki, G. & Stiles, W.S., 1982, *Color Science: Concepts and methods, quantitative data and formulae,* 2nd ed. John Wiley & Sons, New York.

12

ERG in *Drosophila*

Gregor Belušič
University of Ljubljana, Biotechnical faculty
Slovenia

1. Introduction

The fruitfly *Drosophila melanogaster* has been a workhorse of genetics for over a hundred years, following the first report of a white-eyed mutant by T.H. Morgan (Morgan, 1910). Since then, systematic mutagenesis and subsequently, more sophisticated methods of genetic modifications have been implemented to isolate strains with specific defects in various proteins (Ashburner et al., 2005; Greenspan et al., 2004). Finally, the newly developed techniques enabled the researchers to mark, activate or silence specific cells or cell lines (Hampel et al., 2011; Gohl et al., 2011). Genetic modification and elimination of eye-specific proteins have led to fundamental discoveries in the visual pathway and the deciphering of the mechanisms of phototransduction in great detail (Pak, 2011). The prominent compound eyes of *Drosophila* have allowed for an easy selection of the visual mutants on the basis of the eye color, external eye morphology, presence of the deep pseudopupil, phototaxis, and the time course and the amplitude of ERG (Pak, 1995). *Drosophila* ERG is an excellent method for physiological evaluation of genetically induced protein modifications. It is a particularly robust and technically feasible technique which can yield high throughput and reproducible results. The limitations of ERG have become very obvious in the last 20 years due to the development of the whole-cell patch-clamp in isolated ommatidia (Ranganathan et al., 1991; Hardie, 1991) and the advanced application of sharp intracellular electrodes (Juusola and Hardie, 2001). However, ERG in *Drosophila* is an informative and well understood signal. It remains the method of choice in many studies, especially when the molecular genetic tools are extensively applied to studying cellular processes in the photoreceptor model, and when the phenotypes of numerous transgenic fruitfly strains need to be physiologically characterised in a reasonable time.

2. The visual system of *Drosophila*

The visual system of *Drosophila* consists of the three ocelli, the compound eyes and the visual ganglia - the lamina, the medulla, the lobula and the lobula plate. The retina of a compound eye contains ca. 800 ommatidia. Each ommatidium is a cluster of eight photoreceptor cells, supporting cells and pigment cells. The pigment cells contain the red screening pigment which optically isolates the ommatidia. The photoreceptor cells contain an additional, yellow screening pigment which translocates transversely in the photoreceptor soma thus conveying a pupillary response . The yellow and the red screening pigments are absent in commonly used white-eyed mutants.

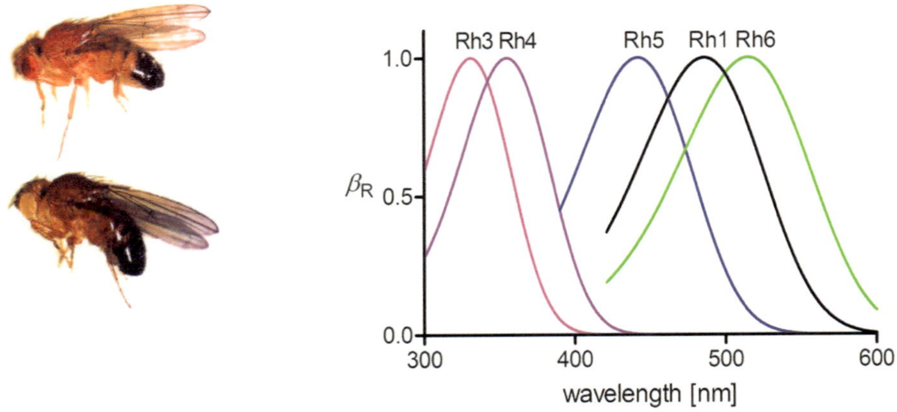

Fig. 1. Left, red and white eyed *Drosophila*. Right, relative absorbance of the five rhodopsins expressed in peripheral photoreceptors (R1-6: Rh1) and in the central photoreceptors (R7y: Rh4; R7p: Rh3; R8y: Rh6; R8p: Rh5). Shown are only the α-bands; Rh1, Rh5 and Rh6 have an additional β-band in the UV (peak height ca. 20% of the α-band peak).

Photoreceptor cells have three morphologically distinct regions: the light sensing *rhabdomere*, the *soma* with the nucleus, endoplasmic reticulum (ER), the mitochondria and other organelles, and the *axon*. The soma and the axon are sometimes referred to as the light-insensitive *basal membrane*, i.e. the membrane portion which is equipped with voltage gated (mostly K^+) channels, which dynamically shape the light response. This is not to be confused with the *basement membrane* (sometimes also the *basal lamina*), an extracellular structure separating the photoreceptor bodies from the higher order neurons in the *lamina*, an optical neuropil.

The light-sensitive part of the photoreceptor cell - the rhabdomere - is composed of ~30.000 microvilli, each 1-2 μm long and 60 nm wide. The microvillus harbours all the molecules that are necessary for the transduction of a successfully captured photon of light to a *quantum bump* – the unitary depolarization of the photoreceptor cell membrane. The microvillar membrane is packed with about 1000 visual pigment (rhodopsin) molecules, making the rhabdomere optically dense and behave as a light guide. The rhabdomeres of an ommatidium together form an open rhabdom. The rhabdomeres of the six outer photoreceptor cells R1-6 function as separate optical waveguides, which surround a central waveguide formed by the superimposed rhabdomeres of the central photoreceptors R7 (positioned distally in the ommatidium) and R8 (positioned proximally). The receptors R1-6 form an achromatic channel for detection of light contrasts and motion, while R7 and R8 receptors mediate colour vision. The R1-6 contain the Rh1 rhodopsin, which absorbs maximally in the blue, at 486 nm, and the R7&8 cells express the rhodopsins Rh3-6, maximally absorbing at 331, 355, 442 and 515 nm; the UV-sensitive rhodopsin Rh2 is expressed in the ocelli (Salcedo et al., 1999). The rhodopsin content in the eyes depends on the amount of carotenoid precursors in the food. Elimination of carotenoids from the feeding media can result in dramatic reduction of rhodopsin in the eyes (Goldsmith et al., 1964; Harris et al., 1977). On the other hand, a carotenoid enriched diet results in high sensitivity of R1-6 cells in the UV, due to the incorporation of an additional chromophore in the opsin molecule which acts as an antenna pigment molecule (Kirschfeld et al., 1983). Maximised rhodopsin content, as well as structural integrity of photoreceptors, can be easily checked by observing the clarity of the deep pseudopupil (optical superposition of rhabdomere images or shadows in the geometrical centre of the eye). Optically, the compound eyes of *Drosophila* are of the apposition type. However, different R1-6 cells in six adjacent ommatidia are arranged so that their visual axes are pointing to the same direction, and their axons project to a common neuron in the lamina. Such information integration, which improves the image quality in dim light, is typical of the higher dipteran insects and is named neural superposition (Kirschfeld and Franceschini, 1968). The central R7 and R8 receptor axons bypass the lamina and form chemical synapses in the medulla (Cajal and Sanchez, 1915; Fischbach and Dittrich, 1989).

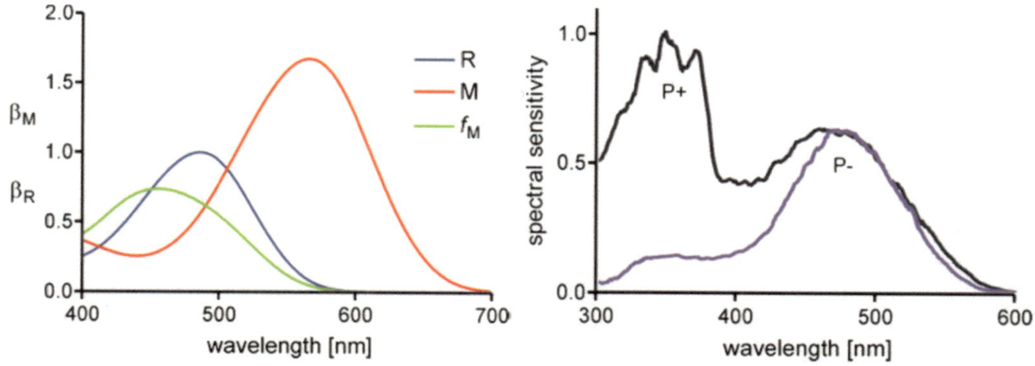

Fig. 2. Left, Spectral properties of the main visual pigment, Rh1, of *Drosophila*. The photosensitivities (β) of the two thermostable states, rhodopsin (R) and metarhodopsin (M), normalized to the rhodopsin peak, and the metarhodopsin fraction f_M in the photoequilibrium created by monochromatic stimuli with wavelenght λ. The spectra were calculated with the template functions of Govardovskii et al. (2000) using peak wavelength values 486 and 566 nm for R and M, respectively. Right, Spectral sensitivities measured via ERG of white-eyed *Drosophila* bred on a carotenoid-rich (P+) and carotenoid-deprived (P-) medium. The spectral sensitivity in P- exhibits the β-peak due to absorption by Rh1 in the UV, while the P+ has an much higher sensitivity in the UV with a fine vibronic structure (triple peaks) due to the incorporation of an additional chromophore into the Rh1 molecule.

Fruitflies are able to detect light photons at wavelengths between 300 nm and 650 nm. Upon photon absorption, their rhodopsins (R) are converted to a thermostabile metarhodopsin (M) isoform. In the case of Rh1, the absorbance peak of M is shifted to longer wavelengths (bathochromic shift) and the absorbance amplitude is higher by a factor of 1.6 (Ostroy et al., 1974; Salcedo et al. 1999). A M molecule can be converted back to R by another photon. The conversion of M to R is facilitated by the leaking of red stray light through the long-pass filtering red screening pigments (Stavenga et al., 1973; Stavenga, 2002). After a sufficient period of time, a photoequilibrium between M and R is created which depends on the spectral composition of the illumination. Short-wavelength monochromatic light can create large amounts of M. M, which triggers phototransduction (Hardie and Raghu, 2001), is quenched by the binding of arrestin. Rhodopsin to arrestin ratio has been estimated as 2.7:1 (Satoh et al., 2010). Thus, high fraction of M can out-titrate the available arrestin (Minke et al., 1975; Hamdorf, 1979; Dolph et al., 1993; Belušič et al., 2010; Satoh et al., 2010). In the white-eyed mutants illuminated with conventional light sources, the photoequilibrium with high metarhodopsin fraction (f_M) can be established within seconds. Thus, a state of maximal receptor depolarization and absolute desensitisation is created, which can persist for many hours in the dark. This phenomenon is called the PDA, prolonged depolarizing afterpotential. A PDA can be abolished with long wavelength light. Usually, the PDA is created with blue light (460-490 nm) and interrupted with orange to red light (580-640 nm). In R7 photoreceptors, PDA can be created with UV and abolished with blue light (Stark, 1977). PDA has never been observed in R8 receptors.

3. The ERG signal

3.1 Recording preparation

The ERG is measured in immobilised living fruitflies. Fruitflies (and other flies) can tolerate extended periods of anoxia without any subsequent changes in the ERG (Agam et al., 2000). Therefore, living animals can be anaestethised by exposure to gaseous CO_2 or N_2 at room temperature or by chilling on ice. Subsequently, they are mounted to a holder, (e.g. a microscope slide or pipette tip) with wax, agarose or putty. Frequently, Krönig's mixture of bees wax and resin (colophony) 3:1 is used due to its excellent adherence to the chitin and its low melting temperature. The waxing is best performed with miniature soldering devices, such as a 12 V soldering needle (Stannol, Germany), driven at 3-4 V. It is important that the animal's abdomen with the stigmata is left untreated during the immobilization procedure in order to avoid suffocation. Suffocation is first indicated by the absence of the neural transient components of the ERG, but a somewhat slowed receptor component can persist for many minutes. The ERG can be recorded in virtually intact animals, and a stable measurement is possible for many hours or even days, if sufficiently high humidity is provided in the air surrounding the animal. The signal is usually recorded with glass micropipettes filled with physiological saline - 0.9% NaCl or insect salines of different compositions, yielding a resistance of a few kΩ to a few MΩ. An ERG can be recorded also with a chlorided silver wire or salinated cotton wicks. Direct illumination of the silver wire must be avoided since a photoelectric artifact of a few mV is easily introduced. The signal is amplified unipolarly in DC mode, with the recording electrode contacting the compound eye dipped into a droplet of EKG gel, or inserted just below the cornea. The grounded reference electrode is dipped into a gel droplet or inserted in a non-illuminated part of the body. Similarly, an ERG can be also obtained from the ocelli.

3.2 Stimulus

The stimulus for obtaining an ERG is typically a simple light pulse, lasting between 10 ms and 10 s. The light source can be a DC operated halogen lamp, a xenon arc lamp, or LED. AC driven lamps and conventional fluorescent bulbs are inadequate since they contain flickering components at 50 Hz or 100 Hz which a fly eye actually perceives as flicker, resulting in oscillations of the signal. The light from the lamps is usually filtered with long-pass (OG515, OG580, Schott, Germany) or short-pass light filters (BG family of filters, Schott, Germany). Monochromators inserted between the light and the preparation can be operated between 300 and 650 nm to produce stimuli for the measurements of spectral sensitivity or for selective light adaptation of different photoreceptor classes. Superluminescent LED sources can deliver light from 300 nm on, capable of saturating any fly photoreceptor. The intensity of the stimuli is adjusted with neutral density filters or metal wedges. In order to cover the entire dynamical working range of the *Drosophila* ERG, the intensity of the light stimuli needs to be adjusted over a range of 6 orders of magnitude, in steps no larger than

0.5 log unit. LED sources can be driven with voltage operated current sources, which allow for fast changes of intensity modulation and thus provide e.g. sinusoidally modulated stimulus or white noise, spectrally flat up to 500 Hz (fast enough even for the fastest insect photoreceptors).

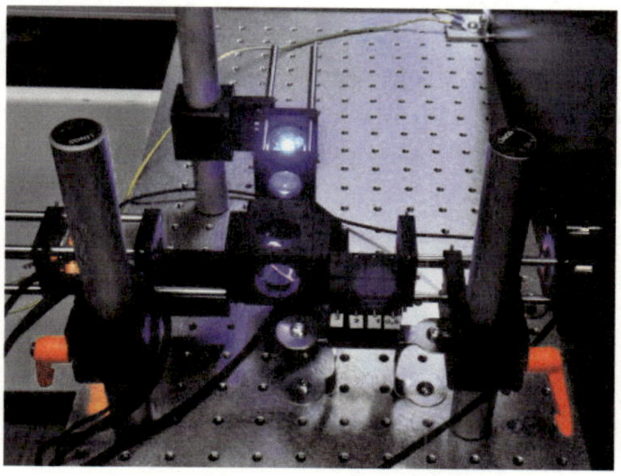

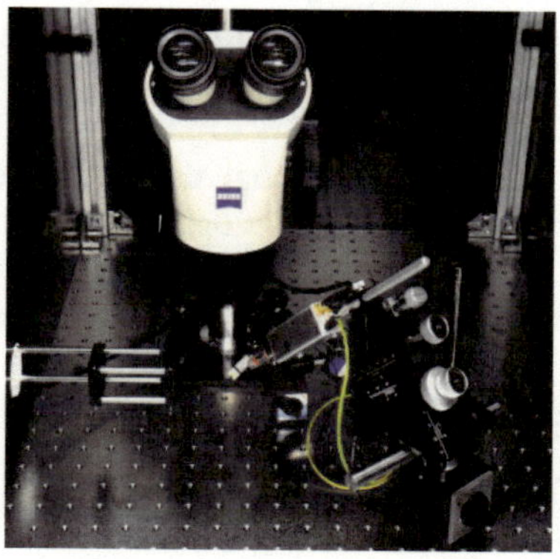

Fig. 3. A simple setup for *Drosophila* ERG, constructed by the author and dr. Olaf Voolstra. Left, Stimulator made of two superluminescent LED sources (480 nm and 580 nm, Roithner Lasertechnik, Austria), three sets of latchable neutral density filters and a 50% neutral density filter (45° inclined) as a beam mixer. Optics and mechanics by Qioptiq, Germany. Right, Faraday cage with an optical breadboard (Thorlabs, Germany), binocular (Zeiss, Germany), a micromanipulator (Märzhauser, Germany) with the recording headstage (NPI, Germany), an improvised *Drosophila* yoke made from a micropipette holder (WPI, USA), with a 50 μm diameter Ag/AgCl wire (Goodfellow, UK) attached as a reference electrode. The objective lens of the stimulus setup protrudes from the left wall of the cage. Photo: O. Voolstra, University of Hohenheim, Stuttgart, Germany.

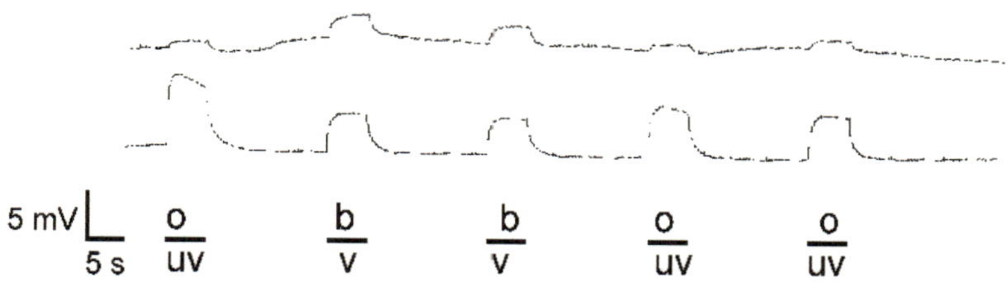

Fig. 4. The photoelectric effect. Signal in a dead animal, recorded with the Ag/AgCl wire directly illuminated with the stimulating light (stimuli corresponding to the upper trace: o - 580 nm; b - 480 nm; stimuli corresponding to the lower trace: uv – 360 nm; v – 420 nm).

3.3 Red-eyed and white-eyed fruitflies

The ERG is usually recorded in a few varieties of white-eyed *Drosophila*. White-eyed fruitflies are preferably used in biochemical experiments since the red pigment from the wild-type eyes colours the homogenates and the gels. In physiological experiments, white-eyed mutants are often preferred because they lack the pupillary response, in wild type mediated by the movement of yellow pigment granules within the photoreceptors. Moreover, uniform »ganzfeld« illumination of the entire compound eye is easily achieved in the translucent retina of white-eyed mutants. The angular sensitivity of the photoreceptors in the white-eyed mutants is extended more than tenfold (Streck, 1972), so that image formation is heavily impaired. The photoreceptor cells of the white-eyed mutants are otherwise physiologically unaffected. However, the red screening pigment in the wild-type flies has an important role as a long-pass, red filter so that illuminations with broadband light allow long wavelength photons reaching the photoreceptors. These photons convert metarhodopsin to rhodopsin so that the metarhodopsin levels in the photoreceptors are kept sufficiently low to be manageable by the limited amount of arrestin molecules. In the white-eyed fruitflies, this is not the case. Under white light, the metarhodopsin levels in white eyes can become so high that the photoreceptors remain depolarized for long periods of time. Furthermore, in physiological experiments, short wavelength light is frequently used as a stimulus. White eyed flies then must be regularly exposed to orange or red light in order to interrupt any possible prolonged depolarizations.

3.4 ERG waveform

The ERG recorded from the retina in the described configuration (DC, unipolar, measuring electrode in the retina, grounded reference in the body) is a rather complex signal, composed of several fast transient components, and several rising and decaying sustained components (Stark and Wasserman, 1972). The photoreceptors contribute a corneal-negative, slow, sustained plateau component at medium light intensities. The second-order neurons L1 and L2 in the lamina contribute fast transient »on« and »off« components, at the beginning and at the end of the stimulus (Coombe, 1986). At light intensities which elicit maximal responses, the ERG is more complex due to fast adaptation processes of the photoreceptor cells. The receptor response is further transformed at the synapse and in the lamina, resulting in additional transients in the ERG (Järvilehto and Zettler, 1971; Laughlin et al., 1987).

In order to understand the nature and origin of the ERG time course in detail, it is necessary to delineate the underlying responses of the photoreceptor cells and second order neurons. All photoreceptor cells (R1-8) respond to a simple light pulse with a sustained depolarization, occurring with a delay as short as 3 ms. This so-called receptor potential lasts as long as the stimulus. Its amplitude is proportional to the logarithm of the stimulus intensity. At high light intensities, the large depolarization of the photoreceptor at the onset of the pulse is reduced after 50-100 ms by fast adaptation mechanisms to a lower level. This results in a sharp spike at the beginning of the receptor potential. In light adapted flies, the fast adaptation is frequently followed by a damped oscillation of the receptor potential plateau. The receptor potential is detected by the ERG electrode in the extracellular space as a corneal-negative signal, with a somewhat smaller amplitude (e.g. -20 mV between the retina and the body, instead of the 40 mV of the transmembrane depolarization), and its time course resembles an inverted receptor potential. The photoreceptors R1-6 convey the receptor potential to second order neurons in the lamina, the L1 and L2. These neurons transform the receptor potential to a sequence of decaying transient components and thus seem to work analogously to the on- and off-bipolar cells in the vertebrate retina (Joesch et al., 2010). The laminar neurons act as high-pass filters with strong amplification at high frequencies, thus greatly amplifying small changes in the receptor potential (Autrum et al., 1970; Uusitalo and Weckström, 2000). The combined signal from L1 and L2 is very well detected by the ERG electrode and contributes a corneal-positive »on« transient at the beginning of the light pulse, and a corneal-negative »off« transient at the end of the pulse.

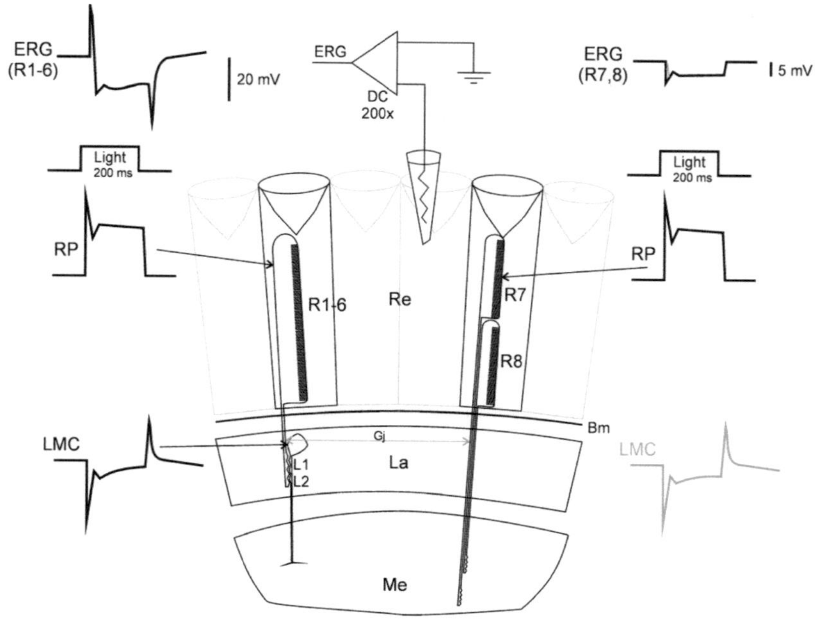

Fig. 5. Origin of the ERG waveform in the retina (Re), recorded in DC mode, unipolarly across the basement membrane (Bm). Left, the ERG from the photoreceptors R1-6, which is an extracellular summation of the inverted receptor potential (RP) from R1-6, and the inverted signal from the large monopolar cells (LMC) L1 and L2 in the lamina (La). Right, the ERG from the photoreceptors R7 and R8, which is a scaled-down, inverted receptor potential from R7 and R8. The large LMC transients are absent because the R7 and R8 form synapses in the medulla (Me). Sometimes, the ERG from R7 and R8 is accompanied with an on-transient (ERG R7,8, grey trace), since R7 and R8 form gap junctions (Gj) with the R1-6 axons in the lamina.

The photoreceptors R7 and R8 form chemical synapses in the medulla and the synapsing higher order interneurons do not contribute any signal to the ERG. Yet, light responses of the R7 and R8 cells are sometimes accompanied by transients, which are presumably due to electrical synapses between the R7 and R8 and the axons of R1-6 and accompanying R1-6 signals to L1 and L2 (Shaw, 1984; Juusola, personal communication).

The *Drosophila* ERG is probably shaped also by the pigment cells which respond to the changes in the ionic composition of the extracellular medium next to the photoreceptors by actively pumping ions (Hamdorf et al., 1978). The receptor potential plateau during long stimuli thus slowly decays, which is reflected in a not fully sustained ERG. The ERG at high light intensities is often accompanied by corneal-positive afterpotentials, in the dark after the stimulus, which is probably due to the hyperpolarizing action of the activated Na^+/K^+ pump in the receptor membrane (Jansonius, 1990).

4. Quantitative analysis of ERG

4.1 ERG amplitude and stimulus-response relationship

The ERG recorded with an electrode in the distal retina and the reference elsewhere in the body is actually measured as a change in the voltage drop across the basement membrane.

The lateral resistance between the ommatidia is low, so that the ERG is not a local phenomenon. The basement membrane separating the retina and the lamina functions as a blood-brain barrier and has a much larger resistance; even in the dark, a voltage drop across the eye of 30-50 mV exists (Heisenberg, 1971). Illumination of only a few ommatidia of a red-eyed fruitfly creates an ERG amplitude of only a few mV, even at high light intensities. In a white-eyed fly, the ERG in a brightly illuminated eye can measure more than 40 mV peak-to-peak, with a sustained (DC) component of as much as 30 mV. The extraordinary large amplitude of the ERG in the uniformly illuminated eye is a result of the concerted activity of a large number of photoreceptors, which produce large currents running across the high resistance of the basement membrane.

Other measuring configurations allow for isolation of specific ERG components. First, if the measuring electrode is advanced into the retina, the basement membrane is penetrated at ca. 120-150 μm from the cornea. This is marked by a sudden voltage drop of ca. 15 mV and a change in the ERG shape. At a depth of between 120-200 μm below the cornea, the receptor component becomes negligible, so that the neuronal transients dominate the ERG response . Further advancement of the electrode leads to a complete loss of the ERG signal. If the reference electrode is placed deep into the receptor layer, just above the basement membrane, the ERG attains the shape of inversed receptor potentials and no neural transients are detectable in the signal. The effects of different recording configurations are described in great detail by Heisenberg (1971).

Both the photoreceptor and the neuronal ERG components are graded with respect to the stimulus intensity. The ERG amplitude is graded over a very wide range of stimulus intensities, spanning more than 6 log units. The relationship between the logarithm of light intensity and the sustained ERG component is very well described by the Hill equation

$$V/V_{max}=I^n/(I^n+I_{50}{}^n) \quad (1)$$

where V/V_{max} is the normalized ERG amplitude, I is the logarithm of the relative light intensity ($\log(I/I_{max})$; at $\log I=0$, $V=V_{max}$,, n is the Hill slope (slope of the sigmoid curve at the half maximum) and I_{50} is the light intensity producing 50% of the maximal ERG amplitude. The Hill coefficient or Hill slope n is used to describe the dynamic working range of a photoreceptor cell. If measured intracellularly, n in *Drosophila* photoreceptors is typically around 0.6 (Wu and Pak, 1978). The Hill slope as estimated from the ERG in white eyed fruitflies in the dark adapted state is as low as 0.49 (Belušič et al., 2010). This means that the estimated photoreceptor dynamic working range via ERG is 5-6 log units or orders of magnitude, and 3-4 log units via intracellular measurements. The dynamic working range via ERG is obviously exaggerated by 2 log units or 100-fold. The difference between the two methods is probably due to the different illumination conditions.

In intracellular measurements, a single cell is illuminated on-axis, and the whole dynamic range of a photoreceptor, from single quantum bumps to saturation is easily studied. In the ERG, oblique illumination with a beam of a limited numerical aperture is most often used, so that a population of the photoreceptors is not illuminated directly, but rather with the scattered light penetrating the retina. The photoreceptors in the white eyed mutant still retain a fraction of directional sensitivity (Streck, 1972) and are progressively recruited as the oblique beam gets stronger. Thus, the saturation state can be reached only at very high light intensities, often higher than available. The problem is even more pronounced in the red eyed flies, but can be overcome by using a hemispherical diffuser around the compound eye, providing real »ganzfeld« illumination. Anyhow, the measurement of the entire dynamic working range is feasible with proper illumination, allowing for very precise estimates of light sensitivity in different populations of the fruitfly.

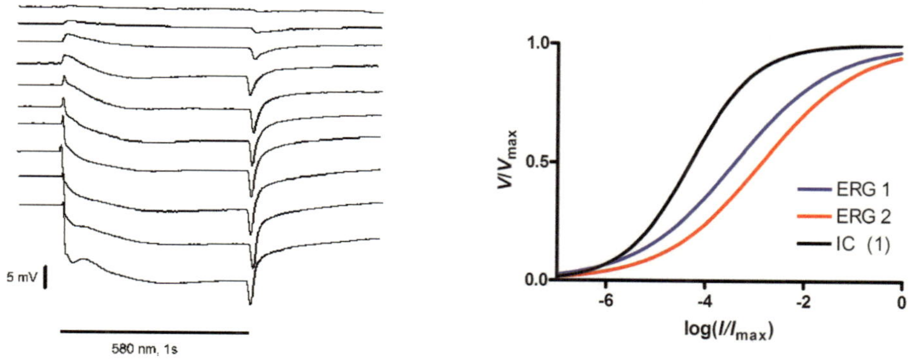

Fig. 6. The stimulus-response relationship. Left, Sequence of ERG recordings from a wild-type, white-eyed fruitfly; stimulus intensity attenuated from -4.5 log ($10^{-4.5}$) to 0 log (full light) in 0.5 log steps. The response is not saturated. Right, The »V-log *I* curve« as obtained with ERG and with intracellular recordings. Curves are plotted with the Hill equation (1) with the Hill slope $n =$ 0.49 (ERG 1,2) and 0.66 (IC (1)), respectively, and $I_{50} = -3.4$ (ERG 1), -2.9 (ERG 2) and -4.3 (IC). The intracellular curve (IC (1)) corresponds to a hypothetical photoreceptor in the most illuminated part of the eye in ERG 1. The ERG curves are shallower than the IC curve due to non-ideal illumination of the retina and the progressive recruitment of the shaded photoreceptors at high light intensities. The working dynamic range of the photoreceptors (3-4 orders of magnitude, IC) as measured intracellularly is exagerrated in the ERG (5-6 orders of magnitude, ERG). The light sensitivity in the flies of ERG 1 is higher than in the flies of ERG 2 by 0.5 log units, i.e. 3.16 fold. Such differences between fly strains can be reliably measured with appropriate instrumentation and skills.

The ERG in *Drosophila* is a very sensitive method. In the white eyed, wild-type flies, the half maximal intensity (I_{50}) corresponds to the photon catch rate of 2.9×10^4 photons s^{-1} per receptor cell (Belušič et al., 2010). Since the signal is detectable already at the light intensities that are three log units lower, i.e. $10^{-3} \times I_{50}$, it follows that at the threshold of the ERG, the rate of photon absorption per receptor is as low as 10 s^{-1}, when the individual quantum bumps are still discernible in the intracellular recordings. The weak supratreshold ERG signal is however characterized only by the neural transients. Namely, the *Drosophila* eye belongs to the neural superposition type, typical of the higher dipteran insects. This means that the axons of the six R1-6 photoreceptors in the adjacent ommatidia which are directed into the same point in the space project to the common neuron in the lamina. Thus, a laminar neuron receives the input from a larger area, covered by six photoreceptors, without much loss in the angular resolving power, and the limited sensitivity of the eye due to the apposition optical design is greatly enhanced. In addition, laminar neurons strongly amplify the small changes in the receptor potential: even the single quantum bumps are faithfully transmitted to the brain (Dubs et al., 1981). Due to the nature of the neural summation of photoreceptor responses, the amplification and the filtering properties of the laminar neurons, i.e. the neuronal component of the ERG signal is detectable even at very dim light, where the photoreceptor response is dominated by single photon absorptions.

4.2 The dynamic properties of ERG

The dynamic properties of the ERG should be treated with great caution. Firstly, *Drosophila* is a poikilothermic animal and the rates of its physiological processes depend strongly on the temperature. The eyes of the flies (*Calliphora vicina, Drosophila melanogaster*) can operate at temperatures of up to 45°C, and the ERG can be detected even at -10°C. The ERG parameters exhibit temperature quotients Q_{10} between 2 and 4 (Hamdorf and Keller, 1962; Stušek et al., 2000). Therefore, it is very important to control the temperature of the preparation and avoid possible heating of the eyes with broadband light sources, which contain infrared light. Secondly, the latencies and rates of depolarization and repolarization depend strongly on the state of the light adaptation and on the effective illumination intensity and tend to become shorter and quicker with the increasing light adaptation. Neural transients are strongly high-pass filtered and amplify the fast components of the receptor response. The amount of the neural ERG transients depends on the quality of the preparation, the ability of the animal to ventilate and on the depth of the electrode within the retina. The visual system of a fruitfly can follow the stimulus flicker of up to 80 Hz at the room temperature, but the signal at the high frequencies originates exclusively in the lamina neurons. If the contribution of the neurons is diminished for any of the aforementioned reasons, the ERG waveform will become slower and the flicker response will cease (flatten) at lower stimulus frequencies.

The speed of repolarization as measured in the ERG seems to reflect the amount of arrestin available in the microvilli (Lee et al., 2003; Satoh et al., 2010) or the ability of arrestin to bind to metarhodopsin (Elsaesser et al., 2010). In the dark adapted state, microvilli contain only 25% of the total arrestin available. With light adaptation, the remaining arrestin is progressively translocated from the soma to the rhabdomere, and the repolarization is accelerated (Satoh et al., 2010).

4.3 The PDA paradigm

Extended or very bright illumination of a fruitfly eye can create any desired fraction of metarhodopsin (f_M) between 0 and 0.7. The easiest way to establish a defined photoequilibrium is to use bright monochromatic light, since the absorbance characteristics of R and M are well known and allow for the precise, wavelength dependent setting of f_M. f_M >0.37 will create a PDA, i.e. maximally depolarize the photoreceptor cell for many hours, even in the dark. PDA can be created with light at wavelengths below 520 nm, and is quickly abolished with orange or red light above 580 nm, which brings the f_M nearly to 0 and leads to repolarization of the photoreceptors. During the blue-light induced PDA, receptors R1-6 are inactivated, but the responses of R7 and R8 can still be elicited with blue, violet or UV pulses (Minke et al., 1975). In the UV-sensitive R7y and R7p receptors, PDA can be created with UV light and abolished with blue light (Stark, 1977). PDA in R8 receptors has never been observed. During the PDA in R1-6, it is not only possible to isolate the ERG of R7 and R8, but also of R8y exclusively in the mutant sevenless (*sev*, lacking R7y, R7p and R8p). PDA represents the maximal metabolic load to photoreceptors and reflects their ability to sustain maximal depolarization for an extended period of time.

The most frequently applied sequence of light pulses presented during a PDA assay is orange - blue - blue - orange - orange (OBBOO), each pulse 5-10 s long, with 10-20 s dark intervals. The first O pulse converts all M to R; the first B creates high f_M and PDA; the second B is to make sure the f_M is maximal or to further increase f_M if the first B was too weak or short; the second O reconverts M back to R and and starts the repolarization; the last O pulse is applied to check if the preceding O was sufficient to bring f_M next to 0. PDA has been traditionally used to characterise the phenotypes of visual mutants. This protocol also allows for separation of the photoreceptor activation from inactivation and deactivation.

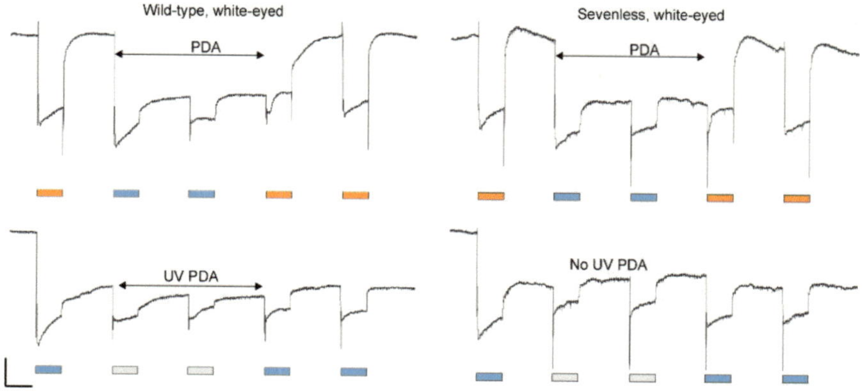

Fig. 7. The PDA paradigm. Left, PDA in the wild-type. Right, PDA in the *sevenless* mutant. Upper row, PDA elicited with blue light (473 nm, 5 s) and abolished with orange light (580 nm, 5 s). Lower row, PDA elicited with blue light (473 nm), additional PDA in R7 cells elicited with UV light (360 nm, 5 s; grey rectangles). In the wild type, PDA isolates the response of R7 and R8; additional UV isolates the ERG of R8y and R8p (lower row, left, second UV pulse). In *sevenless*, R7 and R8p cells are absent; »blue PDA« isolates the response of R8y (upper row, second blue pulse; lower row, UV pulses), which do not enter PDA under any condition. Calibration bars in the lower left corner, 5 s and 5 mV.

Sometimes the blue light pulse cannot provoke a PDA, photoreceptors repolarize vigorously, and the ERG returns back to the baseline. The inability to provoke a PDA can indicate low rhodopsin content due to the lack of carotenoids in the food. Rhodopsin levels are low also in the mutants of the Rh1 gene *nina*E. The *nina*E mutant has been named after its inability to enter a PDA, the property named »neither inactivation, nor activation«, abbreviated into *nina*. PDA is absent also in certain retinal degeneration mutants during early phases of degeneration of photoreceptors R1-6 (such as in the mutant *rdg*C, retinal degeneration C).

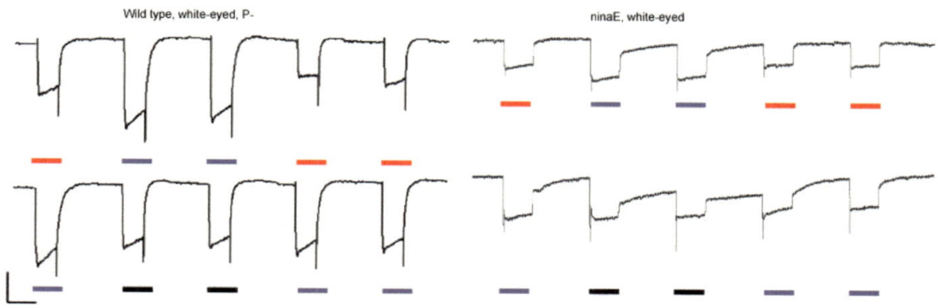

Fig. 8. Left column, absence of PDA in the white-eyed, wild-type fruitfly, reared without the carotenoids in the food. Note the transients indicating that the R1-6 receptors are functional. Right column, same paradigm applied in a *ninaE* fly. The absence of large transients indicates that only receptors R7 and R8 are functional. R7 enter PDA in the UV. Rectangles, 5 s stimuli (orange, 580 nm; blue, 480 nm; black, 360 nm). Calibration bars on the lower left indicate 5 s and 5 mV.

Fruitfly strains can be compared with respect to the amount of blue light, required to enter PDA. The amount can be set by varying pulse intensity or duration. A more precise method is to set a defined f_M in order to provoke PDA with a series of long pulses at different wavelengths. PDA creation depends on the ratio between rhodopsin and arrestin or the ability of arrestin to inactivate metarhodopsin. Thus, the quantity of arrestin can be calculated from the f_M required to provoke a half-maximal PDA (Belušič et al., 2010). PDA is created at low f_M in the mutants of the visual system specific arrestin, *arr*2.
In certain fruitfly mutants, the receptor potential cannot be sustained during the light pulse. The ERG returns to baseline, but a subsequent light pulse does not elicit a response: the photoreceptors are inactivated. Obviously, PDA cannot be created. Such ERG waveform has been named the *transient receptor potential* and was described in the first discovered visual mutant of the fruitfly, *trp* (Cosens and Manning, 1969). The mutant lacks the canonical TRP channel which mediates the major portion of the light-induced current in the photoreceptors. Similar phenotype can be observed in the mutants of the *ina*D class which have mutated or lack the scaffolding protein INAD. This protein anchors TRP and, as a consequence of the mutation, TRP is lost from the microvillar membrane. The abbreviation *ina* denotes the phenotype »inactivation – no afterpotential«, describing the absence of PDA and photoreceptor inactivation.

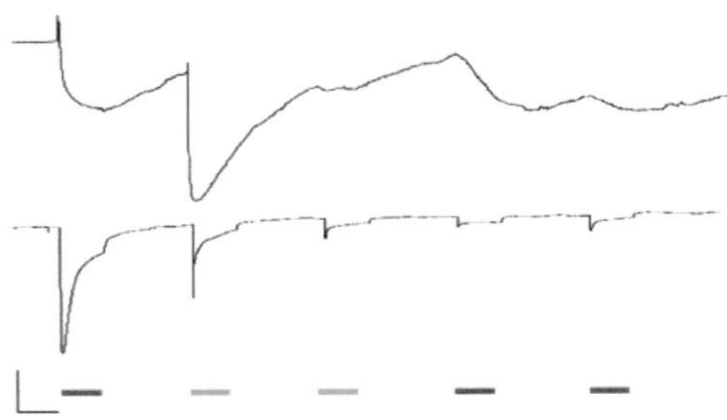

Fig. 9. Transient ERG caused by the transient receptor potential in a *inaD*^{1} mutant (upper trace) and in a *trp*^{P343} mutant (lower trace). Calibration bars, 5s, 3 mV.

All the key players in *Drosophila* phototransduction have been so far studied via mutations which rendered them non-functional. Elimination of certain proteins resulted in very pronounced, easily discernible ERG phenotypes. These were the rhodopsin Rh1 (gene and mutant *ninaE*), the light operated channel TRP (*trp*), the scaffolding protein INAD (*InaD*), and the arrestin 2 (*arr2*). Mutation in the gene *norpA* which eliminated the enzyme phospholypase PLCβ resulted in the absence of receptor potential (no receptor potential; *norp*). However, a number of different mutations have yielded weak ERG phenotypes, converging phenotypes or phenotypes hard to explain. Such were the mutations which eliminated the TRPL channel (resulting e.g. in oscillations of the ERG), yielding an ERG phenotype similar to the one in the flies with arrestin 1 eliminated (Belušič, 2003). Elimination of the protein kinase C (eye specific PKC) gene *inaC* resulted in an inactivation phenotype, similar as in *inaD*.
A number of mutations that include protein eliminations, point mutations or ectopic protein expression result in a general degeneration phenotype. This phenotype is manifested by delayed repolarizations, responses that are diminished over time, and the gradual disappearance of the R1-6 response.

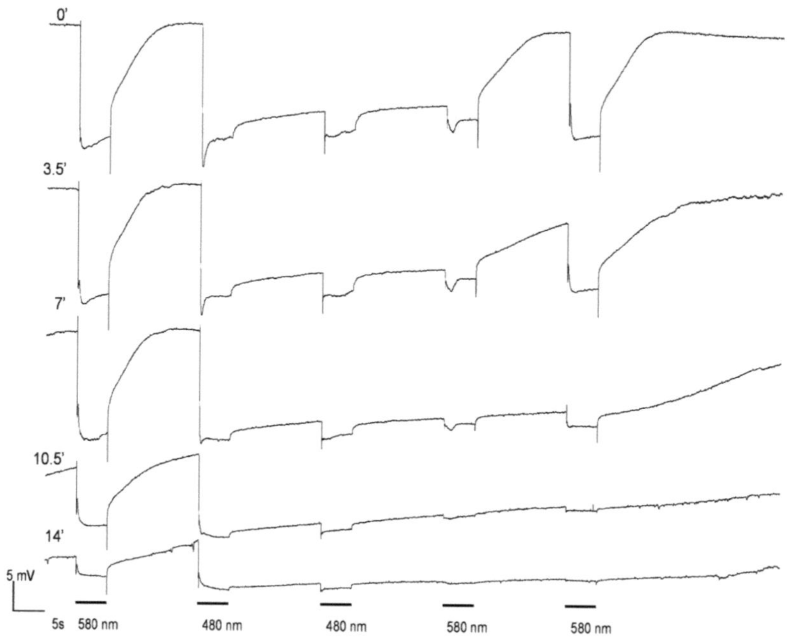

Fig. 10. ERG phenotype in a retinal degeneration mutant *rdgC*. The fly has been dark-raised for a week. Exposure to bright light in the ERG setup elicited rapid decay of the photoreceptors within minutes (numbers at the left of the traces), characterized by progressively slowed repolarization and decreasing amplitude.

5. Future applications of ERG

5.1 ERG in combination with other techniques

ERG in *Drosophila* is a feasible and robust technique that allows for simultaneous measurement of other physiological signals from the eyes. These are the measurement of ionic concentrations with the ion-selective electrodes (Agam et al., 2000), monitoring of pO_2 with carbon fibre electrodes (Meglič et al., 2009), spectrophotometrical measurement of redox states of mitochondria in the photoreceptors (Zupančič, 2003; Meglič and Zupančič, 2011), photometrical estimation of metarhodopsin to rhodopsin ratio (Belušič et al. 2010), or monitoring of GFP marked proteins in the eyes (Meyer et al,. 2006). Exclusive ectopic expression of UV rhodopsin in all functional photoreceptor classes allows for separate photoreceptor stimulation at short wavelengths and optical measurements at long wavelenghts (Liu et al., 2008).

5.2 *Drosophila* as a model for human disease

Drosophila is an animal model for numerous human diseases (Pandey and Nichols, 2011). Nearly 75% of human disease-causing genes are believed to have a functional homolog in the fruitfly. The human diseases available for research in *Drosophila* include Parkinson's disease, Alzheimer's disease, several cardiac diseases, amyotrophic lateral sclerosis, fragile X syndrome, hereditary spastic paraplegia, Huntington disease, hypoparathyroidism-retardation-dysmorphism syndrome, Machado-Joseph Disease, metabolic diseases, diabetes, obesity, microcephaly, neuronal ceroid lipofuscinosis, Niemann-Pick disease, polyglutamine diseases, seizure disorders, epilepsy, spinal muscular atrophy, spinocerebellar ataxia 2, Werner syndrome, and X-linked mental retardation. Several mutations which are lethal if expressed in all somatic cells can be conveniently studied if expressed only in the visual system. This is easily achieved by the driver-reporter genetical systems (Greenspan et al., 2004), and the effects of expression can be elegantly followed by ERG.

6. References

Agam, K., von Campenhausen, M., Levy, S., Ben-Ami, H.C., Cook, B., Kirschfeld, K., Minke, B. (2000). Metabolic Stress Reversibly Activates the Drosophila Light-sensitive Channels TRP and TRPL in vivo. *Journal of Neuroscience*, Vol. 20, No. 15, (August 2000), pp. 5748-5755. ISSN 0270-6474

Ashburner, M., Golic, G. K., Scott, H. R. (2005). *Drosophila: A Laboratory Handbook.* Cold Spring Harbor Laboratory Press, ISBN 978-0879697068, Woodbury, USA.

Autrum, H., Zettler, F. & Jarvilehto, M. (1970). Postsynaptic Potentials From a Single Monopolar Neurone of the Ganglion Opticum of the Blowfly *Calliphora. Zeitschrift fuer Vergleichende Physiologie,* Vol. 70, No. 4, (December 1970), pp. 414-424. ISSN 0044-362X

Belušič, G. (2003). A double role for arrestin 1? In: Proceedings of the 29th Göttingen Neurobiology Conference and the 5th Meeting of the German Neuroscience Society 2003, Elsner, N., Zimmerman, H. (eds.), Georg Thieme Verlag: Stuttgart, Germany; Abstract 459. ISBN 3-13-137351-2

Belušič, G., Pirih, P., Stavenga, D.G. (2010). Photoreceptor Responses of Fruitflies With Normal and Reduced Arrestin Content Studied by Simultaneous Measurements of Visual Pigment Fluorescence and ERG. *Journal of Comparative Physiology A*, Vol. 196, No. 1, (January 2010), pp. 23–35. ISSN 0340-7594

Cajal, S.R., Sanchez, D. (1915). Contribucion al Conocimiento de los Centros Nerviosos de los Insectos (Madrid: Imprenta de Hijos de Nicholas Moja).

Coombe, P.E. (1986). The Large Monopolar Cells L1 and L2 are Responsible for ERG Transients in *Drosophila*. Journal of Comparative Physiology A, Vol. 159, No. 5, (September 1986), pp. 655-665. ISSN 0340-7594

Dolph, P.J., Ranganathan, R., Colley, N.J., Hardy, R.W., Socolich, M., Zuker, C.S. (1993). Arrestin Function in Inactivation of G Protein-Coupled Receptor Rhodopsin *In Vivo. Science,* Vol. 260, No. 5116, (1993), pp. 1910–1916. ISSN 0146-0404.

Dubs, A., Laughlin, S.B., Srinivasan, M.V.. Single Photon Signals in Fly Photoreceptors and First Order Interneurones at Behavioral Threshold. *Journal of Physiology*, Vol. 317, No., (August 1981), pp. 317-334. ISSN 0022-3751

Elsaesser, R., Kalra, D., Li, R., Montell, C. (2010). Light-induced Translocation of *Drosophila* Visual Arrestin2 Depends on Rac2. *Proceedings of the National Academy of Sciences of the U.S.A*, Vol. 107, No. 10, (March 2010), pp. 4740-4745. ISSN 0027-8424

Fischbach, K.F., Dittrich, A.P.M. (1989). The Optic Lobe of *Drosophila melanogaster*. I. A Golgi Analysis of Wild Type Structure. *Cell and Tissue Research,* Vol. 258, , No. 1, (January 1989), pp. 441–475. ISSN 0302-766X

Goldsmith, T.H., Barker, R.J., Cohen, C.F. (1964) Sensitivity of Visual Receptors of Carotenoid-Depleted Flies: A Vitamin A Deficiency in an Invertebrate. *Science,* Vol. 146, No. 3640, (October 1964), pp. 65-67. ISSN 0146-0404

Govardovskii, V.I., Fyhrquist, N., Reuter, T., Kuzmin, D.G., Donner, K. (2000) In Search of the Visual Pigment Template. *Visual Neuroscience,* Vol. 17, No. 4, (September 2000), pp. 509–528. ISSN 0952-5238

Greenspan, R.J. (2004). *Fly Pushing: The Theory and Practice of Drosophila Genetics*. Cold Spring Harbor Laboratory Press, ISBN 978-087969711-2, Woodbury, USA.

Gohl, D.M., Silies, M.A., Gao, X.J., Bhalerao, S., Luongo, F.J., Lin, C.C., Potter, C.J., Clandinin, T.R. (2011). A Versatile *In Vivo* System for Directed Dissection of Gene Expression Patterns. Nature Methods, Vol. 8, No. 3, (March 2011), pp.231-237. ISSN 1548-7091

Hamdorf, K., Höglund, G., Schlecht, P. (1978). Ion Gradient and Photoreceptor Sensitivity. *Journal of Comparative Physiology* A, Vol. 125, No. 3 (September 1978), pp. 237-252. ISSN 0340-7594

Hamdorf, K. (1979). The Physiology of Invertebrate Visual Pigments. In: Autrum H (ed) *Handbook of sensory physiology,* vol VII/6A. Springer, Berlin, pp. 145–224

Hamdorf, K., Keller, L.R. (1962). Das Verhalten des Elektroretinogramms von *Calliphora* im Temperaturbereich von -10°C bis +35°C. *Zeitschrift fuer Vergleichende Physiologie,* Vol.45, No.6, (November 1962), pp. 711-724. ISSN 0044-362X

Hamdorf, K., Razmjoo, S. (1979). Photoconvertible Pigment States and Excitation in *Calliphora;* the Induction and Properties of the Prolonged Depolarizing Afterpotential. *Biophysics of Structure and Mechanism* Vol. 5, pp. 137–161. ISSN 0340-1057

Hampel, S., Chung, P., McKellar, C.E., Hall, D., Looger, L.L., Simpson, J.H. (2011). *Drosophila* Brainbow: a Recombinase-Based Fluorescence Labeling Technique to Subdivide Neural Expression Patterns. *Nature Methods,* Vol. 8, No. 3 (march 2011), pp.253-259. ISSN 1548-7091

Hardie, R.C. (1991). Whole-Cell Recordings of the Light-Induced Current in *Drosophila* Photoreceptors: Evidence for Feedback by Calcium Permeating the Light Sensitive Channels. *Proceedings of the Royal Society of London B,* Vol. 245, No. 1314, (September 1991), pp.203-210. ISSN 0080-4649

Hardie, R.C., Raghu, P. (2001). Visual Transduction in *Drosophila. Nature* Vol. 413, No. 6852, (September 2001), pp. 186–193. ISSN 0028-0836

Harris, W.A., Ready, D.F., Lipson, E.D., Hudspeth, A.J., Stark, W.S.(1977). Vitamin A Deprivation and *Drosophila* Photopigments. *Nature.* Vol. 266, No. 5603, (April 1977), pp. 648-650. ISSN 0028-0836

Heisenberg, M. (1971). Separation of Receptor and Lamina Potentials in the Electroretinogram of Normal and Mutant *Drosophila. Journal of Experimental Biology,* Vol.55, No.1, (August 1971), pp. 85-100, ISSN 0022-0949

Jansonius, N.M. (1990). Properties of the Sodium Pump in the Blowfly Photoreceptor Cell. *Journal of Comparative Physiology A,* Vol. 167, No. 4, (September 1990), pp. 461–467. ISSN 0340-7594

Järviilehto, M., Zettler, F. (1973). Electrophysiological-Histological Studies on Some Functional Properties of Visual Cells and Second Order Neurons of an Insect Retina. *Cell and Tissue Research*, Vol. 136, No. 2, (June 1973), pp. 291-306. ISSN 0340-0336

Joesch, M., Schnell, B., Raghu, S.V., Reiff, D.F., Borst, A. (2010). ON and OFF pathways in *Drosophila* motion vision. *Nature* Vol.468, No.7321, (November 2010), pp. 300-304. ISSN 0028-0836

Juusola, M., Hardie, R.C. (2001). Light Adaptation in *Drosophila* Photoreceptors: I. Response Dynamics and Signaling Efficiency at 25 Degrees C. *Journal of General Physiology*, Vol. 117, No. 1, (January 2001), pp.3-25. ISSN 0022-1295

Kirschfeld, K., Franceschini, N. Optische Eigenschaften der Ommatidien im Komplexauge von *Musca*. *Kybernetik*, Vol. 5, No. 2, (August 1968), pp. 47–52. ISSN 0023-5946

Kirschfeld, K., Feiler, R., Hardie, R., Vogt, K., Franceschini, N. (1983). The Sensitizing Pigment of Fly Photoreceptors. *Biophysics of Structure and Mechanism* Vol. 10, No. 1-2, (April 1983), pp. 81-92. ISSN 0340-1057

Laughlin, S. B. (1987). Form and Function in Retinal Processing. *Trends in Neurosciences* Vol. 10, No. 11, (November 1987), pp. 478-483. ISSN 0166-2236

Lee, S.J., Xu, H., Kang, L.W., Amzel, L.M., Montell, C. (2003). Light Adaptation Through Phosphoinositide-Regulated Translocation of *Drosophila* Visual Arrestin. *Neuron*, Vol. 39, No. 1, (July 2003), pp. 121–132. ISSN 0896-6273

Liu, C.H., Satoh, A.K., Postma, M., Huang, J., Ready, D.F., Hardie, R.C. (2008). Ca^{2+}-dependent Metarhodopsin Inactivation Mediated by Calmodulin and NINAC Myosin III. *Neuron*, Vol. 59, No. 5, (September 2008), pp. 778-789. ISSN 0896-6273

Meglič, A., Belušič, G., Zupančič, G. (2009). Using Carbon Fibre Microelectrodes to Monitor the Oxidative Metabolism of Blowfly Eyes. *Acta biologica slovenica*, Vol. 52, No. 1, pp. 19-28. ISSN 1408-3671

Meglič, A., Zupančič, G. (2011). Changes in Redox States of Respiratory Pigments Recorded From the Eyes of Live Blowflies Exposed to Light Stimuli and Hypoxia. *Journal of Comparative Physiology A*, Vol. 197, No. 3, (March 2011), pp.301-310. ISSN 0340-7594

Meyer, N.E., Joel-Almagor, T., Frechter, S., Minke, B., Huber, A. (2006). Subcellular Translocation of the eGFP-tagged TRPL Channel in *Drosophila* Photoreceptors Requires Activation of the Phototransduction Cascade. *Journal of Cell Science*, Vol. 15, No. 119, (June 2006), pp. 2592-2603. ISSN 0021-9533

Minke, B., Wu, C.F., Pak, W.L. (1975). Isolation of Light-Induced Response of the Central Retinula Cells From the Electroretinogram of *Drosophila*. *Journal of Comparative Physiology A*, Vol. 98, No. 4, (December 1975), pp. 345–355. ISSN 0340-7594

Morgan, T.H. (1910). Sex Limited Inheritance In *Drosophila*. *Science*, Vol. 32, No. 812 (July1910). ISSN 0146-0404

Ostroy, S.E., Wilson, M., Pak, W.L. (1974). *Drosophila* Rhodopsin: Photochemistry, Extraction and Differences in the $NorpA^{P12}$ Phototransduction Mutant. *Biochemichal and Biophysical Research Communications*, Vol. 59, No. 3, (August 1974), pp. 960–966. ISSN 0006-291X

Pak, W.L. (1995). *Drosophila* in Vision Research. The Friedenwald Lecture. *Investigative Ophthalmolgy and Visual Science*, Vol. 36, No. 12 (November 1995), pp. 2340-57. ISSN 0146-0404

Pak, W.L. (2010). Why *Drosophila* to Study Phototransduction? *Journal of Neurogenetics*, Vol. 24, No. 2 (July 2010), pp. 55-66. ISSN 0167-7063

Pandey, U.B., Nichols, C.D (2011). Human Disease Models in *Drosophila melanogaster* and the Role of the Fly in Therapeutic Drug Discovery. *Pharmacological Reviews*, (March 2011). Online ISSN 1521-0081

Ranganathan, R., Harris, G.L., Stevens, C.F., Zuker, C.S. (1991). A *Drosophila* Mutant Defective in Extracellular Calcium-Dependent Photoreceptor Deactivation and Rapid Desensitization. *Nature*, Vol. 354, No. 6350 (November 1991), pp. 230-232. ISSN 0028-0836

Salcedo, E., Huber, A., Henrich, S., Chadwell, L.V., Chou, W.H., Paulsen, R., Britt, S.G. (1999). Blue- and Green-Absorbing Visual Pigments of *Drosophila*: Ectopic Expression and Physiological Characterization of the R8 Photoreceptor Cell-Specific Rh5 and Rh6 Rhodopsins. *Journal of Neuroscience*, Vol. 19, No. (December 1999), pp. 10716–10726. ISSN 0270-6474

Satoh, A.K., Xia, H., Yan, L., Liu, C.H., Hardie, R.C., Ready, D.F (2010). Arrestin Translocation is Stoichiometric to Rhodopsin Isomerization and Accelerated by Phototransduction in *Drosophila* Photoreceptors. *Neuron*, Vol.67, No.6, (September 2010), pp. 997-1008. ISSN 0896-6273

Shaw, S.R. (1984). Early Visual Processing in Insects. *Journal of Experimental Biology*, Vol. 112, No. 1, (September 1984), pp. 225-251. ISSN 0022-0949

Stark, W.S. (1977). Sensitivity and Adaptation in R7, an Ultraviolet Photoreceptor, in the *Drosophila* Retina. *Journal of Comparative Physiology A*, Vol. 115, No. 1, (January 1977), pp. 47-59. ISSN 0340-7594

Stark, W.S., Wasserman, G.S. (1972). Transient and Receptor Potentials in the Electroretinogram of *Drosophila. Vision Research*, Vol. 12, No. 10, (October 1972), pp. 1771-1775. ISSN 0042-6989

Stavenga, D.G. (2002). Colour in the Eyes of Insects. *Journal of Comparative Physiology A*, Vol. 188, No. 5, (June 2002), pp. 337–348. ISSN 0340-7594

Stavenga, D.G., Zantema, A., Kuiper, J.W. (1973) Rhodopsin processes and the function of the pupil mechanism in flies. In: Langer H (ed) *Biochemistry and physiology of visual pigments*. Springer, Berlin, pp. 175–180

Stavenga, D.G., Schwemer, J. (1984). Visual pigments of invertebrates. In: Ali MA (ed) *Photoreception and vision of invertebrates*. Plenum, New York, pp. 11–61

Streck, P. (1972). Der Einfluss des Schirmpigmentes auf das Sehfeld einzelner Sehzellen der Fliege *Calliphora erythrocephala* Meig. *Zeitschrift fuer Vergleichende Physiologie*, Vol.76, No.4, (December 1972), pp. 372-402. ISSN 0044-362X

Stušek, P., Belušič, G., Drašlar, K. (2000). Temperature dependence of photoreceptor signal termination in fruitfly (*Drosophila melanogaster* white eyed mutant). *Pflügers Archiv*, Vol. 439, No. 3, [suppl.] (December 2000), p. R200. ISSN 0031-6768

Uusitalo, R.O., Weckström, M. (2000). Potentiation in the First Visual Synapse of the Fly Compound Eye. *Journal of Neurophysiology*, Vol 83, No. 4, (April 2000), pp. 2103-2112. ISSN 0022-3077

Zupančič G. (2003). A Method For Dynamic Spectrophotometric Measurements *In Vivo* Using Principal Component Analysis-Based Spectral Deconvolution. *Pflügers Archiv*, Vol. 447, No. 1, (October 2003), pp. 109-119. ISSN 0031-6768